Clinical Dermatology

In memory of John Savin, 1935–2006

# Clinical Dermatology

## Richard P.J.B. Weller MD, FRCP (Edin)

*Senior Lecturer*
*Department of Dermatology*
*University of Edinburgh*
*Edinburgh, UK*

## John A.A. Hunter OBE BA MD FRCP (Edin)

*Professor Emeritus of Dermatology*
*University of Edinburgh*
*Edinburgh, UK*

## John A. Savin MA MD ChB FRCP DIH

*Former Consultant Dermatologist*
*The Royal Infirmary*
*Edinburgh, UK*

## Mark V. Dahl BA MD

*Professor of Dermatology and former Chairman*
*College of Medicine*
*Mayo Clinic Arizona*
*Scottsdale, AZ, USA, and*
*Professor Emeritus and former Chairman*
*University of Minnesota Medical School*
*Minneapolis, MN, USA*

## Fourth Edition

**Blackwell**
Publishing

© 1989, 1995, 2002, 2008 Richard Weller, John Hunter, John Savin, Mark Dahl
Blackwell Publishing, Inc., 350 Main Street, Malden, Massachusetts 02148-5020, USA
Blackwell Publishing Ltd, 9600 Garsington Road, Oxford OX4 2DQ, UK
Blackwell Publishing Asia Pty Ltd, 550 Swanston Street, Carlton, Victoria 3053, Australia

First published 1989
Second edition 1995
Third edition 2002
Fourth edition 2008

2   2008

Library of Congress Cataloging-in-Publication Data

Clinical dermatology / Richard Weller . . . [et al.]. — 4th ed.
    p. ; cm.
    Rev. ed. of: Clinical dermatology / J.A.A. Hunter, J.A. Savin, M.V. Dahl. 2nd ed. 1995.
    Includes bibliographical references and index.
    ISBN 978-1-4051-4663-0 (alk. paper)
    1. Skin—Diseases.   2. Dermatology.   I. Weller, Richard, MD.   II. Hunter, J.A.A. Clinical dermatology.
    [DNLM:   1. Skin Diseases—diagnosis.   2. Skin Diseases—therapy.   WR 140 C6413 2007]

    RL71.H934 2007
    616.5—dc22

                                                                        2007018995

ISBN-13: 978-1-4051-4663-0

A catalogue record for this title is available from the British Library

Set in 9/12pt Palatino by Graphicraft Limited, Hong Kong
Printed and bound in Singapore by Markono Print Media Pte Ltd

Commissioning Editor: Martin Sugden
Editorial Assistant: Jennifer Seward
Development Editor: Rob Blundell
Production Controller: Debbie Wyer

For further information on Blackwell Publishing, visit our website:
http://www.blackwellpublishing.com

The publisher's policy is to use permanent paper from mills that operate a sustainable forestry policy,
and which has been manufactured from pulp processed using acid-free and elementary chlorine-free
practices. Furthermore, the publisher ensures that the text paper and cover board used have met
acceptable environmental accreditation standards.

# Contents

# Preface to the fourth edition

Another five years has flown by and more than enough has happened in the world of dermatology to warrant this, the fourth, edition of *Clinical Dermatology*.

The original editorial team felt that our book would be refreshed and energised by a younger co-editor! Richard Weller was approached, as his background bridges clinical and academic dermatology; happily, he agreed to join and even lead the team. We have always felt that our book was a little different from our competitors in that we try to provide more science behind diseases and their treatment than is usual in such short primers. We also make no apologies that we aim to enthuse family doctors (for whom we are primarily writing) to enjoy the challenge of diagnosing and treating skin conditions that they see only too often. At the same time we hope that there is more than enough in the following pages to whet the appetite of budding dermatologists, bright undergraduate students and even physicians looking beyond their own specialty.

2006 was an especially sad year for us. John Savin, our colleague, co-editor and, above all, friend died in August. As usual, he was ahead of the game in rewriting 'his' chapters and editing 'ours'! His name, of course, remains on the front cover of this edition. We miss him enormously but still feel him looking over our shoulders when we struggle to describe some complex problem in simple plain English; we hope that this edition will continue to reflect his way with words.

We have introduced three new chapters into this edition. That on racial skin differences reflects the cosmopolitan world in which we live and should make interpretation of skin disorders in different ethnic groups easier. In chapter 15 we bring together the skin conditions encountered in different age groups, and add two more to Shakespeare's seven ages – those of the foetus and the pregnant woman. Our third newcomer is that on cosmetic dermatology. We hope that this chapter will allow family doctors to keep one step ahead of their patients who, aided by a myriad of TV programmes, seem to know much about keeping ten years younger.

We have also updated every chapter on its own merit and have tried to include important recent advances. The role of the new 'biologicals' in the treatment of psoriasis and their side effects, fillagrin gene mutations in atopic eczema, recently recognized drug eruptions, the science behind the different types of phototherapy and new lasers, the prevention of and protection against infections after dermatological surgery, are but a few.

Finally, we acknowledge that the quickest way that most family doctors can now learn more about a topic is by electronic communication. The first references under 'Further reading' at the end of each chapter therefore provide directions to guidelines, reviews and treatments that can be easily accessed on the internet.

We welcome you to our fourth edition.

R.P.J.B.W., J.A.A.H. and M.V.D.
*Edinburgh and Scottsdale, 2007*

# Preface to the first edition

Some 10% of those who go to their family doctors do so with skin problems. We have seen an improvement in the way these have been managed over the last few years, but the subject still baffles many medical students—on both sides of the Atlantic. They find it hard to get a grip on the soggy mass of facts served up by some textbooks. For them we have tried to create an easily-read text with enough detail to clarify the subject but not enough to obscure it.

There are many doctors too who are puzzled by dermatology, even after years in practice. They have still to learn how to look at the skin with a trained eye. Anyone who denies that clinical dermatology is a visual specialty can never have practised it. In this book we have marked out the route to diagnostic success with a simple scheme for recognizing primary skin lesions using many diagrams and coloured plates.

We hope that this book will help both groups—students and doctors, including some in general medicine and some starting to train as dermatologists—and of course their patients. We make no apologies for our emphasis on diagnosis and management, and accept that we cannot include every remedy. Here, we mention only those preparations we have found to be useful and, to avoid too many trade names, we have tabulated those used in the UK and the USA in a Formulary at the back of the book.

We have decided not to break up the text by quoting lists of references. For those who want to know more there are many large and excellent textbooks on the shelves of all medical libraries.

While every effort has been made to ensure that the doses mentioned here are correct, the authors and publishers cannot accept responsibility for any errors in dosage which may have inadvertently entered this book. The reader is advised to check dosages, adverse effects, drug interactions, and contraindications in the latest edition of the *British National Formulary* or *Drug Information* (American Society of Hospital Pharmacists).

# Acknowledgements

We are grateful to Stuart Taylor and Rob Blundell of Blackwell publishing for their help and encouragement in preparing this book. Dr Gina Pitts provided invaluable feedback on the cosmetic dermatology chapter and Dr Sharnika Abeyakirthi on the leprosy section. Many of the clinical photographs come from the collection of the Department of Dermatology at the Royal Infirmary of Edinburgh and we wish to thank all those who presented them. Dr Kate Coleman (22.1 and 22.2), and Mr Anas Nasaan (22.4 and 22.5) generously provided illustrations for the cosmetic dermatology chapter, as did Q-Med AB (22.3). Dr C. Crutchfield of the University of Minnesota provided all the pictures for Chapter 14. Other colleagues who have kindly supplied pictures are Drs P.K. Buxton (7.12), O.M.V. Schofield (7.14 and 7.17), M.J. Tidman (20.52), E.C. Benton (16.20 and 20.61), G.W. Beveridge (21.17), R. Dawber (27.9) and Mr Auf Quaba (20.14). We are grateful to them all.

## Disclaimer

Although every effort bas been made to ensure that drug doses and other information are presented accurately in this publication, the ultimate responsibility rests with the prescribing physician. Neither the publisher nor the authors can be held responsible for any consequences arising from the use of information contained herein. Any product mentioned in this publication should be used in accordance with the prescribing information prepared by the manufacturers.

# Introduction

Our overall aim in this book has been to make dermatology easy to understand by the many busy doctors who glimpsed it only briefly, if at all, during their medical training. All too often the subject has been squeezed out of its proper place in the under-graduate curriculum, leaving growing numbers who quail before the skin and its reputed 2000 conditions, each with its own diverse presentations. They can see the eruptions clearly enough, but cannot describe or identify them. There are few machines to help them. Even official 'clinical guidelines' for treatment are no use if a diagnosis has not been made. Their patients quickly sense weakness and lose faith. We hope that this book will give them confidence in their ability to make the right diagnosis and then to prescribe safe and effective treatment.

An understanding of the anatomy, physiology and immunology of the skin (Chapter 2) is the bedrock on which all diagnostic efforts must be based. Remembering Osler's aphorism that 'We miss more by not seeing than by not knowing', the identification and description of primary skin lesions and the patterns these have taken up on the skin sur-face follow (Chapter 3) and will lead to a sensible working diagnosis. After this has been achieved, investigations can be directed along sensible lines (Chapter 3) until a firm diagnosis is reached. Then, and only then, will the correct line of treatment snap into place.

General rules for the choice of topical treat-ments are dealt with in Chapter 26, while more specific information on topical and systemic drugs is covered in the chapters on individual conditions. Correct choices here will be repaid by good results. Patients may be quick to complain if they are not doing well; equally they are delighted if their eruptions can be seen to melt rapidly away. Many of them are now joining in the quest for cosmetic perfection that is already well advanced in the USA and becoming more fashionable in the UK. Family doctors who are asked about this topic can find their answers in our new chapter on cosmetic dermatology (Chapter 22).

We do not pretend that all of the problems in the classification of skin diseases have been solved in this book. Far from it; some will remain as long as their causes are still unknown, but we make no apology for trying to keep our terminology as simple as possible. Many doctors are put off by the cumbersome Latin names left behind by earlier

Describe the primary lesion. What is your diagnosis? Turn over the page to find the answer.

A raspberry! 'see and, then reason, but see first.' (W. Osler)

pseudo-botanical classifications. Names like *painful nodule of the ear* or *ear corn* must now be allowed to take over from more traditional ones such as *chondrodermatitis nodularis helicis chronica*.

As well as simplifying the terminology, we have concentrated mainly on common conditions, which make up the bulk of dermatology in developed countries, although we do mention some others which may be rare but which illustrate important general principles. We have also tried to cut out as many synonyms and eponyms as possible. We have included some further reading at the end of each chapter for those wanting more information and, for the connoisseur, the names of some reference books at the end of this section.

We have, wherever possible, grouped together conditions that have the same cause, e.g. fungal infections (Chapter 16) and drug reactions (Chapter 25). Failing this, some chapters are based on a shared physiology, e.g. disorders of keratinization (Chapter 4), or on a shared anatomy, e.g. disorders of hair and nails (Chapter 13), of blood vessels (Chapter 11) or of the sweat glands (Chapter 12). In some chapters we have, reluctantly, been forced to group together conditions that share physical characteristics, e.g. the bullous diseases (Chapter 9) and the papulosquamous disorders (Chapter 6), but this is unsound and brings together some strange bedfellows. Modern research will surely soon reallocate their positions in the dormitory

of dermatology. Finally, we must mention, sooner rather than later, electronic communication and the help that it can offer both patients and doctors. Websites are proliferating almost as rapidly as the epidermal cells in psoriasis; this section deserves its own heading.

## Dermatology on the Internet

Websites come and go, but we hope that the ones we suggest here will last at least as long as this book. The best are packed with useful information; others are less trustworthy. We rely heavily on those of the British Association of Dermatologists (www.bad.org.uk) and the American Academy of Dermatology (www.aad.org) for current guidelines on how to manage a variety of individual skin conditions. They also provide excellent patient information leaflets, and the addresses of patient support groups.

Two other favourite sites are those of the New Zealand Dermatological Society (http://dermnetnz.org which provides both patient information) and a useful pictorial quiz for the budding dermatologist, and DermAtlas (www.dermatlas.com), an online dermatology atlas hosted at Johns Hopkins University.

We are gradually writing our own questions related to this text, and publishing them online at www.derm.med.ed.ac.uk. We hope that this will evolve into a useful addition to *Clinical Dermatology*, allowing readers to check on how much they have learnt from each chapter.

For medical searches, the two main engines we use are the long-standing Pubmed (www.pubmed.gov) which ranks publications by date, and the newer Google Scholar (http://scholar.google.com) which attempts to sort them by relevance. We watch the debate on open access to medical journals with interest. The Public Library of Science (www.plos.org) publishes occasional dermatology papers, and a growing number of journals are allowing free access to their content 12 months after publication. The full text of over half of the world's 200 most cited journals is now available on a website (http://highwire.stanford.edu) that includes the famous 'Topic map': few pleasures exceed that of 'exploding' clinical medicine into its subcategories by a process of simple clicking and dragging.

## Further reading

Braun-Falco O, Plewig G, Wolff HH, Burgdorf WHC & Landthaler M. (eds) (2008) *Dermatology*, 3rd edn. Springer Verlag, Berlin & Heidelberg.

Burns DA, Griffiths CEM, Breathnach SM & Cox N. (eds) (2004) *Textbook of Dermatology*, 7th edn. Blackwell Science, Oxford.

Wolff K, Goldsmith LA, Katz SI, Gilchrest BA, Paller A & Leffell DJ. (eds) (2007) *Fitzpatrick's Dermatology in General Medicine*, 7th edn, McGraw Hill, New York.

Harper J, Oranje A & Prose N. (eds) (2005) *Textbook of Pediatric Dermatology*. 2nd edn. Blackwell Science, Oxford.

Jablonski NG. (2006) *Skin. A Natural History*. University of California Press.

Lebwohl M, Heymann WR, Berth-Jones J & Coulson I. (2005) *Treatment of Skin Diseases. Comprehensive Therapeutic Strategies*, 2nd edn. Mosby, New York.

Shelley WB & Shelley DE. (2001) *Advanced Dermatologic Therapy II*, 2nd edn. Saunders, Philadelphia.

# 1 Skin disease in perspective

This chapter presents an overview of the causes, prevalence and impact of skin disease.

## The many roles of the skin

The skin is the largest organ in the body. It is the boundary between ourselves and the world around us, and its primary role is that of a barrier, preventing the entry of noxious chemicals and infectious organisms, and preventing the exit of water and other chemicals. It is a sort of 'space suit', nicely evolved to house all the other organs and chemicals in our bodies.

Skin has other roles too. It is an important sense organ, and controls heat and water loss. It reflects internal changes (Chapter 21) and reacts to external ones. It can sweat, grow hair, erect its hairs, change colour, smell, grow nails, and secrete sebum. When confronted with insults from outside, it usually adapts easily and returns to a normal state, but sometimes it fails to do so and a skin disorder appears. Some of the internal and external factors that are important causes of skin disease are shown in Fig. 1.1. Often several will be operating at the same time. Just as often, however, no obvious cause for a skin abnormality can be found, and here lies much of the difficulty of dermatology. When a cause is obvious – for example, when the washing of dishes leads to an irritant hand dermatitis, or when episodes of severe sunburn are followed by the development of a melanoma – education and prevention are just as important as treatment.

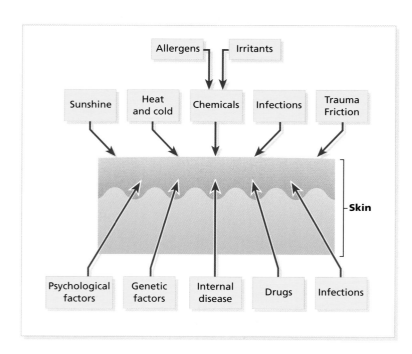

**Fig. 1.1** Some internal and external factors causing skin diseases.

## Prevalence of skin disorders

Skin diseases are very common. Probably everyone has experienced a skin disorder, such as sunburn, irritation, dry skin, acne, warts or pigment changes. The most important skin disorders in the UK are given in Table 1.1. People in other countries and in other environments may also develop skin diseases peculiar to their surroundings, or common skin diseases at different rates. For example, people living in tropical areas develop infectious diseases, such as leishmaniasis, not seen in more temperate climates. Different age groups experience different skin conditions. In the USA, for example, diseases of the sebaceous glands (mainly acne) peak at the age of about 18 years and then decline, while the prevalence of skin tumours steadily mounts with age (Fig. 1.3).

The idea that 'common things occur commonly' is well known to surgeons as an aid to diagnosis. It is equally true of dermatology – an immense subject embracing more than 2000 different conditions. In the UK, some 70% of a dermatologist's work is caused by only nine types of skin disorder (Table 1.1). In the USA, nearly half of all visits to dermatologists are for one of three diagnoses: acne, warts and skin tumours.

Currently, skin disorders account for about 15% of all consultations in general practice in the UK, but this is only the tip of an iceberg of skin disease, the sunken part of which consists of problems that never get to doctors, being dealt with or ignored in the community.

How large is this problem? No one quite knows, as those who are not keen to see their doctors seldom star in the medical literature. People tend to be shy about skin diseases, and many of them settle

**Table 1.1** The most common categories of skin disorder in the UK.

| |
|---|
| Skin cancer |
| Acne |
| Atopic eczema |
| Psoriasis |
| Viral warts |
| Other infective skin disorders |
| Benign tumours and vascular lesions |
| Leg ulcers |
| Contact dermatitis and other eczemas |

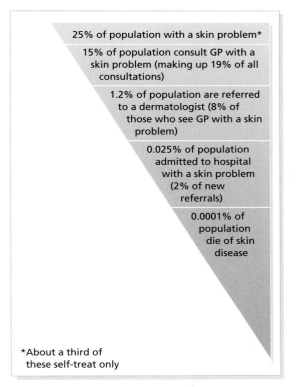

*About a third of these self-treat only

**Fig. 1.2** Skin problems in the UK and how they are dealt within 1 year (derived from Williams 1997). Patients in the USA usually refer themselves to dermatologists.

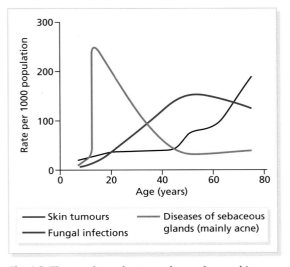

**Fig. 1.3** The age-dependent prevalence of some skin conditions.

**Table 1.2** Responses to minor ailments.

| | |
|---|---|
| Did not use anything | 45% |
| Used a home remedy | 9% |
| Used an over-the-counter remedy | 24% |
| Used a prescription remedy already in the house | 13% |
| Saw a doctor | 13% |

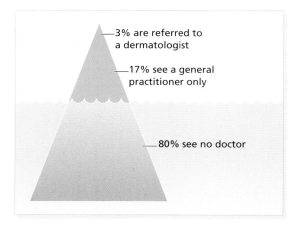

**Fig. 1.4** The 'iceberg' of psoriasis in the UK during a single year.

spontaneously, often before patients seek help. The results of a study of the responses to minor ailments of all types are shown in Table 1.2; clearly, a few patients took more than one course of action. These responses apply to skin disorders too, and form the basis for the 'iceberg' of psoriasis in the UK shown in Fig. 1.4. In the course of a single year most of those with psoriasis do not see a doctor, and only a few will see a dermatologist. Some may have fallen victim to fraudulent practices, such as 'herbal' preparations laced with steroids, and baseless advice on 'allergies'.

Several large studies have confirmed that this is the case with other skin diseases too.

● Of a large representative sample of the US population, 31.2% were found to have significant skin disease that deserved medical attention. Scaled up, these figures suggest that some 80 million of the US population may have significant skin diseases.

● A community study of adults in the UK found 22.5% to have a skin disease needing medical attention: only one in five of these had seen a doctor

within the preceding 6 months. Self-medication was far more common than any treatment prescribed by doctors.

● In another UK study, 14% of adults and 19% of children had used a skin medication during the previous 2 weeks; only one-tenth of these were prescribed by doctors. In a study of several tons of unused medicinal preparations, 7% by weight had been manufactured for topical use on the skin.

● Preparations used to treat skin disease can be found in about half of all homes in the UK; the ratio of non-prescribed to prescribed remedies is about 6 : 1. Skin treatments come second only to painkillers in the list of non-prescription medicines. Even so, in the list of the most commonly prescribed groups of drugs in the UK, those for topical use in skin conditions still come second – behind diuretics.

No one who has worked in any branch of medicine can doubt the importance of diseases of the skin. A neurologist, for example, will know all about the Sturge–Weber syndrome (p. 314), a gastroenterologist about the Peutz–Jeghers syndrome (p. 199) and a cardiologist about the LEOPARD syndrome (lentigines, electrocardiographic conduction abnormalities, ocular hypertelorism, pulmonary stenosis, abnormal genitalia, retardation of growth, and deafness; p. 286); yet paradoxically, even in their own wards, they will see far more of other, more common skin conditions, such as drug eruptions, asteatotic eczema and scabies. They should know about these too. In primary care, skin problems are even more important, and the prevalence of some common skin conditions, such as skin cancer and atopic eczema, is undoubtedly rising.

The pattern of skin disease in a community depends on many other factors, both genetic and environmental; some are listed in Table 1.3. In

**Table 1.3** Some factors influencing the prevalence of skin diseases in a community.

| High level of | High incidence of |
|---|---|
| Ultraviolet radiation | Skin malignancy in Caucasians |
| Heat and humidity | Fungal and bacterial infections |
| Industrialization | Contact dermatitis |
| Underdevelopment | Infestations |
| | Bacterial and fungal infections |

developing countries, for example, overcrowding and poor sanitation play a major part. Skin disorders there are common, particularly in the young, and are dominated by infections and infestations – the so-called 'dermatoses of poverty' – amplified by the presence of HIV infection.

## Impact of skin disorders

Much of this book is taken up with ways in which skin diseases can do harm. Most fit into the five D's shown in Fig. 1.5; others are more subtle. Topical treatment, for example, can seem illogical to those who think that their skin disease is emotional in origin; it has been shown recently that psoriatics with great disability comply especially poorly with topical treatment.

In addition, the problems created by skin disease do not necessarily tally with the extent and severity of the eruption as judged by an outside observer. Quality-of-life studies give a different, patient-based, view of skin conditions. Questionnaires have been designed to compare the impact of skin diseases with those of other conditions; patients with bad psoriasis, for example, have at least as great a disability as those with angina. However, it has recently been shown that surprisingly little information about quality of life is gathered during standard dermatology outpatient consultations. In the background lurk problems brought about by the cost of treatment and time lost from work.

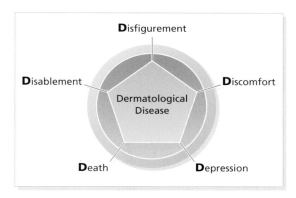

**Fig. 1.5** The five D's of dermatological disease.

### Disfigurement

The possible reactions to disfiguring skin disease are described in Chapter 23. They range from a leper complex (e.g. some patients with psoriasis; p. 54) to embarrassment (e.g. port-wine stains; Fig. 1.6: or androgenetic alopecia in both men and women; p. 181). Disorders of body image can lead those who have no skin disease to think that they have, and even to commit suicide in this mistaken belief (dermatological non-disease; p. 343).

**Fig. 1.6** (a) This patient has a port-wine stain. (b) Her life is transformed by her clever use of modern camouflage cosmetics, which take her less than a minute to apply.

(a)                                    (b)

## Discomfort

Some people prefer pain to itch; skin diseases can provide both. Itchy skin disorders include eczema (p. 79), lichen planus (p. 72), scabies (p. 262) and dermatitis herpetiformis (p. 125). Pain is marked in shingles (p. 240), leg ulcers (p. 152) and glomus tumours (p. 316).

## Disability

Skin conditions are capable of ruining the quality of anyone's life and each carries its own set of problems. At the most obvious level, dermatitis of the hands can quickly destroy a manual worker's earning capacity, as many hairdressers, nurses, cooks and mechanics know to their cost. In the USA, skin diseases account for almost half of all cases of occupational illness and cause more than 50 million days to be lost from work each year.

Disability and disfigurement can blend in a more subtle way, so that, for example, in times of unemployment people with acne find it hard to get jobs. Psoriatics in the USA, already plagued by tactless hairdressers and messy treatments, have been shown to lose thousands of dollars in earnings by virtue of time taken off work. Even trivial psoriasis, if it is on the fingertips of a blind person, can have a huge effect by making it impossible to read Braille.

## Depression

The physical, sensory and functional problems listed above often lead to depression and anxiety, even in the most stable people. Depression also seems to modulate the perception of itching, which becomes much worse. Feelings of stigmatization and rejection are common in patients with chronic skin diseases; up to 10% of patients with psoriasis that they think is bad have had suicidal thoughts. The risk of suicide in patients with severe acne is discussed on p. 169.

## Death

Deaths from skin disease are fortunately rare, but they do occur (e.g. in pemphigus, toxic epidermal necrolysis and cutaneous malignancies). In addition, the stresses generated by a chronic skin disorder such as psoriasis predispose to heavy smoking and drinking, which carry their own risks.

In this context, the concept of skin failure is an important one. It may occur when any inflammatory skin disease becomes so widespread that it prevents normal functioning of the skin, with the results listed in Table 1.4. Its causes include erythroderma (p. 78), toxic epidermal necrolysis (p. 127), severe erythema multiforme (p. 110), pustular psoriasis (p. 59) and pemphigus (p. 120).

**Table 1.4** The consequences of skin failure.

| Function | Skin failure | Treatment |
| --- | --- | --- |
| Temperature control | Cannot sweat when too hot: cannot vasoconstrict when too cold. Hence temperature swings dangerously up and down | Controlled environmental temperature |
| Barrier function | Raw skin surfaces lose much fluid and electrolytes<br>Heavy protein loss<br>Bacterial pathogens multiply on damaged skin | Monitor and replace<br>High protein diet<br>Antibiotic. Bathing/wet compresses |
| Cutaneous blood flow | Shunt through skin may lead to high output cardiac failure in those with poor cardiac reserve | Aggressively treat skin<br>Support vital signs |
| Others | Erythroderma may lead to malabsorption<br>Hair and nail loss later<br>Nursing problems handling patients particularly with toxic epidermal necrolysis (p. 127) and pemphigus (p. 120) | Usually none needed<br>Regrow spontaneously<br>Nurse as for burns |

## Learning points

**1** 'Prevalence' and 'incidence' are not the same thing. Learn the difference and join a small select band.
- The *prevalence* of a disease is the proportion of a defined population affected by it at a particular point in time.
- The *incidence* rate is the proportion of a defined population developing the disease within a specified period of time.

**2** A skin disease that seems trivial to a doctor can still wreck a patient's life.

**3** Remember that many patients, by the time they see you, will have tried many home remedies.

# Further reading

Black M. (1999) Lessons from dermatology: implications for future provision of specialist services. *Journal of the Royal College of Physicians* **33**, 208–211.

David SE, Ahmed Z, Salek MS & Finlay A. (2005) Does enough quality of life-related discussion occur during dermatology outpatient consultations? *British Journal of Dermatology* **153**, 997–1000.

Grob JJ, Stern RS, Mackie RM & Weinstock WA, eds. (1997) *Epidemiology, Causes and Prevention of Skin Diseases*. Blackwell Science, Oxford.

Savin JA. (1993) The hidden face of dermatology. *Clinical and Experimental Dermatology* **18**, 393–395.

Savin JA. (2003) Psychosocial aspects. In: Van De Kerkhof P, ed. *Textbook of Psoriasis*, 2nd edn. Blackwell Science, Oxford: 43–54.

Williams HC. (1997) Dermatology. In: Stevens A & Raftery J, eds. *Health Care Needs Assessment*. Series 2. Radcliffe Medical Press, Oxford.

# 2 The function and structure of the skin

The skin – the interface between humans and their environment – is the largest organ in the body. It weighs an average of 4 kg and covers an area of 2 m$^2$. It acts as a barrier, protecting the body from harsh external conditions and preventing the loss of important body constituents, especially water. A death from destruction of skin, as in a burn or in toxic epidermal necrolysis (p. 127), and the misery of unpleasant acne, remind us of its many important functions, which range from the vital to the cosmetic (Table 2.1).

The skin has three layers. The outer one is the *epidermis*, which is firmly attached to, and supported by connective tissue in the underlying *dermis*. Beneath the dermis is loose connective tissue, the *subcutis / hypodermis*, which usually contains abundant fat (Fig. 2.1).

## Epidermis

The epidermis consists of many layers of closely packed cells, the most superficial of which are flattened and filled with keratins; it is therefore a stratified squamous epithelium. It adheres to the dermis partly by the interlocking of its downward projections (*epidermal ridges* or *pegs*) with upward projections of the dermis (*dermal papillae*) (Fig. 2.1).

The epidermis contains no blood vessels. It varies in thickness from less than 0.1 mm on the eyelids to nearly 1 mm on the palms and soles. As dead surface squames are shed (accounting for some of the dust in our houses), the thickness is kept constant by cells dividing in the deepest (*basal* or *germinative*) layer. A generated cell moves, or is pushed by underlying mitotic activity, to the surface, passing through the *prickle* and *granular cell layers* before dying in the *horny layer*. The journey from the basal layer to the surface (epidermal turnover or transit time) takes 30 to 60 days. During this time the appearance of the cell changes. A vertical section through the epidermis summarizes the life history of a single epidermal cell (Fig. 2.2).

The *basal layer*, the deepest layer, rests on a basement membrane, which attaches it to the dermis. It is a single layer of columnar cells, whose basal surfaces sprout many fine processes and hemidesmosomes, anchoring them to the *lamina densa* of the basement membrane.

In normal skin some 30% of basal cells are preparing for division (growth fraction). Following mitosis, a cell enters the G$_1$ phase, synthesizes RNA and protein, and grows in size (Fig. 2.3). Later, when the cell is triggered to divide, DNA is synthesized

**Table 2.1** Functions of the skin.

| Function | Structure/cell involved |
| --- | --- |
| Protection against: | |
|   chemicals, particles | Horny layer |
|   ultraviolet radiation | Melanocytes |
|   antigens, haptens | Langerhans cells |
|   microbes | Langerhans cells |
| Preservation of a balanced internal environment | Horny layer |
| Prevents loss of water, electrolytes and macromolecules | Horny layer |
| Shock absorber | Dermis and subcutaneous fat |
| Strong, yet elastic and compliant | |
| Temperature regulation | Blood vessels |
| | Eccrine sweat glands |
| Insulation | Subcutaneous fat |
| Sensation | Specialized nerve endings |
| Lubrication | Sebaceous glands |
| Protection and prising | Nails |
| Calorie reserve | Subcutaneous fat |
| Vitamin D synthesis | Keratinocytes |
| Body odour / pheromones | Apocrine sweat glands |
| Psychosocial, display | Skin, lips, hair and nails |

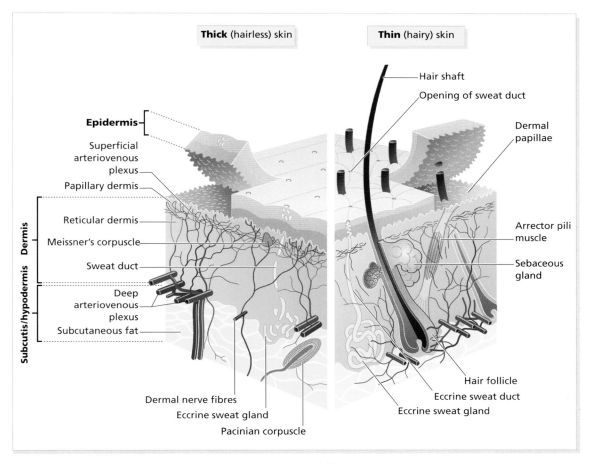

**Fig. 2.1** Three-dimensional diagram of the skin, including a hair follicle.

(S phase) and chromosomal DNA is replicated. A short post-synthetic ($G_2$) phase of further growth occurs before mitosis (M). DNA synthesis continues through the S and $G_2$ phases, but not during mitosis. The $G_1$ phase is then repeated, and one of the daughter cells moves into the suprabasal layer. It then differentiates (Fig. 2.2), having lost the capacity to divide, and synthesizes keratins. Some basal cells remain inactive in a so-called $G_0$ phase but may re-enter the cycle and resume proliferation. The cell cycle time in normal human skin is controversial; estimates of 50–200 h reflect differing views on the duration of the $G_1$ phase. Stem cells reside amongst these interfollicular basal cells and also amongst the cells of the external root sheath at the bulge in the hair follicle at the level of attach-

ment of the arrector pili muscle. Stem cells cannot be identified by histology but experimentally can be identified by their ability to retain radioactive thymidine incorporated into their DNA for long periods of time. These cells divide infrequently, but can generate new proliferative cells in the epidermis and hair follicle in response to damage.

## Keratinocytes

The *spinous* or *prickle cell* layer (Fig. 2.4) is composed of *keratinocytes*. These differentiating cells, which synthesize keratins, are larger than basal cells. Keratinocytes are firmly attached to each other by small interlocking cytoplasmic processes, by abundant desmosomes and by other cadherins p. 26 and

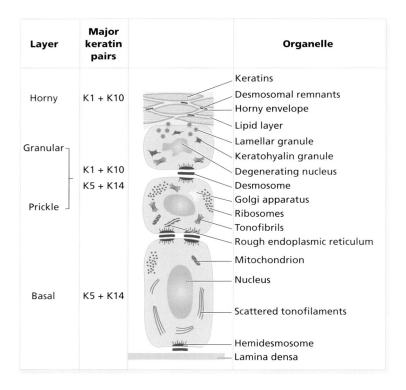

| Layer | Major keratin pairs | Organelle |
|---|---|---|
| Horny | K1 + K10 | Keratins<br>Desmosomal remnants<br>Horny envelope<br>Lipid layer |
| Granular | K1 + K10<br>K5 + K14 | Lamellar granule<br>Keratohyalin granule<br>Degenerating nucleus<br>Desmosome |
| Prickle | | Golgi apparatus<br>Ribosomes<br>Tonofibrils<br>Rough endoplasmic reticulum |
| Basal | K5 + K14 | Mitochondrion<br>Nucleus<br>Scattered tonofilaments<br>Hemidesmosome<br>Lamina densa |

**Fig. 2.2** Changes during keratinization.

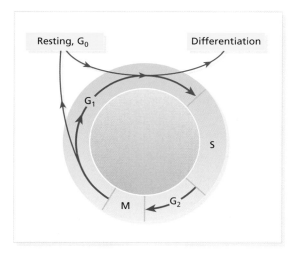

**Fig. 2.3** The cell cycle.

table 2.5 separated by an intercellular layer of glycoproteins and lipoproteins. Under the light microscope, the desmosomes look like 'prickles'. They are specialized attachment plaques that have been characterized biochemically. They contain desmoplakins, desmogleins and desmocollins. Autoantibodies to

these proteins are found in pemphigus (p. 120), when they are responsible for the detachment of keratinocytes from one another and so for intra-epidermal blister formation. Cytoplasmic continuity between keratinocytes occurs at *gap junctions*, specialized areas on opposing cell walls. Tonofilaments are small fibres running from the cytoplasm to the desmosomes. They are more numerous in cells of the spinous layer than of the basal layer, and are packed into bundles called *tonofibrils*. Many *lamellar granules* (otherwise known as membrane-coating granules, Odland bodies or keratinosomes), derived from the Golgi apparatus, appear in the superficial keratinocytes of this layer. They contain polysaccharides, hydrolytic enzymes and stacks of lipid lamellae composed of phospholipids, cholesterol and glucosylceramides. Their contents are discharged into the intercellular space of the granular cell layer to become precursors of the lipids in the intercellular space of the horny layer (p. 13).

Cellular differentiation continues in the granular layer, which normally consists of two or three layers of cells that are flatter than those in the spinous layer, and have more tonofibrils. As the name of

Horny layer
Granular layer
Prickle cell layer
Basal layer
Dermis

(a) (b)

**Fig. 2.4** Layers of the epidermis. (a) Light microscopy and (b) electron micrograph.

the layer implies, these cells contain large irregular basophilic granules of *keratohyalin*, which merge with tonofibrils. These keratohyalin granules contain proteins, including involucrin, loricrin and profilaggrin, which is cleaved into filaggrin by specific phosphatases as the granular cells move into the horny layer.

As keratinocytes migrate out through the outermost layers, their keratohyalin granules break up and their contents are dispersed throughout the cytoplasm. Filaggrin peptides aggregate the keratin cytoskeleton, collapsing it, and thus converting the granular cells to flattened squames. These make up the thick and tough peripheral protein coating of the *horny envelope*. Its structural proteins include loricrin and involucrin, the latter binding to ceramides in the surrounding intercellular space under the influence of transglutaminase. Filaggrin, involucrin and loricrin can all be detected histochemically and are useful as markers of epidermal differentiation.

The *horny layer* (stratum corneum) is made of piled-up layers of flattened dead cells (corneocytes) – the bricks – separated by lipids – the mortar – in the intercellular space. Together these provide an effective barrier to water loss and to invasion by infectious agents and toxic chemicals. The corneocyte cytoplasm is packed with keratin filaments, embedded in a matrix and enclosed by an envel-

ope derived from the keratohyalin granules. This envelope, along with the aggregated keratins that it encloses, gives the corneocyte its toughness, allowing the skin to withstand all sorts of chemical and mechanical insults. Horny cells normally have no nuclei or intracytoplasmic organelles, these having been destroyed by hydrolytic and degrading enzymes found in lamellar granules and the lysosomes of granular cells.

### Keratinization

All cells have an internal skeleton made up of microfilaments (7 nm diameter; actin), microtubules (20–35 nm diameter; tubulin) and intermediate filaments (10 nm diameter). Keratins (from the Greek *keras* meaning 'horn') are the main intermediate filaments in epithelial cells and are comparable to vimentin in mesenchymal cells, neurofilaments in neurones and desmin in muscle cells. Keratins are not just a biochemical curiosity, as mutations in their genes cause a number of skin diseases including simple epidermolysis bullosa (p. 128) and bullous ichthyosiform erythroderma (p. 49).

The keratins are a family of more than 30 proteins, each produced by different genes. These separate into two gene families: one responsible for basic and the other for acidic keratins. The keratin polypeptide has a central helical portion with a non-helical N-terminal head and C-terminal tail. Individual keratins exist in pairs so that their double filament always consists of one acidic and one basic keratin polypeptide. The intertwining of adjacent filaments forms larger fibrils.

Different keratins are found at different levels of the epidermis depending on the stage of differentiation and disease; normal basal cells make keratins 5 and 14, but terminally differentiated suprabasal cells make keratins 1 and 10 (Fig. 2.2). Keratins 6 and 16 become prominent in hyperproliferative states such as psoriasis.

During differentiation, the keratin fibrils in the cells of the horny layer align and aggregate, under the influence of filaggrin. Cysteine, found in keratins of the horny layer, allows cross-linking of fibrils to give the epidermis strength to withstand injury.

### Cell cohesion and desquamation

Firm cohesion in the spinous layer is ensured by 'stick and grip' mechanisms. A glycoprotein intercellular substance acts as a cement, sticking the cells together, and the intertwining of the small cytoplasmic processes of the prickle cells, together with their desmosomal attachments, accounts for the grip. The cytoskeleton of tonofibrils also maintains the cell shape rigidly.

The typical 'basket weave' appearance of the horny layer in routine histological sections is artefactual and deceptive. In fact, cells deep in the horny layer stick tightly together and only those at the surface flake off; this is in part caused by the activity of cholesterol sulphatase. This enzyme is deficient in X-linked recessive ichthyosis (p. 48), in which poor shedding leads to the piling up of corneocytes in the horny layer. Desquamation is normally responsible for the removal of harmful exogenous substances from the skin surface. The cells lost are replaced by newly formed corneocytes; regeneration and turn-over of the horny layer are therefore continuous.

### Epidermal barrier

The horny layer prevents the loss of interstitial fluid from within, and acts as a barrier to the penetration of potentially harmful substances from outside. Solvent extraction of the epidermis leads to an increased permeability to water, and it has been known for years that essential fatty acid deficiency causes poor cutaneous barrier function. These facts implicate ceramides, cholesterol, free fatty acids (from lamellar granules; p. 12), and smaller quantities of other lipids, in cutaneous barrier formation. Natural moisturizing factor (NMF), predominantly made up of amino acids and their metabolites, also helps maintain the properties of the stratum corneum. Barrier function is impaired when the horny layer is removed – experimentally, by successive strippings with adhesive tape, or clinically, by injury or skin disease. It is also decreased by excessive hydration or dehydration of the horny layer and by detergents.

The relative impermeability of the stratum corneum and 'moving staircase' effect of continually shedding the outer corneocytes provide a passive barrier to infective organisms. In addition to this, protection is given by the various antimicrobial peptides (AMPs) found on epithelial surfaces. The two major families of AMPs are the defensins and the cathelicidins which have a broad range of antimicrobial activity and form the first line of immune defence of the body.

The speed at which a substance penetrates through the epidermis is directly proportional to its concentration difference across the barrier layer, and indirectly proportional to the thickness of the horny layer. A rise in skin temperature aids penetration. A normal horny layer is slightly permeable to water, but relatively impermeable to ions such as sodium and potassium. Some other substances (e.g. glucose and urea) also penetrate poorly, whereas some aliphatic alcohols pass through easily. The penetration of a solute dissolved in an organic liquid depends mainly on the qualities of the solvent.

### Epidermopoiesis and its regulation

Both the thickness of the normal epidermis and the number of cells in it remain constant, as cell loss at the surface is balanced by cell production in the basal layer. Locally produced polypeptides (cytokines), growth factors and hormones stimulate or inhibit epidermal proliferation, interacting in complex ways to ensure homoeostasis. Nitric oxide, a gaseous free radical produced on the skin surface by nitrate reduction and also by constitutive enzymes within the

**Table 2.2** Some cytokines produced by keratinocytes.

| Designation | Cytokine | Function |
|---|---|---|
| *Interleukins* | | |
| IL-1 | Interleukin 1 | Lymphocyte activation<br>Langerhans cell activation<br>Acute phase reactions |
| IL-3 | Interleukin 3 | Colony-stimulating factor |
| IL-6 | Interleukin 6 | B-cell differentiation |
| IL-8 | Interleukin 8 | Chemotaxis<br>Angiogenesis |
| IL-10 | Interleukin 10 | Inhibition of Th1 T cells |
| IL-12 | Interleukin 12 | Induction of Th1 T cells |
| *Colony-stimulating factors* | | |
| GM-CSF | Granulocyte–macrophage colony-stimulating factor | Proliferation of granulocytes and macrophages |
| G-CSF | Granulocyte colony-stimulating factor | Proliferation of granulocytes |
| M-CSF | Macrophage colony-stimulating factor | Proliferation of macrophages |
| *Others* | | |
| TGF | Transforming growth factors | Inhibit inflammation |
| TNF-$\alpha$ | Tumour necrosis factor $\alpha$ | Induces inflammatory response and amplifies Th1 response<br>Induces apoptosis |
| IFN-$\alpha$ | $\alpha$-Interferon | Antiviral state |
| IFN-$\gamma$ | $\gamma$-Interferon | Amplification of type IV reactions |

epidermis, affects the balance between keratinocyte differentiation and proliferation. This is dose dependent and involves direct interactions with enzymes containing transition elements such as zinc and iron. Cytokines and growth factors (Table 2.2) are produced by keratinocytes, Langerhans cells, fibroblasts and lymphocytes within the skin. After these bind to high affinity cell surface receptors, DNA synthesis is controlled by signal transduction, involving protein kinase C or inositol phosphate. Catecholamines, which do not penetrate the surface of cells, influence cell division via the adenosine 3′,5′-cyclic monophosphate (cAMP) second messenger system. Steroid hormones bind to receptor proteins within the cytoplasm, and then pass to the nucleus where they influence transcription.

### *Vitamin D synthesis*

The steroid 7-dehydrocholesterol, found in keratino-cytes, is converted by sunlight to cholecalciferol. The vitamin becomes active after 25-hydroxylation in the kidney. Kidney disease and lack of sun, particularly in dark-skinned peoples, can both cause vitamin D deficiency and rickets. A few authors have recently raised concerns that low vitamin D levels may be associated with some internal cancers and suggested that we should encourage more sun exposure. However, the link between sun protection, low vitamin D and cancer remains unproven, and if it were found to be true dietary supplementation raises serum levels of vitamin D without the risks of skin cancer and ageing associated with sunbathing.

### Other cells in the epidermis

Keratinocytes make up about 85% of cells in the epidermis, but three other types of cell are also found there: melanocytes, Langerhans cells and Merkel cells (Fig. 2.5).

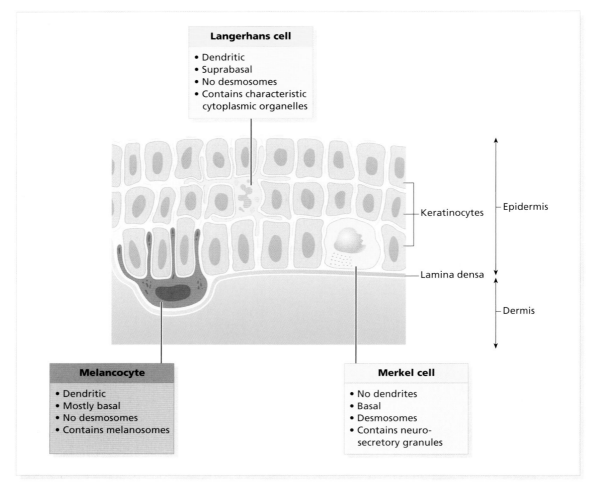

**Langerhans cell**

- Dendritic
- Suprabasal
- No desmosomes
- Contains characteristic cytoplasmic organelles

Keratinocytes

Epidermis

Lamina densa

Dermis

**Melancocyte**

- Dendritic
- Mostly basal
- No desmosomes
- Contains melanosomes

**Merkel cell**

- No dendrites
- Basal
- Desmosomes
- Contains neuro-secretory granules

**Fig. 2.5** Melanocyte, Langerhans cell and Merkel cell.

## Melanocytes

Melanocytes are the only cells that can synthesize melanin. They migrate from the neural crest into the basal layer of the ectoderm where, in human embryos, they are seen as early as 8 weeks' gestation. They are also found in hair bulbs, the retina and pia arachnoid. Each dendritic melanocyte associates with a number of keratinocytes, forming an 'epidermal melanin unit' (Fig. 2.5). The dendritic processes of melanocytes wind between the epidermal cells and end as discs in contact with them. Their cytoplasm contains discrete organelles, the *melanosomes*, containing varying amounts of the pigment melanin (Fig. 2.6). This

is 'injected' into surrounding keratinocytes to provide them with pigmentation to help protect the skin against damaging ultraviolet radiation.

Melanogenesis is described at the beginning of Chapter 19 on disorders of pigmentation.

## Langerhans cells

The Langerhans cell is a dendritic cell (Figs 2.5 and 2.7) like the melanocyte. It also lacks desmosomes and tonofibrils, but has a lobulated nucleus. The specific granules within the cell look like a tennis racket when seen in two dimensions in an electron micrograph (Fig. 2.8), or like a sycamore seed

**Fig. 2.6** Melanocyte (electron micrograph), with melanosomes (inset).

LAMINA DENSA

DERMIS

**Fig. 2.7** Adenosine triphosphatase-positive Langerhans cells in an epidermal sheet: the network provides a reticulo-epithelial trap for contact allergens.

when reconstructed in three dimensions. They are plate-like, with a rounded bleb protruding from the surface.

Langerhans cells come from a mobile pool of precursors originating in the bone marrow. There are approximately 800 Langerhans cells per mm$^2$ in human skin and their dendritic processes fan out to form a striking network seen best in epidermal sheets (Fig. 2.7). Langerhans cells are alone among epidermal cells in possessing surface receptors for C3b and the Fc portions of immunoglobulin G (IgG) and IgE, and in bearing major histocompatibility complex (MHC) class II antigens (HLA-DR, -DP and -DQ). They are best thought of as highly specialized macrophages.

Langerhans cells have a key role in many immune reactions. They take up exogenous antigen, process it and present it to T lymphocytes either in the skin or in the local lymph nodes (p. 31). They probably play a part in immunosurveillance for viral and tumour antigens. In this way, ultraviolet radiation can induce skin tumours both by causing mutations in the epidermal cells, and by decreasing the number of epidermal Langerhans cells, so that cells bearing altered antigens are not recognized or destroyed by the immune system. Topical or systemic glucocorticoids also reduce the density of epidermal Langerhans cells. The Langerhans cell is the principal cell in skin allografts to which the T lymphocytes of the host react during rejection; allograft survival can be prolonged by depleting Langerhans cells.

### Merkel cells

Merkel cells are found in normal epidermis (Fig. 2.5) and act as transducers for fine touch. They are non-dendritic cells, lying in or near the basal layer, and are of the same size as keratinocytes. They are concentrated in localized thickenings of the epidermis near hair follicles (hair discs), and contain membrane-bound spherical granules, 80–100 nm in diameter, which have a core of varying density, separated from

**Fig. 2.8** Langerhans cell (electron micrograph), with characteristic granule (inset).

the membrane by a clear halo. Sparse desmosomes connect these cells to neighbouring keratinocytes. Fine unmyelinated nerve endings are often associated with Merkel cells, which express immunoreactivity for various neuropeptides.

### Epidermal appendages

The skin appendages are derived from epithelial germs during embryogenesis and, except for the nails, lie in the dermis. They include hair, nails and sweat and sebaceous glands. They are described, along with the diseases that affect them, in Chapters 12 and 13, respectively.

## Dermo-epidermal junction

The basement membrane lies at the interface between the epidermis and dermis. With light microscopy it can be highlighted using a periodic acid–Schiff (PAS) stain, because of its abundance of neutral mucopolysaccharides. Electron microscopy (Fig. 2.9) shows that the *lamina densa* (rich in type IV collagen) is separated from the basal cells by an electron-lucent area, the *lamina lucida*. The plasma membrane of basal cells has *hemidesmosomes* (containing bullous pemphigoid antigens, collagen XVII and α6 β4 integrin). The lamina lucida contains the adhesive macromolecules, laminin-1, laminin-5 and entactin.

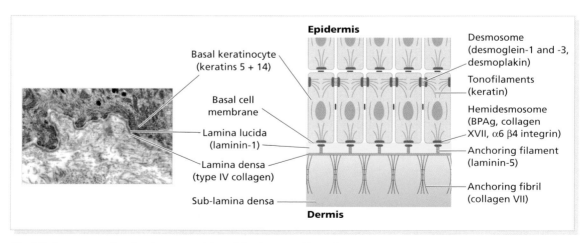

**Fig. 2.9** Structure and molecular composition of the dermo-epidermal junction.

**Table 2.3** Functions of some resident dermal cells.

| | |
|---|---|
| Fibroblast | Synthesis of collagen, reticulin, elastin, fibronectin, glycosaminoglycans, collagenase |
| Mononuclear phagocyte | Mobile: phagocytoses and destroys bacteria<br>Secretes cytokines |
| Lymphocyte | Immunosurveillance |
| Langerhans cell and dermal dendritic cell | In transit between local lymph node and epidermis<br>Antigen presentation |
| Mast cell | Stimulated by antigens, complement components, and other substances to release many inflammatory mediators including histamine, heparin, prostaglandins, leukotrienes, tryptase and chemotactic factors for eosinophils and neutrophils |
| Merkel cell | Acts as transducer for fine touch |

Fine *anchoring filaments* (of laminin-5) cross the lamina lucida and connect the lamina densa to the plasma membrane of the basal cells. *Anchoring fibrils* (of type VII collagen), dermal microfibril bundles and single small collagen fibres (types I and III), extend from the papillary dermis to the deep part of the lamina densa.

Laminins, large non-collagen glycoproteins produced by keratinocytes, aided by entactin, promote adhesion between the basal cells above the lamina lucida and type IV collagen, the main constituent of the lamina densa, below it. The laminins act as a glue, helping to hold the epidermis onto the dermis. Bullous pemphigoid antigens (of molecular weights 230 and 180 kDa) are synthesized by basal cells and are found in close association with the hemidesmosomes and laminin. Their function is unknown but antibodies to them are found in pemphigoid (p. 123), a subcutaneous blistering condition.

The structures within the dermo-epidermal junction provide mechanical support, encouraging the adhesion, growth, differentiation and migration of the overlying basal cells, and also act as a semipermeable filter that regulates the transfer of nutrients and cells from dermis to epidermis.

## Dermis

The dermis lies between the epidermis and the subcutaneous fat. It supports the epidermis structurally and nutritionally. Its thickness varies, being greatest in the palms and soles and least in the eyelids and penis. In old age, the dermis thins and loses its elasticity.

The dermis interdigitates with the epidermis (Fig. 2.1) so that upward projections of the dermis, the dermal papillae, interlock with downward ridges of the epidermis, the rete pegs. This interdigitation is responsible for the ridges seen most readily on the fingertips (as fingerprints). It is important in the adhesion between epidermis and dermis as it increases the area of contact between them.

Like all connective tissues the dermis has three components: cells, fibres and amorphous ground substance.

### Cells of the dermis

The main cells of the dermis are fibroblasts, but there are also small numbers of resident and transitory mononuclear phagocytes, lymphocytes, Langerhans cells and mast cells. Other blood cells (e.g. polymorphs) are seen during inflammation. The main functions of the resident dermal cells are listed in Table 2.3 and their role in immunological reactions is discussed later in this chapter.

### Fibres of the dermis

The dermis is largely made up of interwoven fibres, principally of collagen, packed in bundles. Those in the papillary dermis are finer than those in the deeper reticular dermis. When the skin is stretched, collagen, with its high tensile strength, prevents tearing, and the elastic fibres, intermingled with the collagen, later return it to the unstretched state.

Collagen makes up 70–80% of the dry weight of the dermis. Its fibres are composed of thinner

| Collagen type | Tissue distribution |
|---|---|
| I | Most connective tissues including tendon and bone<br>Accounts for approximately 85% of skin collagen |
| II | Cartilage |
| III | Accounts for about 15% of skin collagen<br>Blood vessels |
| IV | Skin (lamina densa) and basement membranes of other tissues |
| V | Ubiquitous, including placenta |
| VII | Skin (anchoring fibrils)<br>Foetal membranes |

**Table 2.4** Distribution of some types of collagen.

fibrils, which are in turn made up of microfibrils built from individual collagen molecules. These molecules consist of three polypeptide chains (molecular weight 150 kDa) forming a triple helix with a non-helical segment at both ends. The alignment of the chains is stabilized by covalent cross-links involving lysine and hydroxylysine. Collagen is an unusual protein as it contains a high proportion of proline and hydroxyproline and many glycine residues; the spacing of glycine as every third amino acid is a prerequisite for the formation of a triple helix. Defects in the enzymes needed for collagen synthesis are responsible for some skin diseases, including the Ehlers–Danlos syndrome (Chapter 24), and conditions involving other systems, including lathyrism (fragility of skin and other connective tissues) and osteogenesis imperfecta (fragility of bones).

There are many, genetically distinct, collagen proteins, all with triple helical molecules, and all rich in hydroxyproline and hydroxylysine. The distribution of some of them is summarized in Table 2.4.

*Reticulin* fibres are fine collagen fibres, seen in foetal skin and around the blood vessels and appendages of adult skin.

*Elastic* fibres account for about 2% of the dry weight of adult dermis. They have two distinct protein components: an amorphous elastin core and a surrounding 'elastic tissue microfibrillar component'. Elastin (molecular weight 72 kDa) is made up of polypeptides (rich in glycine, desmosine and valine) linked to the microfibrillar component through their desmosine residues. Abnormalities in the elastic tissue cause cutis laxa (sagging inelastic skin) and pseudoxanthoma elasticum (Chapter 24).

## Ground substance of the dermis

The amorphous ground substance of the dermis consists largely of two glycosaminoglycans (hyaluronic acid and dermatan sulphate) with smaller amounts of heparan sulphate and chondroitin sulphate. The glycosaminoglycans are complexed to core protein and exist as proteoglycans.

The ground substance has several important functions:
• it binds water, allowing nutrients, hormones and waste products to pass through the dermis;
• it acts as a lubricant between the collagen and elastic fibre networks during skin movement; and
• it provides bulk, allowing the dermis to act as a shock absorber.

## Muscles

Both smooth and striated muscle are found in the skin. The smooth arrector pili muscles (see Fig. 13.1) are used by animals to raise their fur and so protect them from the cold. They are vestigial in humans, but may help to express sebum. Smooth muscle is also responsible for 'goose pimples' (bumps) from cold, nipple erection, and the raising of the scrotum by the dartos muscle. Striated fibres (e.g. the platysma) and some of the muscles of facial expression are also found in the dermis.

## Blood vessels

Although the skin consumes little oxygen, its abundant blood supply regulates body temperature. The

**Fig. 2.10** Blood vessels of the skin (carmine stain).

blood vessels lie in two main horizontal layers (Fig. 2.10). The deep plexus is just above the subcutaneous fat, and its arterioles supply the sweat glands and hair papillae. The superficial plexus is in the papillary dermis and arterioles from it become capillary loops in the dermal papillae. An arteriole arising in the deep dermis supplies an inverted cone of tissue, with its base at the epidermis.

The blood vessels in the skin are important in thermoregulation. Under sympathetic nervous control, arteriovenous anastomoses at the level of the deep plexus can shunt blood to the venous plexus at the expense of the capillary loops, thereby reducing surface heat loss by convection.

## Cutaneous lymphatics

Afferent lymphatics begin as blind-ended capillaries in the dermal papilla and pass to a superficial lymphatic plexus in the papillary dermis. There are also two deeper horizontal plexuses, and collecting lymphatics from the deeper one run with the veins in the superficial fascia.

## Nerves

The skin is liberally supplied with an estimated 1 million nerve fibres. Most are found in the face and extremities. Their cell bodies lie in the dorsal root ganglia. Both myelinated and non-myelinated fibres exist, with the latter making up an increasing proportion peripherally. Most free sensory nerves end in the dermis; however, a few non-myelinated nerve endings penetrate into the epidermis. Some

of these are associated with Merkel cells (p. 17). Free nerve endings detect the potentially damaging stimuli of heat and pain (nociceptors), while specialized end organs in the dermis, Pacinian and Meissner corpuscles, register deformation of the skin caused by pressure (mechanoreceptors) as well as vibration and touch. Autonomic nerves supply the blood vessels, sweat glands and arrector pili muscles.

Itching is an important feature of many skin diseases. It follows the stimulation of fine free nerve endings lying close to the dermo-epidermal junction. Areas with a high density of such endings (itch spots) are especially sensitive to itch-provoking stimuli. Impulses from these free endings pass centrally in two ways: quickly along myelinated A fibres, and more slowly along non-myelinated C fibres. As a result, itch has two components: a quick localized pricking sensation followed by a slow burning diffuse itching.

Many stimuli can induce itching (electrical, chemical and mechanical). In itchy skin diseases, pruritogenic chemicals such as histamine and proteolytic enzymes are liberated close to the dermo-epidermal junction. The detailed pharmacology of individual diseases is still poorly understood but prostaglandins potentiate chemically induced itching in inflammatory skin diseases.

> **Learning points**
>
> 1 More diseases are now being classified by abnormalities of function and structure rather than by their appearance.
> 2 Today's patients are inquisitive and knowledgeable. If you understand the structure and function of the skin, your explanations to them will be easier and more convincing.

## The skin immune system

The skin acts as a barrier to prevent injury of underlying tissues and to prevent infections from entering the body. Simply put, it keeps the inside in and the outside out. The horny layer is a physical barrier that minimizes the loss of fluid and electrolytes, and also stops the penetration of harmful substances and trauma (p. 10). It is a dry mechanical barrier from which contaminating organisms and chemicals are continually being removed by washing and desquamation. Only when these breach the horny layer do the cellular components, described below, come into play.

The skin is involved in so many immunological reactions seen regularly in the clinic (e.g. urticaria, allergic contact dermatitis, psoriasis, vasculitis) that special mention has to be made of the peripheral arm of the immune system based in the skin – the skin immune system (SIS). It includes the cutaneous blood vessels and lymphatics with their local lymph nodes and contains circulating lymphocytes and resident immune cells. Although it is beyond the scope of this book to cover general immunology, this section outlines some of the intricate ways in which the skin defends itself and the body, and how antigens are recognized by specialized skin cells, mainly the Langerhans cells. It also reviews the ways in which antibodies, lymphocytes, macrophages and polymorphs elicit inflammation in skin.

## Some cellular components of the skin immune system

### *Keratinocytes* (p. 11)

Their prime role is to make the protective horny layer (p. 10) and to support the outermost epithelium of the body, but they also have immunological functions in their own right. Keratinocytes produce large numbers of cytokines (Table 2.2), and can be induced by γ-interferon to express HLA-DR. They release large amounts of interleukin-1 (IL-1) after injury, and this initiates various immune and inflammatory cascades (Fig. 2.11). Keratinocytes play a central part in healing after epidermal injury by self-regulating epidermal proliferation and differentiation (Fig. 2.11). They can also produce α-melanocyte-stimulating hormone (p. 278), which is immunosuppressive.

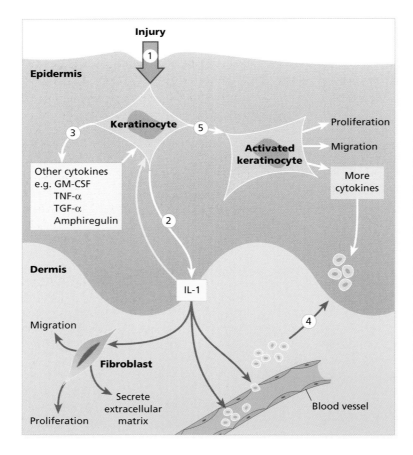

**Fig. 2.11** The keratinocyte and wound healing. The injured keratinocyte turns on wound healing responses. When a keratinocyte is injured (1), it releases interleukin-1 (IL-1) (2). IL-1 activates endothelial cells causing them to express selectins that slow down lymphocytes passing over them. Once lymphocytes stop on the endothelial cells lining the vessels, IL-1 acts as a chemotactic factor to draw lymphocytes into the epidermis (4). At the same time, IL-1 activates keratinocytes by binding to their IL-1 receptors. Activated keratinocytes produce other cytokines (3). Among these is tumour necrosis factor α (TNF-α) that additionally activates keratinocytes and keeps them in an activated state (5). Activation of keratinocytes causes them to proliferate, migrate and secrete additional cytokines.

### Langerhans cells (p. 16)

These dendritic cells come from the bone marrow and move into the epidermis where they remain. Their dendrites intercalate between keratinocytes. They can be identified in tissue sections by demonstrating their characteristic surface markers (e.g. CD1a antigen, MHC class II antigens, adenosine triphosphatase) or S-100 protein in their cytoplasm (also found in melanocytes). Langerhans cells have a key role in antigen presentation.

### Dermal dendritic cells

These poorly characterized cells are found around the tiny blood vessels of the papillary dermis. They bear MHC class II antigens on their surface and, like Langerhans cells, probably function as antigen-presenting cells.

### T lymphocytes

Like T cells elsewhere, these develop and acquire their antigen receptors (T-cell receptors; TCR) in the thymus. They differentiate into subpopulations, recognizable by their different surface molecules (CD meaning cluster of differentiation markers), which are functionally distinct. T lymphocytes that express CD4 on their surfaces work to induce immune reactions and elicit inflammation. T cells that express CD8 are cytotoxic and can lyse infected, grafted and cancerous cells.

Thelper (Th) cells, CD4 (helper) cells are subdivided into Th1 cells that produce IL-2 (T-cell growth factor), $\gamma$-interferon, and other cytokines not produced by Th2 cells. Th2 cells produce other interleukins such as IL-4, IL-5, IL-9 and IL-13. The amounts of IL-12 and IL-4 secreted by antigen-processing cells seem important in determining exactly which path of differentiation is followed. A third subset of CD-4 cells has recently been called, somewhat confusingly, Th17 cells. IL-23 directs these to release IL-17 and IL-22.

Th1 cells induce cell-mediated immune reactions in the skin (e.g. allergic contact dermatitis and delayed hypersensitivity reactions) and are involved in elicitation reactions as well. Th2 cells help B cells produce antibody. Th17 cells are involved in the clearance of infectious agents, and also mediate autoimmune inflammation and psoriasis. Th cells recognize antigen in association with MHC class II molecules (Fig. 2.12) and, when triggered by antigen, release cytokines that attract and activate other inflammatory cells (Fig. 2.13).

Some skin diseases display a predominantly Th1 response (e.g. psoriasis), others a mainly Th2 response (e.g. lepromatous leprosy).

### T-cytotoxic (Tc) cells

These lymphocytes are capable of destroying allogeneic, tumour and virally infected cells, which they recognize by the MHC class I molecules on their surface. They express CD8.

### T-cell receptor (TCR) and T-cell gene receptor rearrangements

Most TCRs are composed of an $\alpha$ and a $\beta$ chain, each with a variable (antigen binding) and a constant domain, which are associated with the CD3 cell surface molecules (Fig. 2.12). The amino acid sequence of the variable portion determines its antigen-binding specificity – different sequences bind different antigens. To provide diversity and the ability to bind almost any antigen, the genes coding for the amino acid sequence undergo rearrangement. Antigenic stimulation results in expansion of appropriate clones carrying TCRs capable of binding to the antigen. Most inflammatory responses are polyclonal. However, malignant transformation is associated with proliferation of a unique clone. In fact, an analysis of the degree of clonality of rearrangements of the gene for the receptor can be used to determine whether a T-cell infiltrate in skin is likely to be malignant or reactive.

### Other (non-T, non-B) lymphocytes

Some lymphocytes express neither CD4 nor CD8. These leucocytes have some properties of T lymphocytes and some properties of myelomonocytic cells. Most have receptors for FcIgG. This subpopulation contains natural killer (NK) and killer (K) cells.

### Natural killer cells

These are large granular leucocytes that can kill virally infected cells, or tumour cells that have not previously been sensitized with antibody. They

**Fig. 2.12** T-lymphocyte activation by (a) antigen and (b) superantigen. When antigen has been processed it is presented on the surface of the Langerhans cell in association with major histocompatibility complex (MHC) class II. The complex formation that takes place between the antigen, MHC class II and T-cell receptor (TCR) provides signal 1, which is enhanced by the coupling of CD4 with the MHC molecule. A second signal for T-cell activation is provided by the interaction between the co-stimulatory molecules CD28 (T cell) and B7 (Langerhans cell). CD2–LFA-3 and LFA-1–ICAM-1 adhesion augment the response to signals 1 and 2. Superantigen interacts with the TCR Vβ and MHC class II without processing, binding outside the normal antigen binding site. Activated T cells secrete many cytokines, including IL-1, IL-8 and γ-interferon, which promote inflammation (Fig. 2.13).

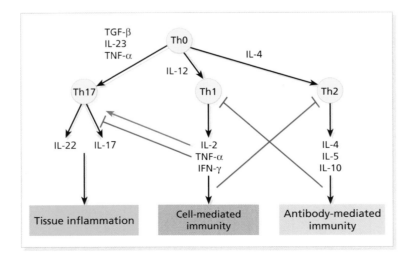

**Fig. 2.13** Characteristics of Th1, Th2 and Th17 responses.

develop in the bone marrow, but have no antigen-specific receptors, reacting instead with self antigens. They especially kill tumour and virally infected cells. These cells can sometimes recognize glycolipid antigens using CD1 surface molecules that do not require presentation by antigen-presenting cells.

### Killer cells

These are cytotoxic T cells, NK cells or monocytic leucocytes that can kill target cells sensitized with antibody. In antibody-mediated cellular cytotoxicity, antibody binds to antigen on the surface of the target cell; the K cell binds to the antibody at its other (Fc) end by its Fc receptor and the target cell is then lysed.

## Mast cells

These are present in most connective tissues, predominantly around blood vessels. Their numerous granules contain inflammatory mediators (see Fig. 8.1). In rodents – and probably in humans – there are two distinct populations of mast cells: connective tissue and mucosal, which differ in their staining properties, content of inflammatory mediators and proteolytic enzymes. Skin mast cells play a central part in the pathogenesis of urticaria (p. 104).

## Molecular components of the skin immune system

### Antigens

Antigens are molecules that are recognized by the immune system thereby provoking an immune reaction, usually in the form of a humoral or cell-mediated immune response. The immune system can usually identify its own molecules, so that it does not direct a reaction against them. If it does, 'autoimmune reactions' occur. Otherwise the skin immune system readily responds to 'non-self' antigens, such as chemicals, proteins, allografted cells and infectious agents. The process of recognizing antigens and developing immunity is called induction or sensitization.

### Superantigens

Some bacterial toxins (e.g. those released by

*Staphylococcus aureus*) are prototypic superantigens. They align with MHC class II molecules of antigen-presenting cells outside their antigen presentation groove and, without any cellular processing, may directly induce massive T-cell proliferation and cytokine production leading to disorders such as the toxic shock syndrome (p. 225). Streptococcal toxins act as superantigens to activate T cells in the pathogenesis of guttate psoriasis.

### Antibodies (immunoglobulins)

Antibodies are immunoglobulins (Ig) that react with antigens.

- IgG is responsible for long-lasting humoral immunity. It can cross the placenta, and binds complement to activate the classic complement pathway. IgG can coat neutrophils and macrophages (by their FcIgG receptors), and acts as an opsonin by cross-bridging antigen. IgG can also sensitize target cells for destruction by K cells.
- IgM is the largest immunoglobulin molecule. It is the first antibody to appear after immunization or infection. Like IgG it can fix complement, but unlike IgG it cannot cross the placenta.
- IgA is the most common immunoglobulin in secretions. It acts as a protective paint in the gastrointestinal and respiratory tracts. It does not bind complement but can activate it via the alternative pathway.
- IgE binds to Fc receptors on mast cells and basophils, where it sensitizes them to release inflammatory mediators in type I immediate hypersensitivity reactions (Fig. 2.14).

### Cytokines

Cytokines are small proteins secreted by cells such as lymphocytes and macrophages, and also by keratinocytes (Table 2.2). They regulate the amplitude and duration of inflammation by acting locally on nearby cells (paracrine action), on those cells that secreted them (autocrine) and occasionally on distant target cells (endocrine) via the circulation. The term cytokine covers interleukins, interferons, colony-stimulating factors, cytotoxins and growth factors. Interleukins are produced predominantly by leucocytes, have a known amino acid sequence and are active in inflammation or immunity.

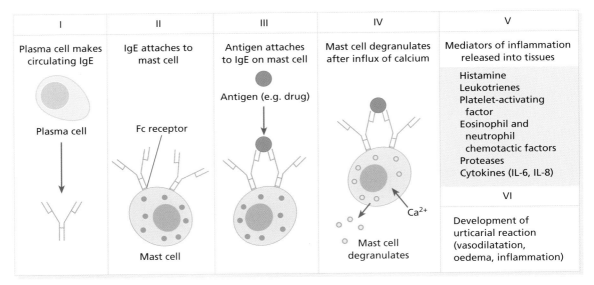

| I | II | III | IV | V |
|---|---|---|---|---|
| Plasma cell makes circulating IgE | IgE attaches to mast cell | Antigen attaches to IgE on mast cell | Mast cell degranulates after influx of calcium | Mediators of inflammation released into tissues |

**Fig. 2.14** Urticaria: an immediate (type I) hypersensitivity reaction.

There are many cytokines (Table 2.2), and each may act on more than one type of cell, causing many different effects. Cytokines frequently have overlapping actions. In any inflammatory reaction some cytokines are acting synergistically while others will antagonize these effects. This network of potent chemicals, each acting alone and in concert, moves the inflammatory response along in a controlled way. Cytokines bind to high-affinity (but not usually specific) cell surface receptors, and elicit a biological response by regulating the transcription of genes in the target cell via signal transduction pathways involving, for example, the Janus protein tyrosine kinase or calcium influx systems. The biological response is a balance between the production of the cytokine, the expression of its receptors on the target cells and the presence of inhibitors.

## Adhesion molecules

Cellular adhesion molecules (CAMs) are surface glycoproteins that are expressed on many different types of cell; they are involved in cell–cell and cell–matrix adhesion and interactions. CAMs are fundamental in the interaction of lymphocytes with antigen-presenting cells (Fig. 2.12), keratinocytes and endothelial cells, and are important in lympho-cyte trafficking in the skin during inflammation (Fig. 2.11). CAMs have been classified into three families: immunoglobulin superfamily, integrins and selectins.

CAMs of special relevance in the skin are listed in Table 2.5.

## Histocompatibility antigens

Like other cells, those in the skin express surface antigens directed by genes. The human leucocyte antigen (HLA) region lies within the major histocompatability (MHC) locus on chromosome 6. In particular, HLA-A, -B and -C antigens (the class I antigens) are expressed on all nucleated cells including keratinocytes, Langerhans cells and cells of the dermis. HLA-DR, -DP, -DQ and -DZ antigens (the class II antigens) are expressed only on some cells (e.g. Langerhans cells and B cells). They are usually not found on keratinocytes except during certain reactions (e.g. allergic contact dermatitis) or diseases (e.g. lichen planus). Helper T cells recognize antigens only in the presence of cells bearing class II antigens. Class II antigens are also important for certain cell–cell interactions. Class I antigens mark target cells for cell-mediated cytotoxic reactions, such as the rejection of skin allografts and the destruction of cells infected by viruses.

**Table 2.5** Cellular adhesion molecules important in the skin.

| Family | Nature | Example | Site | Ligand |
|---|---|---|---|---|
| Cadherins | Glycoproteins Adherence dependent on calcium | Desmoglein | Desmosomes in epidermis | Other cadherins |
| Immunoglobulin | Numerous molecules that are structurally similar to immunoglobulins | ICAM-1 CD2 VCAM-1 | Endothelial cells Keratinocytes Langerhans cells T lymphocytes Some NK cells Endothelial cells | LFA-1 LFA-3 |
| Integrins | Surface proteins comprising two non-covalently bound α and β chains | Very late activation proteins (β1-VLA) LFA-1 Mac-1 | T lymphocyte T lymphocyte Macrophages Monocytes Granulocytes | VCAM ICAM-1 C3b component of complement |
| Selectins | Adhesion molecules with lectin-like domain which binds carbohydrate | E selectin | Endothelial cells | CD15 |

CD2, cluster of differentiation antigen 2; ICAM-1, intercellular adhesion molecule 1; LFA, leucocyte function antigen; Mac-1, macrophage activation 1; VCAM-1, vascular cell adhesion molecule 1.

## Types of immune reactions in the skin

### Innate immune system

The epidermal barrier is the major defence against infection in human skin. When it is breached, cells in the dermis and epidermis can telegraph the danger and engage the innate immunity and inflammatory systems. Innate immunity allows reaction to infectious agents and noxious chemicals, without the need to activate specific lymphocytes or use antibodies. This is fortunate. If an infected person had to wait for immunity to develop, the onset of the reaction might take a week or two, and by then the infection might be widespread or lethal.

For example, defensins in the epidermis inhibit bacterial replication there. Complement can be activated by many infectious agents via the alternative pathway without the need for antigen–antibody interaction. Complement activation generates C5a, which attracts neutrophils, and C3b and C5b, which opsonize the agents so they can be more readily engulfed and killed by the phagocytes when these

arrive. Chemicals such as detergents can activate keratinocytes to produce cytokines, leading to epidermal proliferation and eventual shedding of the toxic agent. After infection or stimulation, certain cells can non-specifically secrete chemokines that bring inflammatory cells to the area. The main effector cells of the innate immune system are neutrophils, monocytes and macrophages.

The antigen-presenting cells have a role in both innate and acquired immunity. They can recognize certain patterns of molecules or chemicals common to many infectious agents. The lipopolysaccharide of Gram-negative bacteria is an example of such a 'pathogen-associated molecular pattern'. The receptors for these reside on cell membranes and are genetically derived.

Toll-like receptors are expressed on Langerhans cells, macrophages and regulatory T cells in the skin and provide the innate immune system with a certain specificity. They are transmembrane proteins, which recognize patterns, and different Toll receptors recognize different patterns and chemicals. For example, Toll-like receptor 2 recognizes lipoproteins, while Toll-like receptor 3 recognizes double-stranded RNA. Toll-like receptors also up-regulate the expression of co-stimulatory molecules that allow appropriate recognition and response of the adaptive immune system.

## Adaptive immune system

Adaptive immunity is not only more specific, but is also long-lasting. It generates cells that can persist in a relatively dormant state. These are ready to react quickly and powerfully when they encounter their antigen again – even years later.

Specific immune responses allow a targeted and amplified inflammatory response. To induce such a response, an antigen must be processed by an antigen-presenting cell such as a Langerhans cell, and then be presented to a T cell, with unique receptor molecules on its surface, that can bind the antigen presented to it. To elicit an inflammatory response, this antigen processing, presentation and binding process is repeated but, this time, with the purpose of bringing in inflammatory, phagocytic and cytotoxic cells to control the inflammation within the area.

It is still helpful, if rather artificial, to separate these elicited specific immune responses into four main types using the original classification of Coombs and Gell. All of these types cause reactions in the skin.

### Type I: immediate hypersensitivity reactions

These are characterized by vasodilatation and an outpouring of fluid from blood vessels. Such reactions can be mimicked by drugs or toxins, which act directly, but immunological reactions are mediated by antibodies, and are manifestations of allergy. IgE and IgG4 antibodies, produced by plasma cells in organs other than the skin, attach themselves to mast cells in the dermis. These contain inflammatory mediators, both in granules and in their cytoplasm. The IgE antibody is attached to the mast cell by its Fc end, so that the antigen-combining site dangles from the mast cell like a hand on an arm (Fig. 2.14). When specific antigen combines with the hand parts of the immunoglobulin (the antigen-binding site or Fab end), the mast cell liberates its mediators into the surrounding tissue. Of these mediators, histamine (from the granules) and leukotrienes (from the cell

membrane) induce vasodilatation, and endothelial cells retract, allowing transudation into the extravascular space. The vasodilatation causes a pink colour, and the transudation causes swelling. Urticaria and angioedema (p. 104) are examples of immediate hypersensitivity reactions occurring in the skin.

Antigen may be delivered to the skin from the outside (as in a bee sting). This will induce a swelling in everyone by a direct pharmacological action. However, some people, with IgE antibodies against antigens in the venom, swell even more at the site of the sting as the result of a specific immunological reaction. If they are extremely sensitive, they may develop wheezing, wheals and anaphylactic shock (see Fig. 25.5), because of a massive release of histamine into the circulation.

Antigens can also reach mast cells from inside the body. Those who are allergic to shellfish, for example, may develop urticaria within seconds, minutes or hours of eating one. Antigenic material, absorbed from the gut, passes to tissue mast cells via the circulation, and elicits an urticarial reaction after binding to specific IgE on mast cells in the skin.

### Type II: humoral cytotoxic reactions

In the main, these involve IgG and IgM antibodies, which, like IgE, are produced by plasma cells and are present in the interstitial fluid of the skin. When they meet an antigen, they fix and activate complement through a series of enzymatic reactions that generate mediator and cytotoxic proteins. If bacteria enter the skin, IgG and IgM antibodies bind to antigens on them. Complement is activated through the classic pathway, and a number of mediators are generated. Amongst these are the chemotactic factor, C5a, which attracts polymorphs to the area of bacterial invasion, and the opsonin, C3b, which coats the bacteria so that they can be ingested and killed by polymorphs when these arrive (Fig. 2.15). Under certain circumstances, activation of complement can kill cells or organisms directly by the 'membrane attack complex' (C5b6789) in the terminal complement pathway. Complement can also be activated by bacteria directly through the alternative pathway; antibody is not required. The bacterial cell wall causes more C3b to be produced by the alternative pathway factors B, D and P

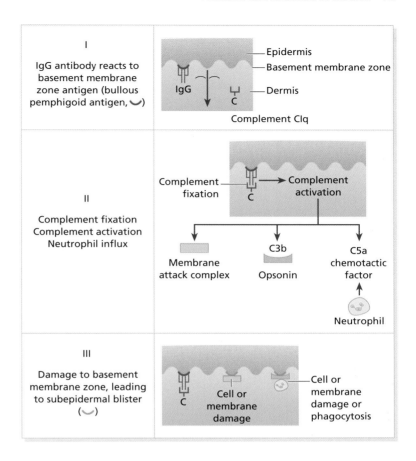

| | |
|---|---|
| **I**<br><br>IgG antibody reacts to basement membrane zone antigen (bullous pemphigoid antigen, ⌣) | Epidermis<br>Basement membrane zone<br>IgG — Dermis<br>C<br>Complement C1q |
| **II**<br><br>Complement fixation<br>Complement activation<br>Neutrophil influx | Complement fixation → Complement activation<br>C<br>Membrane attack complex — C3b Opsonin — C5a chemotactic factor<br>Neutrophil |
| **III**<br><br>Damage to basement membrane zone, leading to subepidermal blister (⌣) | C — Cell or membrane damage<br>Cell or membrane damage or phagocytosis |

**Fig. 2.15** Bullous pemphigoid: a humoral cytotoxic (type II) reaction against a basement membrane zone antigen.

(properdin). Aggregated IgA can also activate the alternative pathway.

Activation of either pathway produces C3b, the pivotal component of the complement system. Through the amplification loop, a single reaction can flood the area with C3b, C5a and other amplification loop and terminal pathway components. Complement is the mediator of humoral reactions.

Humoral cytotoxic reactions are typical of defence against infectious agents such as bacteria. However, they are also involved in certain autoimmune diseases such as pemphigoid (Chapter 9).

Occasionally, antibodies bind to the surface of a cell and activate it without causing its death or activating complement. Instead, the cell is stimulated to produce a hormone-like substance that may mediate disease. Pemphigus (Chapter 9) is a blistering disease of skin in which this type of reaction may be important.

## Type III: immune complex-mediated reactions

Antigen may combine with antibodies near vital tissues so that the ensuing inflammatory response damages them. When an antigen arrives in the dermis (e.g. after a bite or an injection) it may combine with appropriate antibodies on the walls of blood vessels. Complement is activated, and polymorphonuclear leucocytes are brought to the area (an Arthus reaction). Degranulation of polymorphs liberates lysosomal enzymes that damage the vessel walls.

Antigen–antibody complexes can also be formed in the circulation, move to the small vessels in the skin and lodge there (Fig. 2.16). Complement will then be activated and inflammatory cells will injure the vessels as in the Arthus reaction. This causes oedema and the extravasation of red blood cells (e.g. the palpable purpura that characterizes vasculitis; Chapter 8).

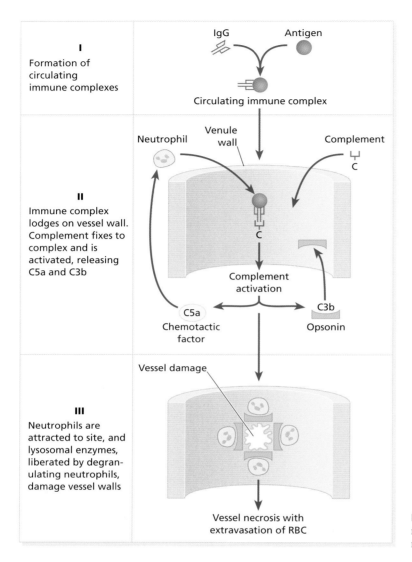

| | |
|---|---|
| **I**<br>Formation of circulating immune complexes | IgG    Antigen<br>Circulating immune complex |
| **II**<br>Immune complex lodges on vessel wall. Complement fixes to complex and is activated, releasing C5a and C3b | Neutrophil   Venule wall   Complement<br>Complement activation<br>C5a Chemotactic factor    C3b Opsonin |
| **III**<br>Neutrophils are attracted to site, and lysosomal enzymes, liberated by degranulating neutrophils, damage vessel walls | Vessel damage<br>Vessel necrosis with extravasation of RBC |

**Fig. 2.16** Immune complex-mediated vasculitis (type III reaction). RBC, red blood cell.

## Type IV: cell-mediated immune reactions

As the name implies, these are mediated by lymphocytes rather than by antibodies. Cell-mediated immune reactions are important in granulomas, delayed hypersensitivity reactions and allergic contact dermatitis. They probably also play a part in some photosensitive disorders, in protecting against cancer and in mediating delayed reactions to insect bites.

During the elicitation phase, most protein and chemical antigens entering the skin are processed by antigen-presenting cells such as macrophages and Langerhans cells (Fig. 2.17) and then interact with sensitized lymphocytes. The lymphocytes are stimulated to enlarge, divide and to secrete cytokines that can injure tissues directly and kill cells or microbes.

## Allergic contact dermatitis

### Induction (sensitization) phase (Fig. 2.17)

When the epidermal barrier is breached, the immune system provides the second line of defence. Among the keratinocytes are Langerhans cells, highly specialized intra-epidermal macrophages with tentacles that intertwine amongst the keratinocytes, providing

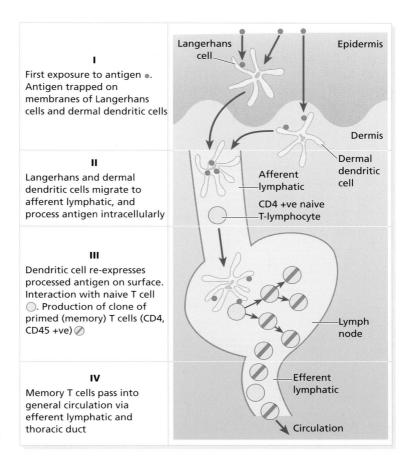

| | |
|---|---|
| **I**<br>First exposure to antigen ●.<br>Antigen trapped on membranes of Langerhans cells and dermal dendritic cells | Langerhans cell / Epidermis / Dermis / Dermal dendritic cell |
| **II**<br>Langerhans and dermal dendritic cells migrate to afferent lymphatic, and process antigen intracellularly | Afferent lymphatic / CD4 +ve naive T-lymphocyte |
| **III**<br>Dendritic cell re-expresses processed antigen on surface. Interaction with naive T cell ○. Production of clone of primed (memory) T cells (CD4, CD45 +ve) ⊘ | Lymph node |
| **IV**<br>Memory T cells pass into general circulation via efferent lymphatic and thoracic duct | Efferent lymphatic / Circulation |

**Fig. 2.17** Induction phase of allergic contact dermatitis (type IV) reaction.

a net (Fig. 2.7) to 'catch' antigens falling down on them from the surface, such as chemicals or the antigens of microbes or tumours. During the initial induction phase, the antigen is trapped by a Langerhans cell which then leaves the epidermis and migrates to the regional lymph node. To do this, it must retract its dendrites and 'swim upstream' from the prickle cell layer of the epidermis towards the basement membrane, against the 'flow' of keratinocytes generated by the epidermal basal cells. Once in the dermis, the Langerhans cell enters the lymphatic system, and by the time it reaches the regional lymph node it will have processed the antigen, which is re-expressed on its surface in conjunction with MHC class II molecules. In the node, the Langerhans cell mingles with crowds of lymphocytes, where it is quite likely to find a T cell with just the right TCR to bind its now processed antigen. Helper (CD4⁺) T lymphocytes recognize antigen only in the presence

of cells bearing MHC class II antigens, such as the Langerhans cell. The interactions between surface molecules on a CD4⁺ T cell and a Langerhans cell are shown in Fig. 2.12. To become activated the T lymphocyte must also bind itself tightly to certain 'accessory molecules', also called co-stimulatory molecules. If these are not engaged, then the immune response does not occur.

When a T cell interacts with an antigen-presenting cell carrying an antigen to which it can react, the T lymphocyte divides many times. This continuing division depends upon the persistence of antigen (and the antigen-presenting cells that contain it) and the T-cell growth factor IL-2. Eventually, a whole cadre of memory T cells is available to return to the skin to attack the antigen that stimulated their proliferation.

CD4⁺, CD45⁺ memory T lymphocytes then leave the node and circulate via lymphatic vessels, the thoracic duct and blood. They return to the skin aided by 'homing molecules' (cutaneous lymphocyte antigen; CLA) on their surfaces that guide their trip so that they preferentially enter the dermis. In the absence of antigen, they merely pass through it, and again enter the lymphatic vessels to return and recirculate. These cells are sentinel cells (Fig. 2.18), alert for their own special antigens. They accumulate in the skin if the host again encounters the antigen that initially stimulated their production. This preferential circulation of lymphocytes into the skin is a special part of the 'skin immune system' and reflects a selective advantage for the body to circulate lymphocytes that react to skin and skin surface-derived antigens.

### Elicitation (challenge) phase (Fig. 2.18)

When a T lymphocyte again encounters the antigen to which it is sensitized, it is ready to react. If the antigen is extracellular, as on an invading bacterium, toxin or chemical allergen, the CD4$^+$ T-helper cells do the work. The sequence of antigen processing by the Langerhans cell in the elicitation reaction is similar to the sequence of antigen processing during the induction phase, described above, that leads to the induction of immunity. The antigens get trapped by epidermal Langerhans cells or dermal dendritic cells, which process them intracellularly before re-expressing the modified antigenic determinant on their surfaces. In the elicitation reaction,

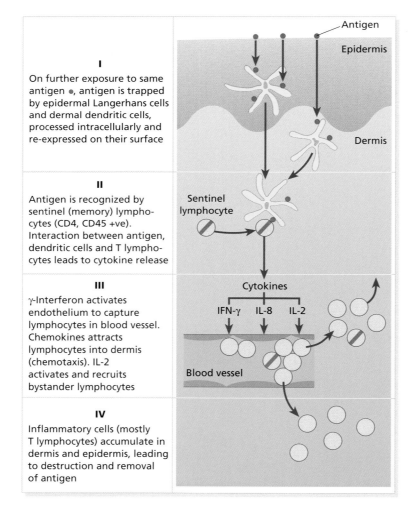

**I**
On further exposure to same antigen •, antigen is trapped by epidermal Langerhans cells and dermal dendritic cells, processed intracellularly and re-expressed on their surface

**II**
Antigen is recognized by sentinel (memory) lymphocytes (CD4, CD45 +ve). Interaction between antigen, dendritic cells and T lymphocytes leads to cytokine release

**III**
γ-Interferon activates endothelium to capture lymphocytes in blood vessel. Chemokines attracts lymphocytes into dermis (chemotaxis). IL-2 activates and recruits bystander lymphocytes

**IV**
Inflammatory cells (mostly T lymphocytes) accumulate in dermis and epidermis, leading to destruction and removal of antigen

Antigen
Epidermis
Dermis
Sentinel lymphocyte
Cytokines
IFN-γ    IL-8    IL-2
Blood vessel

**Fig. 2.18** Elicitation phase of allergic contact dermatitis (type IV) reaction.

the Langerhans cells find appropriate T lymphocytes trafficking through the dermis. In the elicitiation phase, most antigen presentation occurs here. The antigen is presented to CD4+ T cells, which are activated and produce cytokines that cause lymphocytes, polymorphonuclear leucocytes and monocytes in blood vessels to slow as they pass through the dermal blood vessels, then to stop and emigrate into the dermis causing inflammation (Fig. 2.18). Helper or cytotoxic lymphocytes help to stem the infection or eliminate antigen, and polymorphonuclear leucocytes engulf antigens and destroy them. The traffic of inflammatory cells in the epidermis and dermis is determined not only by cytokines produced by lymphocytes, but also by cytokines produced by injured keratinocytes (Fig. 2.11). For example, keratinocyte-derived chemokines bring lymphocytes into the epidermis, and IL-8, also produced by keratinocytes, bring in polymorphonuclear leukocytes, is a potent chemotactic factor for lymphocytes and polymorphs, and brings these up into the epidermis.

## Response to intracellular antigens

Antigens coming from inside a cell, such as intracellular fungi or viruses and tumour antigens, are presented to cytotoxic T cells (CD8+) by the MHC class I molecule. Presentation in this manner makes the infected cell liable to destruction by cytotoxic T lymphocytes or K cells. NK cells can also kill such cells, even though they have not been sensitized with antibody.

## Granulomas

Granulomas form when cell-mediated immunity fails to eliminate antigen. Foreign body granulomas occur because material remains undigested. Immunological granulomas require the persistence of antigen, but the response is augmented by a cell-mediated immune reaction. Lymphokines, released by lymphocytes sensitized to the antigen, cause macrophages to differentiate into epithelioid cells and giant cells. These secrete other cytokines, which influence inflammatory events. Immunological granulomas

of the skin are characterized by Langhans giant cells (not to be confused with Langerhans cells; p. 16), epithelioid cells, and a surrounding mantle of lymphocytes.

Granulomatous reactions also occur when organisms cannot be destroyed (e.g. in tuberculosis, leprosy, leishmaniasis), or when a chemical cannot be eliminated (e.g. zirconium or beryllium). Similar reactions are seen in some persisting inflammations of undetermined cause (e.g. rosacea, granuloma annulare, sarcoidosis and certain forms of panniculitis).

---

**Learning points**

1 Many skin disorders are good examples of an immune reaction at work. The more you know about the mechanisms, the more interesting the rashes become.
2 However, the immune system may not be the only culprit. If *Treponema pallidum* had not been discovered, syphilis might still be listed as an autoimmune disorder.
3 Because skin protects against infections, it has its own unique immune system to cope quickly with infectious agents breaching its barrier.

---

## Further reading

Asadullah K, Sterry W & Volk HD. (2002) Analysis of cytokine expression in dermatology. *Archives of Dermatology* **138**, 1189–1196.

Boehncke WH. (2005) *Lymphocyte Homing to Skin: Immunology, Immunopathology, and Therapeutic Perspectives.* CRC Press, Boca Raton.

Bos JD. (2005) *Skin Immune System: Cutaneous Immunology and Clinical Immunodermatology.* CRC Press, Boca Raton.

Chaplin DD. (2006) Overview of the human immune response. *Journal of Allergy and Clinical Immunology* **117**, S430–S435.

Freinkel RK & Woodley DT. (2001) *The Biology of the Skin.* Parthenon, London.

Kang SSW, Sauls LS & Gaspari AA. (2006) Toll-like receptors: applications to dermatologic disease. *Journal of the American Academy of Dermatology* **54**, 951–983.

Yokoyama WM. (2005) Natural killer cell immune responses. *Immunology Reviews* **32**, 317–326.

# 3 Diagnosis of skin disorders

The key to successful treatment is an accurate diagnosis. You can look up treatments, but you cannot look up diagnoses. Without a proper diagnosis, you will be asking 'What's a good treatment for scaling feet?' instead of 'What's good for tinea pedis?'. Would you ever ask yourself 'What's a good treatment for chest pain?'. Luckily, dermatology differs from other specialties as its diseases can easily be seen. Keen eyes and a magnifying glass are all that are needed for a complete examination of the skin. Sometimes it is best to examine the patient briefly before obtaining a full history; a quick look will often prompt the right questions. However, a careful history is important in every case, as is the intelligent use of the laboratory.

## History

The key points to be covered in the history are listed in Table 3.1 and should include descriptions of the events surrounding the onset of the skin lesions, the progression of individual lesions and the disease in general, including any responses to treatment. Many patients try a few salves before seeing a physician. Some try all the medications in their medicine cabinets, many of which can aggravate the problem. A careful inquiry into drugs taken for other conditions is often useful. Ask also about previous skin disorders, occupation, hobbies and disorders in the family.

## Examination

To examine the skin properly, the lighting must be uniform and bright. Daylight is best. The patient should usually undress so that the whole skin can be examined, although sometimes this is neither desirable (e.g. hand warts) nor possible. Do not be put off this too easily by the elderly, the stubborn,

**Table 3.1** Outline of dermatological history.

*History of present skin condition*
Duration
Site at onset, details of spread
Itch
Burning
Pain
Wet, dry, blisters
Exacerbating factors
Gowth
Bleeding

*General health at present*
Ask about fever

*Past history of skin disorders*

*Past general medical history*
Inquire specifically about asthma and hay fever

*Family history of skin disorders*
If positive, the disorder or the tendency to have it may be inherited. Sometimes family members may be exposed to a common infectious agent or scabies or to a injurious chemical

*Family history of other medical disorders*

*Social and occupational history*
Hobbies
Outdoor versus indoor
Travels abroad
Relationship of rash to work and holidays
Alcohol intake

*Drugs used to treat present skin condition*
Topical
Systemic
Physician prescribed
Patient initiated

*Drugs prescribed for other disorders* (including those taken before onset of skin disorder)

the shy, or the surroundings. The presence of a chaperone, who should be a healthcare professional, and essential if examination of the genitalia is necessary. Sometimes make-up must be washed off or wigs removed. There is nothing more embarrassing than missing the right diagnosis because an important sign has been hidden.

## Distribution

A dermatological diagnosis is based both on the distribution of lesions and on their morphology and configuration. For example, an area of seborrhoeic dermatitis may look very like an area of atopic dermatitis, but the key to diagnosis lies in the location. Seborrhoeic dermatitis affects the scalp, forehead, eyebrows, nasolabial folds and central chest; atopic dermatitis typically affects the antecubital and popliteal fossae.

See if the skin disease is localized, universal or symmetrical. Symmetry implies a systemic origin, whereas unilaterality or asymmetry implies an external cause. Depending on the disease suggested by the morphology, you may want to check special areas, such as the feet in a patient with hand eczema, or the gluteal cleft in a patient who might have psoriasis. Examine as much of the skin as possible. Look in the mouth and remember to check the hair and the nails (Chapter 13). Note negative as well as positive findings (e.g. the way the shielded areas are spared in a photosensitive dermatitis; see Fig. 18.7). Always keep your eyes open for incidental skin cancers which the patient may have ignored.

## Morphology

After the distribution has been noted, next define the morphology of the primary lesions. Many skin diseases have a characteristic morphology, but scratching, ulceration and other events can change this. The rule is to find an early or 'primary' lesion and to inspect it closely. What is its shape? What is its size? What is its colour? What are its margins like? What are the surface characteristics? What does it feel like? Most types of primary lesion have one name if small and a different one if large. The scheme is summarized in Table 3.2.

There are many reasons why you should describe skin diseases properly.
● Skin disorders are often grouped by their morphology. Once the morphology is clear, a differential diagnosis comes easily to mind.
● If you have to describe a condition accurately, you will have to look at it carefully.
● You can paint a verbal picture if you have to refer the patient for another opinion.
● You will sound like a physician and not a homoeopath.
● You will be able to understand the terminology of this book.

## Terminology of lesions (Fig. 3.1)

### Primary lesions

The size in many of the definitions given below (e.g. papule, nodule, macule, patch) is arbitrary and it is often helpful to record the actual measurement.

**Table 3.2** Terminology of primary lesions.

| | Small (<0.5 cm) | Large (>0.5 cm) |
|---|---|---|
| Elevated solid lesion | Papule | Nodule (>0.5 cm in both width and depth)<br>Plaque (>2 cm in width but without substantial depth) |
| Flat area of altered colour or texture | Macule | Large macule (patch) |
| Fluid-filled blister | Vesicle | Bulla |
| Pus-filled lesion | Pustule | Abscess<br>Furuncle |
| Extravasation of blood into skin | Petechia (pinhead size)<br>Purpura (up to 2 mm in diameter) | Ecchymosis<br>Haematoma |
| Accumulation of dermal oedema | Wheal (can be any size) | Angioedema |

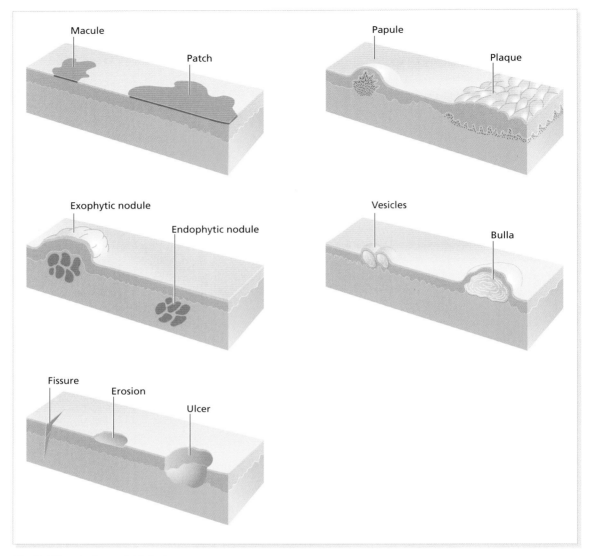

**Fig. 3.1** Terminology of skin lesions.

*Erythema* is redness caused by vascular dilatation.

A *papule* is a small solid elevation of skin, less than 0.5 cm in diameter.

A *plaque* is an elevated area of skin greater than 2 cm in diameter but without substantial depth.

A *macule* is a small flat area, less than 5 mm in diameter, of altered colour or texture.

A *patch* is a large macule.

A *vesicle* is a circumscribed elevation of skin, less than 0.5 cm in diameter, and containing fluid.

A *bulla* is a circumscribed elevation of skin over 0.5 cm in diameter and containing fluid.

A *pustule* is a visible accumulation of pus in the skin.

An *abscess* is a localized collection of pus in a cavity, more than 1 cm in diameter. Abscesses are usually nodules, and the term 'purulent bulla' is sometimes used to describe a pus-filled blister that is situated on top of the skin rather than within it.

A *wheal* is an elevated white compressible evanescent area produced by dermal oedema. It is often surrounded by a red axon-mediated flare. Although usually less than 2 cm in diameter, some wheals are huge.

*Angioedema* is a diffuse swelling caused by oedema extending to the subcutaneous tissue.

A *nodule* is a solid mass in the skin, usually greater than 0.5 cm in diameter, in both width and depth, which can be seen to be elevated (exophytic) or can be palpated (endophytic).

A *tumour* is harder to define as the term is based more correctly on microscopic pathology than on clinical morphology. We keep it here as a convenient term to describe an enlargement of the tissues by normal or pathological material or cells that form a mass, usually more than 1 cm in diameter. Because the word 'tumour' can scare patients, tumours may courteously be called 'large nodules', especially if they are not malignant.

A *papilloma* is a nipple-like projection from the skin.

*Petechiae* are pinhead-sized macules of blood in the skin.

The term *purpura* describes a larger macule or papule of blood in the skin. Such blood-filled lesions do not blanch if a glass lens is pushed against them (Diascopy, p. 39)

An *ecchymosis (bruise)* is a larger extravasation of blood into the skin and deeper structures.

A *haematoma* is a swelling from gross bleeding.

A *burrow* is a linear or curvilinear papule, with some scaling, caused by a scabies mite.

A *comedo* is a plug of greasy keratin wedged in a dilated pilosebaceous orifice. Open comedones are 'blackheads'. The follicle opening of a closed comedo is nearly covered over by skin so that it looks like a pinhead-sized, ivory-coloured papule.

*Telangiectasia* is the visible dilatation of small cutaneous blood vessels.

*Poikiloderma* is a combination of atrophy, reticulate hyperpigmentation and telangiectasia.

*Horn* is a keratin projection that is taller than it is broad.

*Erthyroderma* is a generalized redness of skin that may be scaling (exfoliative erythroderma) or smooth.

## Secondary lesions

These evolve from primary lesions.

A *scale* is a flake arising from the horny layer. Scales may be seen on the surface of many primary lesions (e.g. macules, patches, nodules, plaques).

A *keratosis* is a horn-like thickening of the stratum corneum.

A *crust* may look like a scale, but is composed of dried blood or tissue fluid.

An *ulcer* is an area of skin from which the whole of the epidermis and at least the upper part of the dermis has been lost. Ulcers may extend into subcutaneous fat, and heal with scarring.

An *erosion* is an area of skin denuded by a complete or partial loss of only the epidermis. Erosions heal without scarring.

An *excoriation* is an ulcer or erosion produced by scratching.

A *fissure* is a slit in the skin.

A *sinus* is a cavity or channel that permits the escape of pus or fluid.

A *scar* is a result of healing, where normal structures are permanently replaced by fibrous tissue.

*Atrophy* is a thinning of skin caused by diminution of the epidermis, dermis or subcutaneous fat. When the epidermis is atrophic it may crinkle like cigarette paper, appear thin and translucent, and lose normal surface markings. Blood vessels may be easy to see in both epidermal and dermal atrophy.

*Lichenification* is an area of thickened skin with increased markings.

A *stria* (stretch mark) is a streak-like linear atrophic pink, purple or white lesion of the skin caused by changes in the connective tissue.

*Pigmentation*, either more or less than surrounding skin, can develop after lesions heal.

Having identified the lesions as primary or secondary, adjectives can be used to describe them in terms of their other features.

- Colour (e.g. salmon-pink, lilac, violet).
- Sharpness of edge (e.g. well-defined, ill-defined).
- Surface contour (e.g. dome-shaped, umbilicated, spire-like; Fig. 3.2).
- Geometric shape (e.g. nummular, oval, irregular, like the coast of Maine).
- Texture (e.g. rough, silky, smooth, hard).
- Smell (e.g. foul-smelling).
- Temperature (e.g. hot, warm).

Dermatologists also use a few special adjectives which warrant definition.

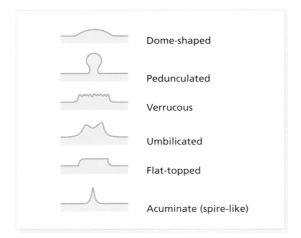

**Fig. 3.2** Surface contours of papules.

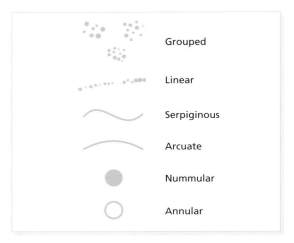

**Fig. 3.3** Configuration of lesions.

- *Nummular* means round or coin-like.
- *Annular* means ring-like.
- *Circinate* means circular.
- *Arcuate* means curved.
- *Discoid* means disc-like.
- *Gyrate* means wave-like.
- *Retiform* and *reticulate* mean net-like.
- *Targetoid* means target-like or 'bull's eye'.
- *Polycyclic* means formed from coalescing circles, or incomplete rings.

To describe a skin lesion, use the term for the primary lesion as the noun, and the adjectives mentioned above to define it. For example, the lesions of psoriasis may appear as 'salmon-pink sharply demarcated nummular plaques covered by large silver polygonal scales'. Try not to use the term 'erythema' as it means a shade of red and therefore is less specific than for example 'fire engine red'.

Try also not to use the terms 'lesion' or 'area'. Why say 'papular lesion' when you can say papule? It is almost as bad as the ubiquitous term 'skin rash'. By the way, there are very few diseases that are truly 'maculopapular'. The term is best avoided except to describe some drug eruptions and viral exanthems. Even then, the terms 'scarlatiniform' (like scarlet fever – punctate, slightly elevated papules) or 'morbilliform' (like measles – a net-like blotchy slightly elevated pink exanthem) are more helpful.

## Configuration

After unravelling the primary and secondary lesions, look for arrangements and configurations that can be, for example, discrete, confluent, grouped, annular, arcuate, segmental or dermatomal (Fig. 3.3). Note that while individual lesions may be annular, several individual lesions may arrange themselves into an annular or polycyclic configuration. Other adjectives, discussed under the morphology of individual lesions, can apply to their groupings too. The Köbner or isomorphic phenomenon is the induction of skin lesions by, and at the site of, trauma such as scratch marks or operative incisions.

## Special tools and techniques

A *magnifying lens* is a helpful aid to diagnosis because subtle changes in the skin become more apparent when enlarged. One attached to spectacles will leave your hand free.

A *Wood's light*, emitting long wavelength ultraviolet radiation, will help with the examination of some skin conditions. Fluorescence is seen in some fungal infections (Chapter 16), erythrasma (p. 221) and *Pseudomonas* infections. Some subtle disorders of pigmentation can be seen more clearly under Wood's light (e.g. the pale patches of tuberous sclerosis, low-grade vitiligo and pityriasis versicolor, and the darker *café au lait* patches of neurofibromatosis). The urine in hepatic cutaneous porphyria (p. 328) often fluoresces coral pink, even without solvent extraction of the porphyrins (see Fig. 21.10).

*Diascopy* is the name given to the technique in which a glass slide or clear plastic spoon is pressed on vascular lesions to blanch them and verify that their redness is caused by vasodilatation and to unmask their underlying colour. Diascopy is also used to confirm the presence of extravasated blood in the dermis (i.e. petechia and purpura, the appearance of which do not change on pressure).

*Photography*, mostly digital nowadays, helps to record the baseline appearance of a lesion or rash, so that change can be assessed objectively at later visits. Small changes in pigmented lesions can be detected by analysing sequential digital images stored in computerized systems.

## Dermatoscopy (also known as dermoscopy, epiluminescence microscopy, skin surface microscopy)

This non-invasive technique for distinguishing pigmented lesions *in vivo* has come of age in the last few years. It provides a link between macroscopic clinical dermatology and microscopic histology. Many structures can be identified that are not visible to the naked eye. The lesion is covered with ultrasound gel, mineral oil, alcohol or water and then illuminated and observed at 10× magnification with a hand-held dermatoscope (Fig. 3.4). The gel or fluid eliminates surface reflection and makes the horny layer translucent so that pigmented structures in the

**Fig. 3.4** A dermatoscope.

epidermis and superficial dermis, and the superficial vascular plexus (p. 20), can be assessed. The glass plate of the dermatoscope should be regularly cleaned and disinfected to prevent nosocomial infection.

The first (and easiest) step is to distinguish non-melanocytic lesions, including seborrhoeic warts, haemangiomas, angiokeratomas and pigmented basal cell carcinomas, from melanocytic ones – primarily melanocytic naevi and malignant melanomas. Set criteria exist for each diagnosis although distinguishing some suspicious melanocytic naevi from melanomas (Fig. 3.5) by dermatoscopy alone may be beyond the reach of even the most experienced expert. Images can be recorded digitally and sequential changes assessed. With formal training and practice, the use of dermatoscopy improves the accuracy with which pigmented lesions are diagnosed.

Irregular pigmentation = 1 point

Irregular streaks = 1 point

Irregular dots/globules = 1 point

Blue-whitish veil = 2 points

Atypical pigment network = 2 points

**Fig. 3.5** Dermatoscopic appearance of a malignant melanoma.

A dermatoscope can also be used to identify scabies mites in their burrows (p. 262) and, used without oil, it is handy for diagnosing abnormalities of hair shafts.

## Assessment

Next try to put the disease into a general class; the titles of the chapters in this book are representative. Once classified, a differential diagnosis is usually forthcoming. Each diagnosis can then be considered on its merits, and laboratory tests may be used to confirm or refute diagnoses in the differential list. At this stage you must make a working diagnosis or formulate a plan to do so.

> ### Learning points
>
> **1** As Osler said: 'See and then reason, but see first'.
> **2** A correct diagnosis is the key to correct treatment.
> **3** The term 'skin rash' is as bad as 'gastric stomach'.
> **4** Avoid using too many long Latin descriptive names as a cloak for ignorance.
> **5** The history is especially important when the diagnosis is difficult.
> **6** Undress the patient and use a lens, even if it only gives you more time to think.
> **7** A modern dermatologist without a dermatoscope is like a cardiologist without a stethoscope.
> **8** Remember the old adage that if you do not look in the mouth you will put your foot in it.

## Side-room and office tests

A number of tests can be performed in the practice office so that their results will be available immediately.

### Potassium hydroxide preparations for fungal infections

If a fungal infection is suspected, scales or plucked hairs can be dissolved in an aqueous solution of 20% potassium hydroxide (KOH) containing 40% dimethyl sulphoxide (DMSO). The scale from the edge of a scaling lesion is vigorously scraped on to a glass slide with a No. 15 scalpel blade or the edge of a second glass slide. Other samples can include nail

**Fig. 3.6** Preparing a skin scraping for microscopy by adding potassium hydroxide (KOH) from a pipette.

**Fig. 3.7** Fungal hyphae in a potassium hydroxide (KOH) preparation. The polygonal shadows in the background are horny layer cells.

clippings, the roofs of blisters, hair pluckings and the contents of pustules when a candidal infection is suspected. A drop or two of the KOH solution is run under the cover slip (Fig. 3.6). After 5–10 min the mount is examined under a microscope with the condenser lens lowered to increase contrast. Nail clippings take longer to clear – up to a couple of hours. With experience, fungal and candidal hyphae can be readily detected (Fig. 3.7). No heat is required if DMSO is included in the KOH solution.

### Detection of a scabies mite

Burrows in an itchy patient are diagnostic of scabies. Retrieving a mite from the skin will confirm the diagnosis and convince a sceptical patient of the infestation. The burrow should be examined under a magnifying glass or dermatoscope; the acarus is seen as a tiny black or grey dot at the most recent, least scaly end (see Fig. 17.5. It can be removed by a sterile needle and placed on a slide within a marked circle. Alternatively, if mites are not seen, possible burrows can be vigorously scraped with a No. 15 scalpel blade, moistened with liquid paraffin or vegetable oil, and the scrapings transferred to a slide. Patients never argue the toss when confronted by a magnified mobile mite.

## Cytology (Tzanck smear)

Cytology can aid the diagnosis of viral infections such as herpes simplex and zoster, and of bullous diseases such as pemphigus. A blister roof is removed and the cells from the base of the blister are scraped off with a No. 10 or 15 surgical blade. These cells are smeared on to a microscope slide, air-dried and fixed with methanol. They are then stained with Giemsa, toluidine blue or Wright's stain. Acantholytic cells (Chapter 9) are seen in pemphigus, and multinucleate giant cells are diagnostic of herpes simplex or varicella zoster infections (Chapter 16). Practice is needed to obtain good preparations. The technique has fallen out of favour as histology, virological culture and PCR have become more accessible.

## Patch tests

Patch tests are invaluable in detecting the allergens responsible for allergic contact dermatitis (Chapter 7). A patch test involves applying a chemical to the skin and then watching for dermatitis to develop 48–96 h later.

Either suspected individual antigens or a battery of antigens which are common culprits can be tested. Standard dilutions of the common antigens in appropriate bases are available commercially (Fig. 3.8). The test materials are applied to the back under aluminium discs or patches; the occlusion encourages penetration of the allergen. The patches are left in place for 48 h and then, after careful marking, are removed. The sites are inspected 10 min later, again 2 days later and sometimes even later if doubtful reactions require further assessment. The test detects type IV delayed hypersensitivity reactions

**Fig. 3.8** Patch testing equipment. Syringes contain commercially prepared antigens, to be applied in aluminium cups.

(Chapter 2). The readings are scored according to the reaction seen:

NT  Not tested.
−  No reaction.
±  Doubtful reaction (minimal erythema).
+  Weak positive reaction (erythema and maybe papules).
++  Strong reaction (palpable erythema and/or vesicles; Fig. 3.9).
+++  Extreme reaction (intense palpable erythema, coalescing vesicles and/or bullae).
IR  Irritant reaction (variable, but often sharply circumscribed, with a glazed appearance and increased skin markings).

**Fig. 3.9** A strong positive reaction to a rubber additive.

A positive patch test does not prove that the allergen in question has caused the current episode of contact dermatitis; the results must be interpreted in the light of the history and possible previous exposure to the allergen.

Patch testing requires attention to detail in applying the patches properly and skill and experience in interpreting the results. The concentration of allergen must be sufficient to penetrate the thick skin of the back and yet not so high as to create a false positive irritation reaction.

## Prick testing

Prick testing is much less helpful in dermatology. It detects immediate (type I) hypersensitivity (Chapter 2) and patients should not have taken systemic antihistamines for at least 48 h before the test. Commercially prepared diluted antigens and a control are placed as single drops on marked areas of the forearm. The skin is gently pricked through the drops using separate sterile fine (e.g. 25 gauge, or smaller) needles. The prick should not cause bleeding. The drops are then removed with a tissue wipe. After 10 min the sites are inspected and the diameter of any wheal measured and recorded. A result is considered positive if the test antigen causes a wheal of 4 mm or greater (Fig. 3.10) and the control elicits a negligible reaction.

**Fig. 3.10** Prick testing: many positive results in an atopic individual.

Like patch testing, prick testing should not be undertaken by those without formal training in the procedure. Although the risk of anaphylaxis is small, resuscitation facilities including adrenaline (epinephrine) and oxygen must be available. The relevance of positive results to the cause of the condition under investigation – usually urticaria or atopic dermatitis – is often debatable. Positive results should correlate with positive radio-allergosorbent tests (RAST; p. 84) used to measure total and specific immunoglobulin E (IgE) levels to inhaled and ingested allergens. RAST tests, although more expensive, pose no risk of anaphylaxis and take up less of the patient's time in the clinic. They are now used more often than prick tests.

## Skin biopsy

Biopsy (from the Greek *bios* meaning 'life' and *opsis* 'sight') of skin lesions is useful to establish or confirm a clinical diagnosis. A piece of tissue is removed surgically for histological examination and sometimes for other tests (e.g. culture for organisms). When used selectively, a skin biopsy can solve the most perplexing problem but, conversely, will be unhelpful in conditions without a specific histology (e.g. most drug eruptions, pityriasis rosea, reactive erythemas).

Skin biopsies may be *incisional*, when just part of a lesion is removed for laboratory examination, or *excisional*, when the whole lesion is cut out. Excisional biopsy is preferable for most small lesions (up to 0.5 cm diameter) but incisional biopsy is chosen when the partial removal of a larger lesion is adequate for diagnosis, and complete removal might leave an unnecessary and unsightly scar. Ideally, an incisional biopsy should include a piece of the surrounding normal skin (Fig. 3.11), although this may not be possible if a small punch is used.

The main steps in skin biopsy are:
**1** Obtain written and informed consent from the patient before starting the procedure;
**2** Administration of local anaesthesia; and
**3** Removal of all (excision) or part (incision) of the lesion and repair of the defect made by a scalpel or punch.

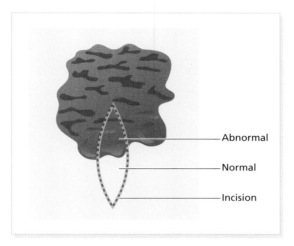

Abnormal

Normal

Incision

**Fig. 3.11** Incision biopsy. This should include adjacent normal skin.

### Local anaesthetic

Lidocaine (lignocaine) 1–2% is used. Sometimes adrenaline (epinephrine) 1 : 200 000 is added. This causes vasoconstriction, reduced clearance of the local anaesthetic and prolongation of the local anaesthetic effect. Plain lidocaine should be used on the fingers, toes and the penis as the prolonged vasoconstriction produced by adrenaline can be dangerous here. Adrenaline is also best avoided in diabetics with small vessel disease, in those with a history of heart disease (including dysrhythmias), in patients taking non-selective α-blockers and tricyclic antidepressants (because of potential interactions) and in uncontrolled hyperthyroidism. There are exceptions to these general rules and, undoubtedly, the total dose of local anaesthetic and/or adrenaline is important. Nevertheless, the rules should not be broken unless the surgeon is quite sure that the procedure that he or she is about to embark on is safe.

It is wise to avoid local anaesthesia during early pregnancy and to delay non-urgent procedures until after the first trimester.

As 'B' follows 'A' in the alphabet, get into the habit of checking the precise concentration of the lidocaine ± added adrenaline on the label *before* withdrawing it into the syringe and then, *before* injecting it, confirm that the patient has not had any previous allergic reactions to local anaesthetic.

Infiltration of the local anaesthetic into the skin under and around the area to be biopsied is the most widely used method. If the local anaesthetic is injected into the subcutaneous fat, it will be relatively pain-free, will produce a diffuse swelling of the skin and will take several minutes to induce anaesthesia. Intradermal injections are painful and produce a discrete wheal associated with rapid anaesthesia. The application of EMLA cream (eutectic mixture of local anaesthesia) to the operation site 2 h before giving a local anaesthetic to children helps to numb the initial prick.

### Scalpel biopsy

This provides more tissue than a punch biopsy. It can be used routinely, but is especially useful for biopsying disorders of the subcutaneous fat, for obtaining specimens with both normal and abnormal skin for comparison (Fig. 3.11) and for removing small lesions *in toto* (excision biopsy; p. 371). After selecting the lesion for biopsy, an elliptical piece of skin is excised. The specimen should include the subcutaneous fat. Removing the specimen with forceps may cause crush artefact, which can be avoided by lifting the specimen with either a Gillies hook or a syringe needle. The wound is then sutured; firm compression for 5 min stops oozing. Non-absorbable 3/0 sutures are used for biopsies on the legs and back, 5/0 for the face and 4/0 for elsewhere. Stitches are usually removed from the face in 4 days, from the anterior trunk and arms in 7 days, and from the back and legs in 10 days. Some guidelines for skin biopsies are listed in Table 3.3.

### Punch biopsy

The skin is sampled with a small (3–4 mm diameter) tissue punch. Lidocaine 1% is injected intradermally first, and a cylinder of skin is incised with the punch by rotating it back and forth (Fig. 3.12). The skin is lifted up carefully with a needle or forceps and the base is cut off at the level of subcutaneous fat. Be careful not to crush the specimen as this will render interpretation difficult. The defect is cauterized or repaired with a single suture.

**Table 3.3** Guidelines for skin biopsies.

Sample a fresh lesion
Obtain your specimen from near the lesion's edge
Avoid sites where a scar would be conspicuous
Avoid the upper trunk or jaw line where keloids are most
    likely to form
Avoid the legs, where healing is slow
Avoid lesions over bony prominences, where infection is
    more likely
Use the scalpel technique for scalp disorders and diseases
    of the subcutaneous fat or vessels
Do not crush the tissue
Place in appropriate fixative*, usually 10% formalin for
    routine histology
If two lesions are sampled, be sure they do not get mixed
    up or mislabelled. Label specimen containers before the
    biopsy is placed in them
Make sure that the patient's name, age and sex are clearly
    indicated on the pathology form
Provide the pathologist with a legible summary of the
    history (including laboratory numbers of previous
    relevant biopsies), the site of the biopsy and a
    differential diagnosis
Discuss the results with the pathologist

* Specimens for immunofluorescence should be immediately
frozen or placed in special transport medium. Transport of
specimens for microbiology should be discussed with the
laboratory. Preservative-free lidocaine may be indicated to
prevent the local anaesthesic from killing organisms during the
process of biopsy.

If a lesion is superficial, a shave biopsy may be
preferred (p. 372).

The tissue can be sent to the pathologist with a
summary of the history, a differential diagnosis and
the patient's age. Close liaison with the pathologist
is essential, because the diagnosis may only become
apparent with knowledge of both the clinical and
histological features.

> **Learning points**
>
> 1 A biopsy is the refuge of a bankrupt mind when dealing
>   with conditions that do not have a specific histology.
>   Here, a return to the history and examination is more
>   likely to reveal diagnostic clues than a pathologist.
> 2 If you do not remember the three essential checks before
>   injecting local anaesthetic then read p. 43 again.

## Laboratory tests

The laboratory is vital for the accurate diagnosis of
many skin disorders. Tests include various assays of
blood, serum and urine, bacterial, fungal and viral
culture from skin and other specimens, immuno-
fluorescent and immunohistological examinations
(Figs 3.13 and 3.14), radiography, ultrasonography
and other methods of image intensification. Specific
details are discussed as each disease is presented.

## Conclusions

Clinical dermatology is a visual specialty. You must
see the disease, and understand what you are seeing.
Look closely and thoroughly. Take time. Examine
the whole body. Locate primary lesions and check
configuration and distribution. Ask appropriate questions, especially if the diagnosis is difficult. Classify
the disorder and list the differential diagnoses. Use
the history, examination and laboratory tests to
make a diagnosis if this cannot be made by clinical

(a)          (b)          (c)

**Fig. 3.12** Steps in taking a punch biopsy.

**Fig. 3.13** Direct immunofluorescence detects antibodies in a patient's skin. Here immunoglobulin G (IgG) antibodies are detected by staining with a fluorescent dye attached to antihuman IgG.

Fluorescent dye attached to antibody raised against human immunoglobulin

Section of patient's skin

Microscope slide

Ultraviolet source

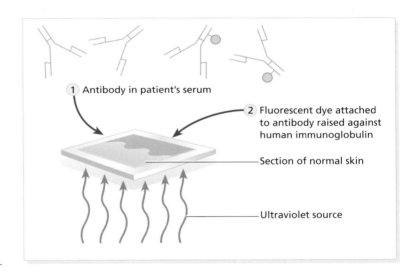

**Fig. 3.14** Indirect immunofluorescence detects antibodies in a patient's serum. There are two steps. (1) Antibodies in this serum are made to bind to antigens in a section of normal skin. (2) Antibody raised against human immunoglobulin, conjugated with a fluorescent dye can then be used to stain these bound antibodies (as in the direct immunofluorescence test).

1 Antibody in patient's serum

2 Fluorescent dye attached to antibody raised against human immunoglobulin

Section of normal skin

Ultraviolet source

features alone. Then treat. Refer the patient to a dermatologist if:

- You cannot make a diagnosis;
- The disorder does not respond to treatment;
- The disorder is unusual or severe; or
- You are just not sure.

## Further reading

British Association of Dermatologists (2007) Guidelines to clinicians on the handling of skin biopsies for histopathology. http://www.bad.org.uk/healthcare guidelines

Cox NH & Lawrence CM. (1998) *Diagnostic Problems in Dermatology*. Mosby Wolfe, Edinburgh.

Dermatology Lexicon Project (2007) The morphology of skin lesions. http://www.futurehealth.rochester.edu/dlp2/morphHome.html

Lawrence CM & Cox NM. (2001) *Physical Signs in Dermatology*, 2nd edn. Mosby, Edinburgh.

Mutasim DF & Adams BB. (2001) Immuno-fluorescence in dermatology. *Journal of the American Academy of Dermatology* **45**, 803–822.

Savin JA, Hunter JAA & Hepburn NC. (1997) *Skin Signs in Clinical Medicine: Diagnosis in Colour*. Mosby Wolfe, London.

Shelley WB & Shelley ED. (1992) *Advanced Dermatologic Diagnosis*. W.B. Saunders, Philadelphia, PA.

Shelley WB & Shelley ED. (2006) *Consultations in Dermatology. Studies of Orphan and Unique Patients*. Cambridge University Press, New York.

Stolz W, Landthaler M, Braun Falco O, *et al.* (2002) *Color Atlas of Dermatoscopy*, 2nd edn. Blackwell Science, Oxford.

White GM & Cox NH. (2005) *Diseases of the Skin*, 2nd edn. Mosby, London.

# 4 Disorders of keratinization

The complex but orderly processes of keratinization, and of cell cohesion and proliferation within the epidermis, have been described in Chapter 2. As they proceed, the living keratinocytes of the deeper epidermis change into the dead corneocytes of the horny layer, where they are stuck together by intercellular lipids. They are then shed in such a way that the surface of the normal skin does not seem scaly to the naked eye. Shedding balances production, so that the thickness of the horny layer does not alter. However, if keratinization or cell cohesion is abnormal, the horny layer may become thick or the skin surface may become dry and scaly. Such changes can be localized or generalized.

In this chapter we describe a variety of skin disorders that have as their basis a disorder of keratinization. During the last few years the molecular mechanisms underlying many of these have become clearer, including abnormal genetic coding for keratins, the enzymes involved in cell cohesion in the horny layer, and the molecules that are critical in the signalling pathway governing cell cohesion in the spinous layer.

## The ichthyoses

The word ichthyosis comes from the Greek word for a fish. It is applied to disorders that share, as their main feature, a dry rough skin with marked scaling but no inflammation. Strictly speaking, the scales lack the regular overlapping pattern of fish scales, but the term is usefully descriptive and too well entrenched to be discarded. There are several types.

### Ichthyosis vulgaris

#### Cause

Inherited as an autosomal semi-dominant disorder, this condition is common and affects about 1 person in 250. Mutations in the filaggrin gene lead to loss or reduction of profilaggrin. This is the major component of the keratohyalin granules and when cleaved to filaggrin is responsible for aggregating keratin filaments in the cornified cell envelope. Mutant alleles have a frequency of 4% in European populations, which accounts for this being such a common disorder. Heterozygotes have milder disease than homozygotes.

#### Presentation

The dryness is usually mild and symptoms are few. The scales are small and branny, being most obvious on the limbs and least obvious in the major flexures. The skin creases of the palm may be accentuated. Keratosis pilaris (p. 50) is often present on the limbs.

#### Clinical course

The skin changes are not usually present at birth but develop over the first few years of life. Some patients improve in adult life, particularly during warm weather, but the condition seldom clears completely.

#### Complications

The already dry skin chaps in the winter and is easily irritated by degreasing agents. This should be taken into account in the choice of a career. Ichthyosis of this type is apt to appear in a stubborn combination with atopic eczema, as mutations in the filaggrin gene are strong predisposing factors for atopic eczema (p. 91).

#### Differential diagnosis

It can usually be distinguished from less common types of ichthyosis on the basis of the pattern of inheritance and of the type and distribution of the scaling.

### Investigations

None are usually needed.

### Treatment

This is palliative. The dryness can be helped by the regular use of emollients, which are best applied after a shower or bath. Emulsifying ointment, soft white paraffin, E45 and Unguentum Merck are all quite suitable (Formulary 1, p. 381) and the selection depends on the patient's preference. Many find proprietary bath oils and creams containing humectants such as glycerin, urea or lactic acid helpful also (Formulary 1, p. 381).

## X-linked recessive ichthyosis

### Cause

This less common type of ichthyosis is inherited as an X-linked recessive trait and therefore, in its complete form, is seen only in males, although some female carriers show mild scaling. The condition affects about 1 in 6000 males in the UK and is associated with a deficiency of the enzyme steroid sulphatase, which hydrolyses cholesterol sulphate. The responsible gene has been localized to the end of the short arm of the X chromosome, at Xp 22.3 (Chapter 24).

### Presentation and course

In contrast to the delayed onset of the dominantly inherited ichthyosis vulgaris, scaling appears early, often soon after birth, and always by the first birthday. The scales are larger and browner (Fig. 4.1), involve the neck, and to a lesser extent the popliteal and antecubital areas, as well as the skin generally. The palms and soles are normal. There is no association with atopy or keratosis pilaris. The condition persists throughout life.

### Complications

Affected babies may be born after a prolonged

**Fig. 4.1** Ichthyosis: large rather dark scales suggest the less common type inherited as a sex-linked recessive trait.

labour. Corneal opacities may appear in adult life. Kallmann's syndrome is caused by the deletion of a part of the X chromosome that includes the gene for X-linked recessive ichthyosis, which is therefore one of its features. Other features of this contiguous gene disorder are hypogonadism, anosmia and neurological defects.

### Differential diagnosis

This is as for ichthyosis vulgaris. It is helpful to remember that only males are affected. Bear Kallmann's syndrome in mind if there are other congenital abnormalities.

### Investigations

None are usually needed. A few centres can measure steroid sulphatase in fibroblasts cultured from a skin biopsy.

### Treatment

Oral aromatic retinoids are probably best avoided. Topical measures are as for ichthyosis vulgaris.

**Fig. 4.2** A collodion baby who had an underlying non-bullous ichthyosiform erythroderma.

## Collodion baby (Fig. 4.2)

This is a description and not a diagnosis. The bizarre skin charges are seen at birth. At first the stratum corneum is smooth and shiny, and the skin looks as though it has been covered with cellophane or collodion. Its tightness may cause ectropion and feeding difficulties. The shiny outer surface is shed within a few days leaving behind red scaly skin. This is most often caused by non-bullous ichthyosiform erythroderma, and less often lamellar ichthyosis – both being caused by mutations in the trans-glutaminase-1 gene. Problems with temperature regulation and high water loss through the skin in the early days of life are best dealt with by the use of a high-humidity incubator. Regular applications of a greasy emollient also limit fluid loss and make the skin supple. The much rarer 'harlequin fetus' (resulting from loss of function mutations in the *ABCA12* gene that normally has a role in forming the skin lipid barrier) is covered with thick fissured hyperkeratosis. Ectropion is extreme and most affected infants die early.

## Lamellar ichthyosis and non-bullous ichthyosiform erythroderma

These rare conditions have often been confused in the past, because they look so similar. Both may be inherited as an autosomal recessive trait, and in both the skin changes at birth are those of a collodion baby (see above). Later the two condi-tions can be distinguished by the finer scaling and more obvious redness of non-bullous ichthyosiform erythroderma and the plate-like scales of lamellar ichthyosis. Both last for life and are sufficiently disfiguring for the long-term use of acitretin to be justifiable (Formulary 2, p. 401). Lamellar ichthyosis shows genetic heterogeneity: the most severe type is caused by mutations in the gene for keratinocyte transglutaminase-1, an enzyme that cross-links the cornified cell envelope, lying on chromosome 14q11.2.

## Epidermolytic hyperkeratosis (bullous ichthyosiform erythroderma)

This rare condition is inherited as an autosomal dominant disorder. Shortly after birth the baby's skin becomes generally red and shows numerous blisters. The redness fades over a few months, and the tendency to blister also lessens, but during childhood a gross brownish warty hyperkeratosis appears, sometimes in a roughly linear form and usually worst in the flexures. The diseased skin often becomes secondarily infected and painful, and develops a foul odour. For many patients this is as socially disabling as the skin disease. The histology is distinctive: a thickened granular cell layer contains large granules, and clefts may be seen in the upper epidermis. The condition is caused by mutations in the genes (on chromosomes 12q13 and 17q21) controlling the production of keratins 1 and 10. A few patients with localized areas of hyper-keratosis with the same histological features have gonadal mosaicism, and so their children are at risk of developing the generalized form of the disorder. Treatment is symptomatic. Antibacterial washes and masking fragrances are helpful. Antibiotics may be needed from time to time but should not be used for prolonged periods. Acitretin (Formulary 2, p. 401) has helped in severe cases.

## Other ichthyosiform disorders

Sometimes, ichthyotic skin changes are a minor part of a multisystem disease, but such associ-ations are very rare. *Refsum's syndrome*, an autosomal recessive trait, is caused by deficiency of a single enzyme concerned in the breakdown of phytanic acid, which then accumulates in the tissues. The other features (retinal degeneration, peripheral neuropathy and ataxia) overshadow the minor dryness of the skin.

*Rud's syndrome* is an ichthyosiform erythroderma in association with mental retardation and epilepsy. In *Netherton's syndrome*, brittle hairs, with a so-called 'bamboo deformity', are present as well as a curious gyrate and erythematous hyperkeratotic eruption (ichthyosis linearis circumflexa). Other conditions are identified by confusing acronyms: IBIDS (also known as trichothiodystrophy) stands for ichthyosis, brittle hair, impaired intelligence, decreased fertility and short stature; the KID syndrome consists of keratitis, ichthyosis and deafness.

## Acquired ichthyosis

It is unusual for ichthyosis to appear for the first time in adult life but, if it does, an underlying disease should be suspected. The most frequent is Hodgkin's disease. Other recorded causes include other lymphomas, leprosy, sarcoidosis, malabsorption and a poor diet. The skin may also appear dry in hypothyroidism.

## Other disorders of keratinization

### Keratosis pilaris

#### Cause

This common condition is inherited as an autosomal dominant trait, and is possibly caused by mutations in a gene lying on the short arm of chromosome 18. Heterozygote carriers of an abnormal profilaggrin gene often have keratosis pilaris. The abnormality lies in the keratinization of hair follicles, which become filled with horny plugs.

#### Presentation and course

The changes begin in childhood and tend to become less obvious in adult life. In the most common type, the greyish horny follicular plugs, sometimes with red areolae, are confined to the outer aspects of the thighs and upper arms, where the skin feels rough. Less often, the plugs affect the sides of the face; perifollicular erythema and loss of eyebrow hairs may

then occur. There is an association with ichthyosis vulgaris.

#### Complications

Involvement of the cheeks may lead to an ugly pitted scarring. Rarely, the follicles in the eyebrows may be damaged with subsequent loss of hair there.

#### Differential diagnosis

A rather similar pattern of widespread follicular keratosis (phrynoderma) can occur in severe vitamin deficiency. The lack is probably not just of vitamin A, as was once thought, but of several vitamins.

#### Investigations

None are needed.

#### Treatment

Treatment is not usually needed, although keratolytics such as salicylic acid or urea in a cream base may smooth the skin temporarily (Formulary 1, p. 386). Ultraviolet radiation also provides temporary benefit. A move to a more humid climate is helpful.

### Keratosis follicularis (Darier's disease)

#### Cause

This rare condition is inherited as an autosomal dominant trait. Fertility tends to be low and many cases represent new mutations. The abnormal gene (on chromosome 12q24.1) encodes for a molecule important in a pump that keeps a high concentration of calcium in the endoplasmic reticulum.

#### Presentation

The first signs usually appear in the mid-teens, sometimes after overexposure to sunlight. The characteristic lesions are small pink or brownish papules with a greasy scale (Fig. 4.3). These coalesce into warty plaques in a 'seborrhoeic' distribution (Fig. 4.4). Early lesions are often seen on the sternal and interscapular areas, and behind the ears. The

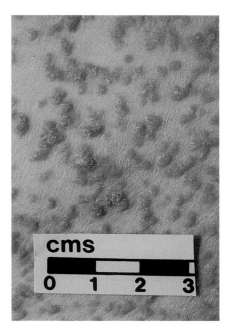

**Fig. 4.3** The typical yellow–brown greasy papules of Darier's disease.

**Fig. 4.4** Extensive Darier's disease, in this case made worse by sun exposure.

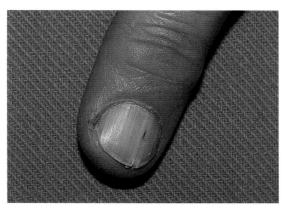

**Fig. 4.5** The nail in Darier's disease. One or more longitudinal pale or pink stripes run over the lunule to the free margin where they end in a triangular nick.

severity of the condition varies greatly from person to person; sometimes the skin is widely affected. The abnormalities remain for life, often causing much embarrassment and discomfort.

Other changes include lesions looking like plane warts on the backs of the hands, punctate keratoses or pits on the palms and soles, cobblestone-like irregularities of the mucous membranes in the mouth, and a distinctive nail dystrophy. White or pinkish lines or ridges run longitudinally to the free edge of the nail where they end in triangular nicks (Fig. 4.5).

### Complications

Some patients are stunted. In some families, Darier's disease runs with bipolar mood disorder. Personality disorders, including antisocial behaviour, are seen more often than would be expected by chance. An impairment of delayed hypersensitivity may be the basis for a tendency to develop widespread herpes simplex and bacterial infections. Bacterial overgrowth is responsible for the unpleasant smell of some severely affected patients.

### Differential diagnosis

The distribution of the lesions may be similar to that of seborrhoeic eczema, but this lacks the warty papules of Darier's disease. The distribution differs from that of acanthosis nigricans (mainly flexural) and of keratosis pilaris (favours the outer upper arms and thighs). Other forms of folliculitis and Grover's disease (p. 123) can also cause confusion.

### Investigations

The diagnosis should be confirmed by a skin biopsy, which will show characteristic clefts in the epidermis, and dyskeratotic cells.

## Treatment

Severe and disabling disease can be dramatically alleviated by long-term acitretin (Formulary 2, p. 401). Milder cases need only topical keratolytics, such as salicylic acid, and the control of local infection (Formulary 1, p. 384).

## Keratoderma of the palms and soles

### Inherited types

Many genodermatoses share keratoderma of the palms and soles as their main feature; they are not described in detail here. The clinical patterns and modes of inheritance vary from family to family. Punctate, striate, diffuse and mutilating varieties have been documented, sometimes in association with metabolic disorders such as tyrosinaemia, or with changes elsewhere. The punctate type is caused by mutations in the keratin 16 gene on chromosome 17q12-q21; the epidermolytic type by mutations in the gene for keratin 9, found only on palms and soles.

The most common pattern is a diffuse one, known also as tylosis (Fig. 4.6), which is inherited as an autosomal dominant trait linked to changes in chromosome region 12q11-q13, which harbours the type 11 keratin gene cluster. In a few families these changes have been associated with carcinoma of the oesophagus, but in most families this is not the case.

Treatment tends to be unsatisfactory, but keratolytics such as salicylic acid and urea can be used in higher concentrations on the palms and soles than elsewhere (Formulary 1, p. 384).

### Acquired types

It is not uncommon for normal people to have a few inconspicuous punctate keratoses on their palms, and it is no longer thought that these relate to internal malignancy, although palmar keratoses caused by arsenic may have this association. Black patients are prone to keratotic papules along their palmar creases.

Keratoderma of the palms and soles may be part of the picture of some generalized skin diseases such as pityriasis rubra pilaris (p. 75) and lichen planus (p. 72).

A distinctive pattern (keratoderma climactericum) is sometimes seen in middle-aged women at about the time of the menopause. It is most marked around the borders of the heels where painful fissures form and interfere with walking (Fig. 4.7). Regular paring and the use of keratolytic ointments are often more helpful than attempts at hormone replacement. Many improve with applications of 40% urea in cream or ointment bases. Acitretin in low doses may be worth a trial, especially when the disorder interferes with walking. The condition tends to settle over a few years.

**Fig. 4.6** Tylosis.

**Fig. 4.7** Keratoderma climactericum – thickly keratotic skin, especially around the heels. Painful fissures are a problem.

## Knuckle pads

### Cause

Sometimes these are familial; usually they are not. Trauma seems not to be important.

### Presentation

Fibromatous and hyperkeratotic areas appear on the backs of many finger joints, usually beginning in late childhood and persisting thereafter. There may be an association with Dupuytren's contracture.

### Differential diagnosis

Occupational callosities (e.g. in carpet layers), granuloma annulare and viral warts should be considered.

### Investigations

A biopsy may be helpful in the few cases of genuine clinical difficulty.

### Treatment

None, including surgery, is satisfactory.

## Callosities and corns

Both are responses to pressure. A *callosity* is a more diffuse type of thickening of the keratin layer, which seems to be a protective response to widely applied repeated friction or pressure. Callosities are often occupational (e.g. they are seen on the hands of manual workers). Usually painless, they need no therapy.

*Corns* have a central core of hard keratin, which can hurt if forced inwards. They appear where there is high local pressure, often between bony prominences and shoes. Favourite areas include the under surface of the toe joints, and the soles under prominent metatarsals. 'Soft corns' arise in the third or fourth toe clefts when the toes are squeezed together by tight shoes; such corns are often macerated and may present as eroded nodules, causing diagnostic confusion.

The main differential is from hyperkeratotic warts, but these will show tiny bleeding points when pared down, whereas a corn has only its hard compacted avascular core surrounded by a more diffuse thickening of opalescent keratin.

The right treatment for corns is to eliminate the pressure that caused them, but patients may be slow to accept this. While regular paring reduces the symptoms temporarily, well-fitting shoes are essential. Corns under the metatarsals can be helped by soft spongy soles, but sometimes need orthopaedic surgery to alter weight bearing. Special care is needed with corns on ischaemic or diabetic feet, which are at greater risk of infection and ulceration.

## Further reading

Cooper SM & Burge SM. (2003) Darier's disease: epidemiology, pathophysiology and management. *American Journal of Clinical Dermatology* **4**, 97–105.

Dunnill MG. (1998) The molecular basis of inherited disorders of keratinization. *Hospital Medicine* **59**, 17–22.

Hernandez-Martin A, Gonzalez-Sarmiento R & De Unamuno P. (1999) X-linked ichthyosis: an update. *British Journal of Dermatology* **141**, 617–627.

Ishida-Yamamoto A, Tanaka H, Nakane H, Takahashi H & Iizuka H. (1998) Inherited disorders of epidermal keratinization. *Journal of Dermatological Science* **18**, 139–154.

Ratnavel RC & Griffiths WAD. (1997) The inherited palmoplantar keratodermas. *British Journal of Dermatology* **137**, 485–490.

Rugg EL & Leigh IM. (2004) The keratins and their disorders. *American Journal of Medical Genetics. Clinical Seminar of Medical Genetics* **131C**, 4–11.

Sakuntbhai A, Burge S, Monk S & Hovnanian A. (1999) Spectrum of novel ATP2A2 mutations in patients with Darier's disease. *Human Molecular Genetics* **8**, 1611–1619.

Shwayder T. (2004) Disorders of keratinisation. *American Journal of Clinical Dermatology* **5**, 17–29.

# 5 Psoriasis

Psoriasis is a chronic, non-infectious, inflammatory skin disorder, characterized by well-defined salmon-pink plaques bearing large adherent silvery centrally attached scales. One to three per cent of most populations have psoriasis, which is most prevalent in European and North American white people, uncommon in American black people and almost non-existent in American Indians. It can start at any age but is rare under 10 years, and appears most often between 15 and 40 years. Its course is unpredictable but is usually chronic with exacerbations and remissions.

## Cause and pathogenesis

The precise cause of psoriasis is still unknown. However, there is often a genetic predisposition, and sometimes an obvious environmental trigger.

There are two key abnormalities in a psoriatic plaque: hyperproliferation of keratinocytes; and an inflammatory cell infiltrate in which neutrophils, tumour necrosis factor and probably Th17 type T lymphocytes predominate. Both of these abnormalities can induce the other, leading to a vicious cycle of keratinocyte proliferation and inflammatory reaction, but it is still not clear which is the primary defect. Perhaps the genetic abnormality leads first to keratinocyte hyperproliferation that, in turn, produces a defective skin barrier (p. 14) allowing the penetration by, or unmasking of, hidden antigens to which an immune response is mounted. Alternatively, the psoriatic plaque might reflect a genetically determined reaction to different types of trauma (e.g. physical wounds, environmental irritants and drugs) in which the healing response is exaggerated and uncontrolled.

To prove the primary role of an immune reaction, putative antigens (e.g. bacteria, viruses or autoantigens) that initiate the immune response will have to be identified. This theory postulates that the increase in keratinocyte proliferation is caused by inflammatory cell mediators or signalling. Theories about the pathogenesis of psoriasis tend to tag along behind fashions in cell biology, and this idea is currently in vogue.

## Genetics

There are two inheritance modes. One type has onset in youth and a more common family history of psoriasis, and the other has onset in late adulthood in patients without obvious family history. Psoriasis does not usually follow a simple Mendelian pattern of inheritance. The mode of inheritance is genetically complex, implying a polygenic inheritance. A child with one affected parent has a 16% chance of developing the disease, and this rises to 50% if both parents are affected. Genomic imprinting (p. 349) may explain why psoriatic fathers are more likely to pass on the disease to their children than are psoriatic mothers. If non-psoriatic parents have a child with psoriasis, the risk for subsequent children is about 10%. In one study, the disorder was concordant in 70% of monozygotic twins but in only 20% of dizygotic ones.

Early-onset psoriasis shows a genetic linkage (p. 348) with a psoriasis susceptibility locus (PSOR-1) located on 6p21 within the major histocompatibility complex class I (MHC-I) region, very near the HLA-C locus, and possibly HLA-Cw6 itself. The risk of those with the HLA-Cw6 genotype developing psoriasis is 20 times that of those without it; 10% of Cw6+ individuals will develop psoriasis. The hereditary element and the HLA associations are much weaker in late-onset psoriasis.

While PSORS-1 is the most important locus in psoriasis, accounting for up to 50% of genetic susceptibility to the disease, at least eight other loci (PSORS-2 to 9) have been identified. At present perhaps it is best to consider psoriasis as a multi-factorial disease with a complex genetic trait. An individual's predisposition to it is determined by a large number of genes, each of which has only a low penetrance. Clinical expression of the disease may result from environmental stimuli including antigen exposure.

## Epidermal cell kinetics

The epidermis of psoriasis replicates too quickly. Keratinocytes proliferate out of control, and an excessive number of germinative cells enter the cell cycle. This 'out of control' proliferation is rather like a car going too fast because the accelerator is stuck, and cannot be stopped by putting a foot on the brake. The growth fraction (p. 10) of epidermal basal cells is greatly increased to almost 100% compared with 30% in normal skin. The epidermal turnover time (p. 11) is greatly shortened, to less than 10 days compared with 30 to 60 days in normal skin. This epidermal hyperproliferation accounts for many of the metabolic abnormalities associated with psoriasis. It is not confined to obvious plaques: similar but less marked changes also occur in the apparently normal skin of psoriatics.

The exact mechanism underlying this increased epidermal proliferation is uncertain, but the skin behaves as though it were trying to repair a wound. Cyclic guanosine monophosphate (cGMP), inducible nitric oxide synthase, arachidonic acid metabolites, polyamines, calmodulin and plasminogen activator are all increased in psoriatic plaques, but theories based on their prime involvement have neither stood the test of time nor provided useful targets for therapeutic intervention. Perhaps the underlying abnormality is a genetic defect in the control of keratinocyte growth, such that the skin defaults to a wound-healing phenotype. γ-Interferon (IFN-γ) inhibits growth and promotes the differentiation of normal keratinocytes by the phosphorylation and activation of the transcription factor STAT-1α but IFN-γ fails to activate STAT-1α in psoriatic keratinocytes. Subnormal activation of another transcription factor, NFκB, may also be important for the formation of psoriatic plaques, as the absence of NFκB activity in gene knock-out mice leads to epidermal hyperproliferation.

Some people think that psoriasis is caused by a genetic defect of retinoid signalling and that is why it improves with retinoid treatment. Receptor-specific retinoids are now available that bind to retinoic acid A receptors (RARs), reduce keratinocyte proliferation, normalize differentiation and reduce infiltration by inflammatory cells.

## Inflammation

Psoriasis differs from the ichthyoses (p. 47) in its accumulation of inflammatory cells, and this could be an immunological response to as yet unknown antigens. Certain interleukins and growth factors are elevated, and adhesion molecules are expressed or up-regulated in the lesions. Immune events may well have a primary role in the pathogenesis of the disease of psoriasis and a hypothetical model might run as follows.

Keratinocytes are stimulated by various insults (e.g. trauma, infections, drugs, ultraviolet radiation) to release interleukin-1 (IL-1), IL-8 and IL-18. IL-1 up-regulates the expression of intercellular adhesion molecule-1 (ICAM-1) and E selectin on vascular endothelium in the dermal papillae. CLA positive memory T lymphocytes accumulate in these papillary vessels because their lymphocyte function-associated antigen (LFA-1) sticks to adhesion molecules that are expressed on the vascular endothelium (p. 26).

IL-8 and chemokines from keratinocytes attract T lymphocytes into the epidermis where they are held by adhesion of their LFA-1 to ICAM-1 on keratinocytes. T cells are further activated by their interactions with Langerhans cells or other antigen-presenting cells (possibly presenting unmasked retroviral or mycobacterial antigens or antigens shared by streptococci and keratinocytes; p. 25). Activated T cells release type I and 17 cytokines including IL-2, IL-17, IL-22, IFN-γ and tumour necrosis factor-α (TNF-α). IL-2 ensures proliferation of the local T cells.

IFN-γ and TNF-α induce keratinocytes to express HLA-DR, to up-regulate their ICAM-1 expression and to produce further IL-6, IL-8, transforming growth factor-α (TGF-α) and TNF-α.

Inflammation results. Chemical mediators include polyamines and leukotrienes. TNF-α is important.

Genes controlling types of TNF-α are located near the psoriais gene PSOR-1 at Cw6, and treatment with biological agents targeting TNF quietens the inflammation dramatically. TGF-α acts as an autocrine mediator and attaches to epidermal growth factor (EGF) receptors inducing keratinocyte proliferation. IL-6 and TGF-α also have keratinocyte mitogenic properties.

Neutrophils have also attracted attention. Some believe that psoriasis is a neutrophil-driven disease. They postulate that infiltrating neutrophils cause microinjuries that shift the skin into a wound-healing mode of hyperproliferation. In this model, IL-8 and chemokines also attract neutrophils from the papillary dermis to move into the epidermis where they create microinjuries, perpetuating the healing response phenotype. Circulating neutrophils are activated, particularly in acute flares. They accumulate in the skin after sticking to endothelial cells (ICAM-1–MAC-1 family interaction). They then migrate through the layers of the epidermis up to the horny layer forming (Munro's) microabscesses, under the influence of chemotactic factors produced by activated keratinocytes, including IL-8, Gro-α and leukotriene-B4. Scales of psoriasis also contain chemotactic factors and these provoke visible collections of subcorneal neutrophils as seen in pustular psoriasis (p. 59).

### The dermis

The dermis is abnormal in psoriasis. If psoriatic skin is grafted on to athymic mice, both epidermis and dermis must be present for the graft to sustain its psoriasis. The dermal capillary loops in psoriatic plaques are abnormally dilated and tortuous, and these changes come before epidermal hyperplasia in the development of a new plaque. Fibroblasts from psoriatics replicate more rapidly *in vitro* and produce more glycosaminoglycans than do those from non-psoriatics.

### Precipitating factors

**1** *Trauma* If the psoriasis is active, lesions can appear in skin damaged by scratches or surgical wounds (the Köbner phenomenon; Fig. 5.1).

**Fig. 5.1** The Köbner phenomenon seen after a recent thoracotomy operation.

**2** *Infection* Tonsillitis caused by β-haemolytic streptococci often triggers guttate psoriasis. Bacterial exotoxins produced by *Staphylococcus aureus* and certain streptococci can act as superantigens (p. 25) and promote polyclonal T-cell proliferation. AIDS depresses cell-mediated immunity, so one might expect HIV infection to ameliorate psoriasis. Actually, HIV infection often worsens psoriasis, or precipitates explosive forms. For now this paradox challenges current assumptions related to pathogenesis.

**3** *Hormonal* Psoriasis frequently improves in pregnancy only to relapse postpartum. Hypocalcaemia secondary to hypoparathyroidism is a rare precipitating cause.

**4** *Sunlight* Improves most psoriatics but 10% become worse.

**5** *Drugs* Antimalarials, beta-blockers, IFN-α and lithium may worsen psoriasis. Psoriasis may 'rebound' after withdrawal of treatment with efalizumab, systemic steroids or potent topical steroids. The case against non-steroidal anti-inflammatory drugs (NSAIDs) remains unproven.

**6** *Cigarette smoking and alcohol* Psoriasis is more common in smokers and ex-smokers but cause and effect relationships are uncertain.

**7** *Emotion* Emotional upsets seem to cause some exacerbations.

### Histology (Fig. 5.2)

The main changes are the following.

**1** Parakeratosis (nuclei retained in the horny layer).

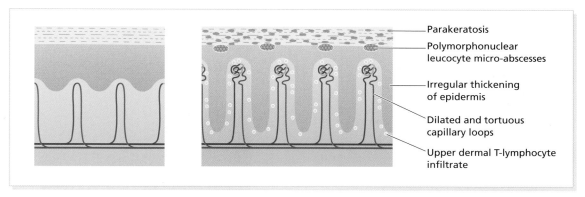

Parakeratosis

Polymorphonuclear leucocyte micro-abscesses

Irregular thickening of epidermis

Dilated and tortuous capillary loops

Upper dermal T-lymphocyte infiltrate

**Fig. 5.2** Histology of psoriasis (right) compared with normal skin (left).

**2** Irregular thickening of the epidermis over the rete ridges, but thinning over dermal papillae. Bleeding may occur when scale is scratched off (Auspitz's sign).
**3** Epidermal polymorphonuclear leucocyte infiltrates and micro-abscesses (described originally by Munro).
**4** Dilated and tortuous capillary loops in the dermal papillae.
**5** T-lymphocyte infiltrate in upper dermis.

## Presentation

### Common patterns

#### *Plaque pattern*

This is the most common type. Lesions are well demarcated and range from a few millimetres to many centimetres in diameter (Fig. 5.3). The lesions are pink or red with large, centrally adherent, silvery-white, polygonal scales. Symmetrical sites on the elbows, knees, lower back and scalp are sites of predilection (Fig. 5.4).

**Fig. 5.3** Psoriasis: extensive plaque psoriasis.

#### *Guttate pattern*

This is usually seen in children and adolescents and may be the first sign of the disease, often triggered by streptococcal tonsillitis. The word 'guttate' means 'drop-shaped'. Numerous small round red macules come up suddenly on the trunk and soon become scaly (Fig. 5.5). The rash often clears in a few months but plaque psoriasis may develop later.

#### *Scalp*

The scalp is often involved. Areas of scaling are interspersed with normal skin; their lumpiness is sometimes more easily felt than seen (Fig. 5.6). Frequently, the psoriasis overflows just beyond the scalp margin. Significant hair loss is rare.

**Fig. 5.4**  Psoriasis favours the extensor aspects of the knees and elbows.

**Fig. 5.5**  Guttate psoriasis.

## Nails

Involvement of the nails is common, with 'thimble pitting' (Fig. 5.7), onycholysis (separation of the nail from the nail bed; Fig. 5.8) and sometimes sub-ungual hyperkeratosis.

## Flexures

Psoriasis of the submammary, axillary and anogenital folds is not scaly although the glistening sharply demarcated red plaques (Fig. 5.9), often with fissuring

**Fig. 5.6**  Untreated severe and extensive scalp psoriasis.

**Fig. 5.7**  Thimble-like pitting of nails with onycholysis.

in the depth of the fold, are still readily recognizable. Flexural psoriasis is most common in women and in the elderly, and is more common among HIV-infected individuals than uninfected ones. Many patients with plaque psoriasis harbour psoriasis in their gluteal fold. Sometimes, when the diagnosis is in doubt, it pays to check for this and for relatively scaleless red papules on the penis.

## Palms and soles

Palmar psoriasis may be hard to recognize, as its lesions are often poorly demarcated and barely ery-thematous. The fingers may develop painful fissures. At other times lesions are inflamed and studded with 1–2 mm pustules (palmoplantar pustulosis)

**Fig. 5.8** Onycholysis.

**Fig. 5.9** Sharply defined glistening erythematous patches of flexural psoriasis.

**Fig. 5.10** Pustular psoriasis of the sole.

**Fig. 5.11** A closer view of pustules on the sole.

(Figs 5.10 and 5.11). The pustulosis are followed by brown macules or scales. Some consider this recalcitrant, often painful, condition an entity separate from psoriasis. Psoriasis of the palms and soles may be disabling.

## Less common patterns

### Napkin psoriasis

A psoriasiform spread outside the napkin (nappy/diaper) area may give the first clue to a psoriatic tendency in an infant (Fig. 5.12). Usually it clears quickly but there is an increased risk of ordinary psoriasis developing in later life.

### Acute generalized pustular psoriasis

This is a rare but serious condition, with fever and recurrent episodes of pustulation within areas of erythema.

### Erythrodermic psoriasis

This is also rare and can be sparked off by the

**Fig. 5.12**  An irritant napkin rash now turning into napkin psoriasis.

irritant effect of tar or dithranol, by a drug eruption or by the withdrawal of potent topical or systemic steroids. The skin becomes universally and uniformly red with variable scaling (Fig. 5.13). Malaise is accompanied by shivering and the skin feels hot and uncomfortable.

**Fig. 5.13**  Erythrodermic psoriasis.

**Fig. 5.14**  Fixed flexion deformity of distal interphalangeal joints following arthropathy.

**Fig. 5.15**  Rheumatoid-like changes associated with severe psoriasis of hands.

## Complications

### Psoriatic arthropathy

Arthritis occurs in about 5–20% of psoriatics. Several patterns are recognized. Distal arthritis involves the terminal interphalangeal joints of the toes and fingers, especially those with marked nail changes (Fig. 5.14). Other patterns include involvement of a single large joint; one that mimics rheumatoid arthritis and may become mutilating (Fig. 5.15); and one where the brunt is borne by the sacroiliac joints and spine. Tests for rheumatoid factor are negative and nodules are absent. In patients with spondylitis and sacroiliitis there is a strong correlation with the presence of HLA-B27. Other patients develop painful inflammation where tendons meet bones (enthetitis).

## Differential diagnosis

### Discoid eczema (p. 99)

Lesions are less well defined and may be exudative or crusted, lack thick scales and may be extremely itchy. Lesions do not favour the scalp or extensor aspects of elbows and knees but rather the trunk and proximal parts of the extremities.

### Seborrhoeic eczema (p. 97)

Scalp involvement is more diffuse and less lumpy. Intervening areas of normal scalp skin are unusual. Plaques are not so sharply marginated.

Flexural plaques are also less well defined and more exudative. There may be signs of seborrhoeic eczema elsewhere, such as in the eyebrows, naso-labial folds or on the chest.

### Pityriasis rosea (p. 71)

This may be confused with guttate psoriasis but the lesions, which are oval rather than round, tend to run along rib lines. Scaling is of collarette type and a herald plaque may precede the rash. Lesions are mostly confined to the upper trunk.

### Secondary syphilis (p. 226)

There is usually a history of a primary chancre. The scaly lesions are brownish and characteristically the palms and soles are involved. Oral changes, patchy alopecia, condylomata lata and lymphadenopathy complete the picture.

### Cutaneous T-cell lymphoma (p. 319)

The lesions, which tend to persist, are not in typical locations and are often annular, arcuate, kidney-shaped or show bizarre outlines. Atrophy or poikilo-derma may be present and individual lesions may vary in their thickness. About half of patients report

that somebody wrongly diagnosed psoriasis, so tread carefully here. Erythrodermic psoriasis mimics the erythroderma of Sézary syndrome

### Tinea unguium (p. 248)

The distal subungual form is often confused with nail psoriasis but is more asymmetrical and there may be obvious tinea of neighbouring skin. Uninvolved nails are common. Pitting is not seen and nails tend to be crumbly and discoloured at their free edge.

## Investigations

**1** Biopsy is seldom necessary. Usually, the diagnosis of common plaque psoriasis is obvious from its clinical appearance. Treated psoriasis and variant forms may pose diagnostic problems, made worse because atypical clinical forms are also frequently atypical histologically.
**2** Throat swabbing for β-haemolytic streptococci is needed in guttate psoriasis.
**3** Skin scrapings and nail clippings may be required to exclude tinea.
**4** Radiology and tests for rheumatoid factor are helpful in assessing arthritis.

## Treatment

The need for this depends both on the patient's own perception of his or her disability, and on the doctor's objective assessment of how severe the skin disease is. The two do not always tally. The cosmetic disfigurement and psychological disability may be severe. Who is worse and needs treatment more – a woman with localized plaque psoriasis who will not go out and who becomes reclusive, or a man with generalized psoriasis who would rather wear shorts than cover up his more numerous plaques?

The effect of psoriasis on the quality of life as perceived by the patient can be scored with such measures as the Dermatology Life Quality Instrument (DLQI). The questionnaire asks questions such as 'Over the past week, how itchy, painful or stinging has your psoriasis been?' and 'Over the past week, how embarrassed or self-conscious have you been?'. The questionnaire tallies 3 points for 'very much', 2 points for 'a lot', 1 point for 'some' and 0 points for 'not at all'. Scores for the 10 questions are summed. A DLQI of 10 or more implies disease markedly affecting life.

Meanwhile, the severity of psoriasis can be scored on the Psoriasis Area and Severity Index (PASI), which quantifies the scaliness, erythema, thickness and extent. Although very useful and reproducible for clinical research studies, the PASI is cumbersome for use in the clinic. Both physician and patient know the extent and severity without the need to score. However, the time may come when third parties will require certain PASI and DLQI scores before they will pay for expensive drugs such as biological agents. Although the maximum score is 72, most dermatologists would interpret a PASI of 12 as severe disease.

## General measures

Explanations and reassurances must be geared to the patient's or the parent's intelligence. Information leaflets help to reinforce verbal advice. The doctor as well as the patient should keep the disease in perspective, and treatment must never be allowed to be more troublesome than the disease itself. The disease is not contagious. In the end, the treatment is one that is chosen by patient and doctor together after an informed and frank discussion of treatment options, including risks, mess, cost, compliance and co-morbidities.

At present there is no cure for psoriasis; all treatments are suppressive and aimed at either inducing a remission or making the condition more tolerable. However, spontaneous remissions will occur in 50% of patients. Treatment for patients with chronic stable plaque psoriasis is relatively simple and may be safely administered by the family practitioner. However, systemic treatment for severe psoriasis should be monitored by a dermatologist. No treatment, at present, alters the overall course of the disease.

Physical and mental rest help to back up the specific management of acute episodes. Concomitant anxiety and depression should be treated on their own merits (Table 5.1).

## Main types of treatment

These can be divided into four main categories: topical, ultraviolet radiation, systemic and combined.

Broad recommendations are listed in Table 5.1, but most physicians will have their own favourites. In many ways it is better to become familiar with a few remedies than dabble with many. The management of patients with psoriasis is an art as well as a science and few other skin conditions benefit so much from patience and experience – of both patients and doctors.

### Local treatments

#### Vitamin D analogues

Calcipotriol (calcipotriene, USA), calcitriol and tacalcitol are analogues of chlolecalciferol, which do not cause hypercalcaemia and calciuria when used topically in the recommended dosage. All can be used for mild to moderate psoriasis affecting less than 40% of the skin. They work by influencing vitamin D receptors in keratinocytes, reducing epidermal proliferation and restoring a normal horny layer. They also inhibit the synthesis of polyamines (p. 55).

Patients like calcipotriol because it is odourless, colourless and does not stain. It seldom clears plaques of psoriasis completely, but does reduce their scaling and thickness. Local and usually transient irritation may occur with the recommended twice-daily application. One way of lessening this is to combine the use of calcipotriol with that of a moderately potent steroid, the calcipotriol being applied in the evening and the steroid in the morning (p. 64). Calcipotriol should not be used on the face. Up to 100 g/week calcipotriol may be used but the manufacturer's recommendations should be consulted when used in children under 6 years old. Calcitriol appears less irritant than calcipotriol. Tacalcitol ointment is applied sparingly once daily at bedtime, the maximum amount being 10 g/day. As with calcipotriol, irritation – often transient – may occur. The drug should not be used for longer than a year at a time and is not yet recommended for children.

#### Local retinoids

Tazarotene is a topically active retinoid. It has a selective affinity for Retinoic acid receptors (RAR) and, when bound to these, improves psoriasis by reducing keratinocyte proliferation, normalizing the

**Table 5.1** Treatment options in psoriasis.

| Type of psoriasis | Treatment of choice | Alternative treatments |
|---|---|---|
| Stable plaque | Vitamin D analogue<br>Local retinoid<br>Local steroid<br>Dithranol<br>Salicylic acid | Coal tar |
| Extensive stable plaque (>30% surface area) recalcitrant to local therapy | Broadband UVB<br>Narrowband UVB<br>PUVA<br>PUVA + acitretin | Methotrexate<br>Ciclosporin<br>Acitretin<br>Sulfasalazine<br>Mycophenolate mofetil<br>Biological agents |
| Widespread small plaque | UVB | Vitamin D analogue<br>Coal tar<br>Systemic therapies |
| Guttate | Systemic antibiotic<br>Emollients while erupting; then UVB | Weak tar preparation<br>Mild local steroids |
| Facial | Tacrolimus<br>Mild to moderately potent local steroid | |
| Flexural | Tacrolimus<br>Vitamin D analogue (caution: may irritate. Calcitriol less irritant than calcipotriol)<br>Mild to moderately potent local steroid + anticandidal/fungal | |
| Pustular psoriasis of hands and feet | Moderately potent or potent local steroid<br>Local retinoid | Acitretin<br>Topical PUVA |
| Acute erythrodermic, unstable or generalized pustular | Inpatient treatment with ichthammol paste<br>Local steroid may be used initially with or without wet compresses | Gentle phototherapy (UVB)<br>Acitretin<br>Methotrexate<br>Ciclosporin<br>Biologic agents |

disturbed differentiation and lessening the infiltrate of dermal inflammatory cells. It is recommended for chronic stable plaque psoriasis on the trunk and limbs covering up to 20% of the body. It is applied sparingly once a day, in the evening, and can be used for courses of up to 12 weeks. It works slowly and can reduce durable emissions. More often it reduces the induration, scaling and redness of plaques. It is available as either a 0.05% or 0.1% gel. Like the vitamin D analogues, its main side-effect is irritation. If this occurs, the strength should be reduced to 0.05%; if irritation persists, applications should be cut to alternate days and a combination treatment with a local steroid considered.

In the USA, tazarotene is licensed for children aged 12 years and over; in Europe it is currently licensed only for adults over 18 years old. The drug should not be used in pregnancy or during lactation. Females of child-bearing age should use adequate contraception during therapy.

*Topical corticosteroids*

Practice varies from centre to centre and from country to country. Many dermatologists, particularly in the USA, find topical corticosteroids most helpful and use them as the mainstay of their long-term management of stable plaque psoriasis. Patients like them because they are clean and reduce scaling and redness.

**Fig. 5.16** Unstable psoriasis following long-term use of a potent topical steroid.

In our view, such usage is safe, but only under proper supervision by doctors well aware of problems such as dermal atrophy, tachyphylaxis, early relapses, the occasional precipitation of unstable psoriasis (Fig. 5.16) and, rarely, in extensive cases, of adrenal suppression caused by systemic absorption. A commitment by the prescriber to keep the patient under regular clinical review is especially important if more than 50 g/week of a moderately potent topical corticosteroid preparation is being used. Combined tar–steroid preparations may also be helpful (Formulary 1, p. 386).

The regular use of topical corticosteroids is less controversial under the following circumstances.

**1** In 'limited choice' areas such as the face, ears, genitals and flexures where tar and dithranol are seldom tolerated (mildly potent steroid preparations should be used if possible).

**2** For patients who cannot use vitamin D analogues, tar or dithranol because of allergic or irritant reactions (moderately potent preparations, except for 'no choice' areas where mildly potent ones should be used if possible).

**3** For unresponsive psoriasis on the scalp, palms and soles (moderately potent, potent and very potent – but only in the short term – preparations).

**4** For patients with minor localized psoriasis (moderately potent or potent preparations).

A combination ointment of calcipotriol and betamethasone diproprionate (a potent corticosteroid) is available. The maximum dose should not exceed 15 g/day or 100 g/week and the ointment should not be applied for longer than 4 weeks.

### Dithranol (anthralin)

Dithranol is rarely used in the USA nowadays but remains popular in the UK. Like coal tar it inhibits DNA synthesis, but some of its benefits may be brought about by the formation of free radicals of oxygen.

Dithranol is more tricky to use than coal tar. It has to be applied carefully, to the plaques only; often it needs to be covered with gauze dressings to prevent movement onto uninvolved skin and clothing, which it stains a rather indelible purple colour. Dithranol also stains normal skin, but the purple–brown discoloration peels off after a few days. It also stains bathtubs, which need to be scrubbed down. It is irritant, so treatment should start with a weak (0.1%) preparation; thereafter the strength can be stepped up at weekly intervals. Dithranol stronger than 1% is seldom necessary. Irritation of the surrounding skin can be lessened by the application of a protective bland paste (e.g. zinc paste). One popular regimen is to apply dithranol daily for 5 days in the week; after 1 month many patients will be clear.

Short-contact therapy, in which dithranol is applied for no longer than 30 min, is also effective. Initially, a test patch of psoriasis is treated with a 0.1% dithranol cream, left on for 20 min and then washed off. If there is no undue reaction, the application can be extended the next day and, if tolerated, can be left on for 30 min. After the cream is washed off, a bland application such as soft white paraffin or emulsifying ointment is applied. Depending on response, the strength of the dithranol can be increased from 0.1% to 2% over 2–3 weeks. Suitable preparations are listed in Formulary 1 (p. 390).

Dithranol is too irritant to apply to the face, the inner thighs, genital region or skin folds. Special care must be taken to avoid contact with the eyes.

### Coal tar preparations

Crude coal tar and its distillation products have been used to treat psoriasis for many years. Their precise mode of action is uncertain but tar does inhibit DNA synthesis and photosensitizes the skin.

Many preparations are available but it is wise to become familiar with a few. The less refined tars are smelly, messy and stain clothes, but are more effective than the cleaner refined preparations. Tar emulsions can also be added to the bath. Suitable preparations are listed in Formulary 1 (p. 390). Despite its reputation as a carcinogen, no increase in skin cancer has been found in patients treated for long periods with tar preparations.

### Salicylic acid

This is a common constituent of psoriasis remedies sold without prescriptions, usually at 2% concentrations. Dermatologists often use 3–6% concentrations. Salicylic acid débrides scales that contain chemotactic factors, enhances the penetration of other topical therapies and may have anti-inflammatory effects. It is best used for short periods (e.g. 2 days) at the beginning of a course of treatment.

### Calcineurin inhibitors (topical immunomodulators)

Both tacrolimus and pimecrolimus have been used, but they are usually too weak to do much except for psoriasis on the face, genitals or intertriginous areas.

### Ultraviolet radiation

Most patients improve with natural sunlight and should be encouraged to sunbathe. During the winter, courses of artificial ultraviolet radiation (UVB), as an outpatient or at home, may help (Fig. 5.17). Both broadband and narrowband UVB can be used. Narrowband UVB uses intense ultraviolet radiation at wavelength 311 nm. This wavelength of ultraviolet radiation is especially effective for clearing psoriasis while minimizing exposure to potentially carcinogenic wavelengths less than 300 nm.

Treatments should be given by an expert, twice to three times weekly for 8 weeks. Goggles should be

**Fig. 5.17** Ultraviolet radiation therapy.

worn. The initial dose is calculated either by establishing the skin type (p. 268) or by determining the minimal dose of UVB that causes erythema in a test patch 24 h after radiation. The initial small dose is increased incrementally after each exposure providing it is well tolerated. The number of treatments and dosage employed should be recorded. The main risk of UVB therapies in the short term is acute phototoxicity (sunburn-like reaction) and, in the long term, the induction of photodamage and skin cancer.

### Special situations

#### Scalp psoriasis

This is often recalcitrant. Oily preparations containing 3–6% salicylic acid are useful (Formulary 1, p. 391). They should be rubbed into the scalp three times a week and washed out with a tar shampoo 4–6 h later. If progress is slow, they can be left on for one or two nights before shampooing. Salicylic acid and tar combinations are also effective.

#### Guttate psoriasis

A course of penicillin V or erythromycin is indicated

for any associated streptococcal throat infection. Bland local treatment is often enough as the natural trend is towards remission. Suitable preparations include emulsifying ointment and zinc and ichthammol cream. Tar–steroid preparations are reasonable alternatives. A course of ultraviolet therapy (UVB) may be helpful after the eruptive phase is over.

### Eruptive or unstable psoriasis

Bland treatment is needed and rest is important. Tar, dithranol and UVB are best avoided. Suitable preparations include oilated baths, mild or moderately potent topical steroids, emulsifying ointment and zinc and ichthammol cream. Refer these patients to dermatologists.

### Systemic treatment

A systemic approach should be considered for extensive psoriasis (more than 20% of the body surface) that fails to improve with prolonged courses of tar or dithranol, and for patients whose quality of life is low. As the potential side-effects are sometimes great, local measures should be given a good trial first. The most commonly used systemic treatments are photochemotherapy with psoralen and ultraviolet A (PUVA) treatment, retinoids, methotrexate, hydroxyurea (hydroxycarbamide), ciclosporin, mycophenolate mofetil, sulfasalazine, and an array of biological agents.

### Photochemotherapy (PUVA)

In this ingenious therapy, a drug is photo-activated in the skin by ultraviolet radiation. An oral dose of 8-methoxypsoralen (8-MOP) or 5-methoxypsoralen (5-MOP) is followed by exposure to long-wave ultraviolet radiation (UVA: 320–400 nm). The psoralen reaches the skin and, in the presence of UVA, forms photo-adducts with DNA pyrimidine bases and cross-links between complementary DNA strands; this inhibits DNA synthesis and epidermal cell division.

The 8-MOP (crystalline formulation 0.6–0.8 mg/kg body weight or liquid formulation 0.3–0.4 mg/kg) or 5-MOP (1.2–1.6 mg/kg) is taken 1–2 h before exposure to a bank of UVA tubes mounted in a cabinet similar to that seen in Fig. 5.17. Psoralens may also be administered in bath water for those unable to tolerate the oral regimen. The initial exposure is calculated either by determining the patient's minimal phototoxic dose (the least dose of UVA that after ingestion of 8-MOP produces a barely perceptible erythema 72 h after testing) or by assessing skin colour and ability to tan. Treatment is given two or three times a week with increasing doses of UVA, depending on erythema production and the therapeutic response. Protective goggles are worn during radiation and UVA opaque plastic glasses must be used after taking the tablets and for 24 h after each treatment. All phototherapy equipment should be serviced and calibrated regularly by trained personnel. An accurate record of each patient's cumulative dosage and number of treatments should be kept.

Clearance takes 5–10 weeks. Thereafter it is often possible to keep the skin clear by PUVA once a fortnight or every 3 weeks. However, as the side-effects of PUVA relate to its cumulative dose (see below), maintenance therapy should not be used unless alternative treatments prove to be unsatisfactory. As far as possible, PUVA therapy is avoided in younger patients.

*Side-effects* Painful erythema is the most common side-effect but the risk of this can be minimized by careful dosimetry. One-quarter of patients itch during and immediately after radiation; fewer feel nauseated after taking 8-MOP. 5-MOP, not yet available in the USA, is worth trying if these effects become intolerable. Long-term side-effects include premature ageing of the skin (with mottled pigmentation, scattered lentigines, wrinkles and atrophy), cutaneous malignancies (usually after a cumulative dose greater than 1000 J or after more than 250 treatments) and, theoretically at least, cataract formation. The use of UVA-blocking glasses for 24 h after each treatment should protect against the latter. The long-term side-effects relate to the total amount of UVA received over the years; this must be recorded and kept as low as possible, without denying treatment when it is clearly needed.

### Retinoids

Acitretin (10–25 mg/day; Formulary 2, p. 401) is an

analogue of vitamin A, and is one of the few drugs helpful in pustular psoriasis. It is also used to thin down thick hyperkeratotic plaques. Minor side-effects are frequent and dose related. They include dry lips, mouth, vagina and eyes, peeling of the skin, pruritus and unpleasant paronychia. All settle on stopping or reducing the dosage of the drug, but the use of emollients and artificial tears is often recommended. Hair thinning or loss is common. Occasionally, all hair is lost when acetretin is used as monotherapy at higher doses of 0.5–1 mg/kg/day. Hair regrows when treatment is stopped, but meanwhile patients generally hate their baldness.

Acitretin can be used for long periods, but regular blood tests are needed to exclude abnormal liver function and the elevation of serum lipids (mainly triglycerides but also cholesterol). Yearly X-rays should detect bone spurs and ossification of ligaments, especially the paraspinal ones (disseminated interstitial skeletal hyperostosis [DISH] syndrome). Monitor too for depression, although a causal relationship between retinoids and depression has not been proved. Children, and those with persistently abnormal liver function tests or hyperlipidaemia, should not be treated.

The most important side-effect is teratogenicity, so acitretin should not normally be prescribed to women of child-bearing age. If, for unavoidable clinical reasons, it is still the drug of choice, effective oral contraceptive measures must be taken and, in view of the long half-life of its metabolite, these should continue for 2 years after treatment has ceased. Blood donation should be avoided for a similar period.

Retinoids and PUVA act synergistically and are often used together in the so-called Re-PUVA regimen. This clears plaque psoriasis quicker than PUVA alone, and needs a smaller cumulative dose of UVA. The standard precautions for both PUVA and retinoid treatment should, of course, still be observed. Low doses of acitretin are often used in combination with other topical therapies for palmoplantar psoriasis.

### Methotrexate

Methotrexate, at the doses used for the treatment of psoriasis, inhibits proliferating lymphoid cells by its effects on purine biosynthesis. These effects are brought about by inhibition of both dihydrofolate reductase, and 5-aminoimidazole-4-carboxamide ribonucleotide (AICAR) transferase. AICAR accumulation reduces adenosine deaminase activity causing adenosine to accumulate in T cells and inhibit their effects. Folate supplementation may reduce methotrexate toxicity, but does not appear to greatly reduce its therapeutic effectiveness.

After an initial trial dose of 2.5 mg, in an adult of average weight, the drug is given orally once a week and the dose increased gradually to a maintenance one of 7.5–20 mg/week. This often controls even aggressive psoriasis. The drug is eliminated largely by the kidneys and so the dose must be reduced if renal function is poor. Aspirin and sulphonamides displace the drug from binding with plasma albumin, and furosemide decreases its renal clearance: note must therefore be taken of concurrent drug therapy (Formulary 2, p. 400) and the dose reduced accordingly. Minor and temporary side-effects, such as nausea and malaise, are common in the 48 h after administration. The most serious drawback to this treatment is hepatic fibrosis, the risk of which is greatly increased in those who drink alcohol. Unfortunately, routine liver function tests and scans cannot predict this reliably, and a liver biopsy to exclude active liver disease has hitherto been advised for those with risk factors, and repeated after every cumulative dose of 1.5–2 g, especially in less than perfectly healthy drinking adults. Liver biopsy is now being replaced in the UK by serial assays of serum procollagen III aminopeptide (PIIINP), which appears to be an adequately sensitive marker for hepatic fibrosis. Blood checks to exclude marrow suppression, and to monitor renal and liver function, should also be performed – weekly at the start of treatment, with the interval being slowly increased to monthly or every third month depending on when stable maintenance therapy is established.

The drug is teratogenic and should not be given to females in their reproductive years. Oligospermia has been noted in men and fertility may be lowered; however, a child fathered by a man on methotrexate can be expected to be normal. Folic acid, 5 mg/day, taken on days when the patient does not have methotrexate, can lessen nausea and reduce marrow suppression. Methotrexate should not be taken at the same time as retinoids or ciclosporin.

*Ciclosporin*

Ciclosporin inhibits cell-mediated immune reactions. It blocks resting lymphocytes in the $G_0$ or early $G_1$ phase of the cell cycle and inhibits lymphokine release, especially that of IL-2.

Ciclosporin is effective in severe psoriasis, but patients needing it should be under the care of specialists. Most prefer to use the drug only for short periods to stabilize disease or to buy time while other therapies are started. The initial daily dose is 3–4 mg/kg/day and not more than 5 mg/kg/day. With improvement the dose can often be reduced but the side-effects of long-term treatment include hypertension, kidney damage and persistent viral warts with a risk of skin cancer. Blood pressure and renal function should be assessed carefully before starting treatment. The serum creatinine should be measured two or three times before starting therapy to be sure of the baseline and then every other week for the first 3 months of therapy. Thereafter, if the results are stable, the frequency of testing will depend on the dosage (monthly for >2.5 mg/kg/day or every other month for <2.5 mg/kg/day). The dosage should be reduced if the serum creatinine concentration rises to 30% above the baseline level on two occasions within 2 weeks. If these changes do not reverse themselves when the dosage has been reduced for 1 month, then the drug should be stopped.

Hypertension is a common side-effect of ciclosporin: nearly 50% of patients develop a systolic blood pressure over 160 mmHg and/or a diastolic blood pressure over 95 mmHg. Usually, these rises are mild or moderate, and respond to concomitant treatment with a calcium-channel blocker, such as nifedipine. If this cannot be tolerated, an angiotensin-converting enzyme inhibitor should be used under specialist supervision. Diuretics, which may themselves worsen renal function, and beta-blockers, which may worsen psoriasis, should probably be avoided. Ciclosporin interacts with a number of drugs (Formulary 2, p. 399). It is also advisable to watch levels of cholesterol, triglycerides, potassium and magnesium, and advise patients that they will become hirsute and that they may develop gingival hyperplasia. Treatment with ciclosporin should not continue for longer than 1 year without careful assessment and close monitoring.

*Other systemic drugs*

Antimetabolites such as mycophenolate mofetil, 6-tioguanine, azathioprine and hydroxyurea help psoriasis, but less than methotrexate; they tend to damage the marrow rather than the liver. Regular blood monitoring is again essential. Fumaric acid esters, although unlicensed, have been effective in some patients with treatment-resistant psoriasis, but with a high incidence of gastrointestinal upset. Sulfasalazine occasionally helps psoriasis.

### Biological agents

The idea of using a weekly injection to control psoriasis is no longer a pipe dream. The immunologically based pathogenesis of psoriasis presents many targets for therapeutic exploitation (Fig. 5.18). Pharmaceutical companies have synthesized monoclonal antibodies that bind key molecules. Some of these have proved very effective and safe, but also very expensive.

Etanercept is a fusion protein of immunoglobulin G (IgG) and the extracellular TNF-$\alpha$ receptor, so that it effectively mops up free TNF-$\alpha$, preventing its action. Infliximab is a chimeric antibody against TNF-$\alpha$ that binds both soluble and bound TNF-$\alpha$. Adalimumab is a recombinant IgG monoclonal antibody against TNF-$\alpha$ with similar action.

Alefacept (not licensed for use in the UK) and efalizumab do not bind TNF-$\alpha$. Alefacept is a fusion protein of human LFA-3 and IgG that inhibits T-cell activation by blocking the action of accessory molecules needed for lymphocyte activation (Fig. 2.12). Efalizumab is a humanized murine IgG that binds to CD11a. This inhibits both T-cell activation and adhesion.

Both dermatologists and patients often ponder when to use biological treatments, and then which agent to use. As with other therapies, the choice depends upon type of psoriasis, co-morbidities (including arthritis), insurance coverage, cost, efficacy, mode of administration and safety.

In the UK, guidelines have been produced by the British Association of Dermatologists (BAD) and also by the National Institute for Health and Clinical Excellence (NICE). Patients must have severe psoriasis and have failed, or been intolerant of, standard

**Fig. 5.18** Therapeutic targets of the major biological agents used in psoriasis. Etanercept is a soluble receptor for TNF-$\alpha$, while infliximab and adalimumab are antibodies to TNF-$\alpha$. ICAM-1, intercellular adhesion molecule; IL, interleukin; LFA, lymphocyte function-associated antigen; MHC, major histocompatibility complex; TCR, T-cell receptor; TNF, tumour necrosis factor.

systemic therapy and phototherapy for biological therapy to be considered (Table 5.2). Etanercept is generally recommended as the first line biological, with efalizumab being used if this is ineffective. For psoriatic arthritis, etanercept is used first, with infliximab in reserve.

**Table 5.2** Elements suggesting the need for treatment with biological agents.

PASI score more than 10
DLQI score more than 10
Globally severe disease
Life-threatening psoriasis
Unstable psoriasis
Unresponsive to other therapies
Intolerant to other therapies
Would otherwise need hospitalization
Significant co-morbidities
Associated significant psoriatic arthritis

DLQI, Dermatology Life Quality Instrument.
PASI Psoriasis Area and Severity Index

In the USA, many dermatologists first choose etanercept, because of its good safety profile, relative efficacy and relative ease of administration (it can be injected at home by the patient). There are worries about opportunistic infections and about precipitating multiple sclerosis, congestive heart failure, lupus-like syndromes and lymphomas. It can be used in children.

Treatment with efalizumab is rarely associated with thrombocytopenias, and with rebound worsening and instability of psoriasis when the drug is stopped. Infliximab probably works fastest of all the biological agents, but requires intravenous infusions and may allow reactivation of dormant tuberculosis. Alefacept requires weekly counts of CD4 lymphocytes, because it can cause lymphopenias. It is given in courses.

All the biological agents are expensive. Patients who pay could buy a car each year for the money they will spend. However, the treatments are very effective and relatively safe. They minimize costs of laboratory test monitoring, physician visits, phototherapies, and costs associated with long-term side-effects of other choices such as liver disease (methotrexate), renal disease (ciclosporin) and heart disease (hyperlipidaemias from retinoids).

## Combination therapy

If psoriasis is resistant to one treatment, a combination of treatments used together may be the answer. Combination treatments can even prevent side-effects by allowing less of each drug to be used. Common combinations include topical vitamin D analogues with either local steroids or UVB, dithranol following a tar bath and UVB (Ingram regimen) and coal tar following a tar bath and UVB (Goeckerman regimen). Combination therapy with biological agents is possible, but experience is limited.

Rotational therapy may also minimize the toxicity of some treatments – an example would be PUVA, methotrexate, acitretin and ciclosporin, each used separately for a while before moving on to the next treatment.

---

**Learning points**

- Discuss a treatment plan with the patient. Consider disability, cost, time, mess and risk of systemic therapy to general health
- The treatment must not be worse than the disease
- Do not aggravate eruptive psoriasis
- Never use systemic steroids
- Avoid the long-term use of potent or very potent topical corticosteroids
- Never promise a permanent cure, but be encouraging
- Great advances have been made over the last 20 years in the treatment of severe psoriasis, but patients taking modern systemic agents require careful monitoring

---

## Further reading

Bowcock AM. (2005) The genetics of psoriasis and autoimmunity. *Annual Review of Genomics and Human Genetics* **6**, 93–122.

Gaspari AA. (2006) Innate and adaptive immunity and the pathophysiology of psoriasis. *Journal of the American Academy of Dermatology* **54**, S67–80.

Koo J, Lee E, Lee CS & Lebwohl M. (2004) Psoriasis (Periodic synopsis). *Journal of the American Academy of Dermatology* **50**, 613–622.

Lebwohl M. (2005) A clinican's paradigm in the treatment of psoriasis. *Journal of the American Academy of Dermatology* **53**, S59–69.

Lebwohl M & Ali S. (2001) Treatment of psoriasis. I. Topical therapy and phototherapy. *Journal of the American Academy of Dermatology* **45**, 487–498.

Lebwohl M & Ali S. (2001) Treatment of psoriasis. II. Systemic therapies. *Journal of the American Academy of Dermatology* **45**, 649–661.

Mease PJ & Mentor MA. (2006) Quality of life issues in psoriasis and psoriatic arthritis: outcome measures and therapies from a dermatological perspective. *Journal of the American Academy of Dermatology* **54**, 685–704.

Nelson AA, Pearce DJ, Fleisher AB, Balkrishnan R & Feldman SR. (2006) New treatments for psoriasis: which biologic is best? *Journal of Dermatologic Treatment* **17**, 96–107.

Schon MP & Boehncke WH. (2005) Psoriasis. *New England Journal of Medicine* **352**, 1899–1912.

Smith CH, Anstey AV, Barker JN, *et al.* (2005) British Association of Dermatologists guidelines for use of biological interventions in psoriasis 2005. *British Journal of Dermatology* **153**, 486–497.

Thomas VD, Yang EC & Kvedar JC. (2005) Biologics in psoriasis: a quick reference guide. *Journal of the American Academy of Dermatology* **53**, 346–351.

van der Kerkhof PCM. (1999) *Textbook of Psoriasis.* Blackwell Science, Oxford.

van der Kerkhof PC & Kragballe K. (2005) Recommendations for the topical treatment of psoriasis. *Journal of the European Academy of Dermatology and Venerology* **19**, 495–499.

# 6 Other papulosquamous disorders

Psoriasis is not the only skin disease that is sharply marginated and scaly; Table 6.1 lists some of the most common ones. Eczema can also be raised and scaly, but is usually poorly marginated with fissures, crusts or lichenification and signs of epidermal disruption such as weeping, and yellow scaling (Chapter 7). Psoriasis is discussed in Chapter 5.

## Pityriasis rosea

### Cause

Pityriasis rosea may be caused by reactivation of either human herpes virus 7 or human herpes virus 6. The disease may occur in clusters, both geographical and temporal, and seems not to be contagious.

### Presentation

Pityriasis rosea is common, particularly during the winter. It mainly affects children and young adults,

**Table 6.1** Some important papulosquamous diseases.

Psoriasis
Pityriasis rosea
Lichen planus
Pityriasis rubra pilaris
Parapsoriasis
Mycosis fungoides (cutaneous T-cell lymphoma)
Pityriasis lichenoides
Discoid lupus erythematosus
Subacute cutaneous lupus erythematosus
Tinea corporis
Pityriasis versicolor
Nummular eczema
Seborrhoeic dermatitis
Secondary syphilis
Drug eruptions
Extramammary Paget's disease
Squamous cell carcinoma *in situ*

and second attacks are rare. Most patients develop one plaque (the 'herald' or 'mother' plaque) before the others (Fig. 6.1). It is larger (2–5 cm diameter) than later lesions, and is rounder, redder and more scaly. After several days many smaller plaques appear, mainly on the trunk, but some also on the neck and extremities. About half of patients complain of itching. An individual plaque is oval, salmon pink and shows a delicate scaling, adherent peripherally as a collarette. The configuration of such plaques is often characteristic. Their longitudinal axes run down and out from the spine in a 'fir tree' pattern (Fig. 6.2), along the lines of the ribs. Purpuric lesions are rare.

**Fig. 6.1** The herald plaque of pityriasis rosea is usually on the trunk and is larger than the other lesions. Its annular configuration is shown well here.

**Fig. 6.2** Extensive pityriasis rosea showing a 'fir tree' distribution on the back.

## Course

The herald plaque precedes the generalized eruption by several days. Subsequent lesions enlarge over the first week or two. A minority of patients have systemic symptoms such as aching and tiredness. The eruption lasts 2–10 weeks and then resolves spontaneously, sometimes leaving hyperpigmented patches that fade more slowly.

## Differential diagnosis

Although herald plaques are often mistaken for ringworm (tinea corporis), the two disorders most likely to be misdiagnosed early in the general eruption are guttate psoriasis and secondary syphilis. Tinea corporis and pityriasis versicolor can be distinguished by the microscopical examination of scales (p. 40), and secondary syphilis by its other features (mouth lesions, palmar lesions, condylomata lata, lymphadenopathy, alopecia) and by serology. Gold and captopril are the drugs most likely to cause a pityriasis rosea-like drug reaction, but barbiturates, penicillamine, some antibiotics and other drugs can also do so.

## Investigations

Because secondary syphilis can mimic pityriasis rosea so closely, testing for syphilis is usually wise.

## Treatment

No treatment is curative, and active treatment is seldom needed. A moderately potent topical steroid or calamine lotion will help the itching. One per cent salicylic acid in soft white paraffin or emulsifying ointment reduces scaling. Sunlight or artificial UVB often relieves pruritus and may hasten resolution. So far, treatment with antiviral agents has not been helpful.

> **Learning points**
>
> - Check serology for syphilis if in doubt about the diagnosis
> - Revise the diagnosis if the rash lasts for longer than 3 months

## Lichen planus

### Cause

The precise cause of lichen planus is unknown, but the disease seems to be mediated immunologically. It has been postulated that CD8$^+$ cytotoxic T cells (p. 23) recognize an antigen (unknown at present) associated with major histocompatibility complex (MHC) class I (p. 26) on basal keratinocytes in lesions, and the keratinocytes are then lysed. Chronic graft-vs.-host disease can cause an eruption rather like lichen planus in which histoincompatibility causes lymphocytes to attack the epidermis. There may be a genetic susceptibility to idiopathic lichen planus although an abnormal gene has not yet been identified. Rarely, familial cases are reported. Lichen planus is also associated with autoimmune disorders, such as alopecia areata, vitiligo and ulcerative colitis, more commonly than would be expected by chance. Contact allergy to mercury compounds (in dental amalgam fillings) seems to be an important cause of oral lichen planus, especially if there is close contact with the amalgam and if there is no concomitant cutaneous lichen planus. Drugs too can cause lichen planus (see below). Some patients with lichen planus also have a hepatitis C infection – but lichen planus itself is not infectious.

## Presentation

Typical lesions are violaceous or lilac-coloured, intensely itchy, flat-topped papules that usually arise on the extremities, particularly on the volar aspects of the wrists and legs (Fig. 6.3). A close look is needed to see a white streaky pattern on the surface of these papules (Wickham's striae). White asymptomatic lacy lines, dots, and occasionally small white plaques, are also found in the mouth, particularly inside the cheeks, in about 50% of patients (Fig. 6.4), and oral lesions may be the sole manifestation of the disease. The genital skin may be similarly affected (see Fig. 13.37). Variants of the classic pattern are rare and often difficult to diagnose (Table 6.2). Curiously, although the skin plaques are usually itchy, patients rub rather than scratch, so that excoriations are uncommon. As in psoriasis, the Köbner phenomenon may occur (Fig. 6.5). The nails are usually normal, but in about 10% of patients show changes ranging from fine longitudinal grooves to destruction of the entire nail fold and bed (see Fig. 13.26). Scalp lesions can cause a patchy scarring alopecia.

**Fig. 6.4** Lichen planus: classic white lacy network lying on the buccal mucosa.

**Table 6.2** Variants of lichen planus.

Annular
Atrophic
Bullous
Follicular
Hypertrophic (Fig. 6.6)
Ulcerative

**Fig. 6.5** Lichen planus: striking Köbner effect on the forearm.

## Course

Individual lesions may last for many months and the eruption as a whole tends to last about 1 year. However, the hypertrophic variant of the disease, with thick warty lesions usually around the ankles (Fig. 6.6), often lasts for many years. As lesions resolve, they become darker, flatter and leave discrete brown or grey macules. About one in six patients will have a recurrence.

**Fig. 6.3** Shiny flat-topped papules of lichen planus. Note the Wickham's striae.

**Fig. 6.6** The thickened purplish lesions characteristic of hypertrophic lichen planus on the shins.

## Complications

Nail and hair loss can be permanent. The ulcerative form of lichen planus in the mouth may lead to squamous cell carcinoma. Ulceration, usually over bony prominences, may be disabling, especially if it is on the soles. Any association with liver disease may be caused by a coexisting hepatitis C infection, as mentioned above.

## Differential diagnosis

Lichen planus should be differentiated from the other papulosquamous diseases listed in Table 6.1. Lichenoid drug reactions can mimic lichen planus closely. Gold and other heavy metals have often been implicated. Other drug causes include antimalarials, beta-blockers, non-steroidal anti-inflammatory drugs, para-aminobenzoic acid, thiazide diuretics and penicillamine. Contact with chemicals used to develop colour photographic film can also produce similar lesions. It may be hard to differentiate lichen planus from generalized discoid lupus erythematosus if only a few large lesions are present, or if the eruption is on the palms, soles or scalp. Wickham's striae or oral lesions favour the diagnosis of lichen planus. Oral candidiasis (pp. 196, 253) can also cause confusion.

## Investigations

The diagnosis is usually obvious clinically. The histology is characteristic (Fig. 6.7), so a biopsy will confirm the diagnosis if necessary.

## Treatment

Treatment can be difficult. If drugs are suspected as the cause, they should be stopped and unrelated ones substituted. Potent topical steroids will sometimes relieve symptoms and flatten the plaques. Systemic steroid courses work too, but are recommended only in special situations (e.g. unusually

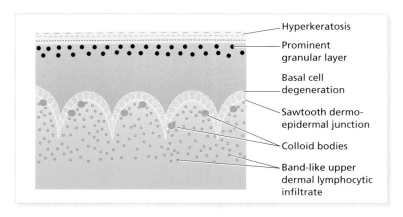

Hyperkeratosis

Prominent granular layer

Basal cell degeneration

Sawtooth dermo-epidermal junction

Colloid bodies

Band-like upper dermal lymphocytic infiltrate

**Fig. 6.7** Histology of lichen planus.

extensive involvement, nail destruction or painful and erosive oral lichen planus). Treatment with photochemotherapy with psoralen and ultraviolet A (PUVA; p. 66) or with narrowband UVB (p. 65) may reduce pruritus and help to clear up the skin lesions. Oral ciclosporin (Formulary 2, p. 399) or acitretin (Formulary 2, p. 401) have also helped some patients with stubborn lichen planus. Antihistamines may blunt the itch. Mucous membrane lesions, both oral and genital, are usually asymptomatic and do not require treatment; if they do, then applications of a corticosteroid or calcineurin inhibitor such as tacrolimus in a gel base may be helpful.

**Fig. 6.8** Pityriasis rubra pilaris. Note the red plugged follicles, seen even in the 'spared' areas.

---

**Learning points**

- A good diagnostic tip is to look for light reflected from shiny papules
- Always look in the mouth
- If you can recognize lichen planus, you have pulled ahead of 75% of your colleagues

---

## Pityriasis rubra pilaris

This heading describes a group of uncommon skin disorders characterized by fine scaling (pityriasis), redness (rubra) and involvement of hair follicles (pilaris). It is unclear if the different presentations of this combination of signs are separate conditions or variants of one disease. The prevalence of pityriasis rubra pilaris, including all types, is very low at around 1 in 400,000 of the population in the UK.

### Cause

No cause has been identified for any type. There is epidermal hyperproliferation in lesional skin and the epidermal turnover time (p. 10) is decreased, but not to the extent seen in psoriasis. A defect in vitamin A metabolism was once suggested but has been disproved. The familial type has an autosomal dominant inheritance.

### Presentation

The familial type develops gradually in childhood. A circumscribed juvenile type affects the palms and soles, and fronts of the knees and backs of the elbows in children. The most common acquired type begins in adult life with erythema and scaling of the face and scalp. Later, red or orange plaques grow quickly and merge, so that patients with pityriasis rubra pilaris are often erythrodermic. Perifollicular papules and keratinous follicular plugs develop at this stage. Small islands of skin may be 'spared' from this general erythema, but even here the follicles may be red and plugged with keratin (Fig. 6.8). Equally striking may be the relative sparing of the peri-areolar and axillary skin. The generalized plaques, although otherwise rather like psoriasis, may also show follicular plugging. The palms and soles become thickened, smooth and yellow. Fissures are common there. The nails also thicken, as a result of an accumulation of keratin under them without pitting of the nail plate (cf. psoriasis), appearing as 'half and half' nails (p. 326). The scalp becomes covered with fine bran-like scales in contrast to the larger scales of psoriasis and the greasier ones of seborrhoeic dermatitis. The ability to sweat is often impaired.

### Course

The most common acquired form generally resolves within 3 years, but may recur. Even when the plaques have gone, the skin may retain a rough scaly texture with persistent small scattered follicular plugs. The familial type, developing in childhood, persists throughout life. The juvenile circumscribed type usually clears in the teens.

## Complications

There are usually few complications although ectropion may be a problem. Accompanying arthritis, as seen in psoriasis, is not a feature. Erythroderma causes patients to tolerate cold poorly.

## Differential diagnosis

Psoriasis is the disorder closest in appearance to pityriasis rubra pilaris, but lacks its slightly orange tinge. The thickening of the palms and soles, the follicular erythema in islands of uninvolved skin, and follicular plugging within the plaques, especially over the knuckles, are other features – besides those mentioned already – that help to separate them.

## Investigations

A biopsy may help to distinguish psoriasis from pityriasis rubra pilaris. There are no polymorphonuclear leucocyte micro-abscesses of Munro, less parakeratosis and broader rete pegs in pityriasis rubra pilaris. Even so, the two disorders share many histological features.

## Treatment

Most patients require copious topical treatment and many prefer this to systemic treatment. Emollients (Formulary 1, p. 381) and keratolytics (Formulary 1, p. 384) for the palms and soles are the mainstay of this. About 50% of patients respond slowly to systemic retinoids such as acitretin (in adults, 25–50 mg/day for 6–8 months; p. 401). Oral methotrexate in low doses, taken once a week, may also help a similar percentage (p. 400). Phototherapies do not help much unless given concomitantly with orally administered retinoids. A recent report of treatment with the tumour necrosis factor α (TNF-α) inhibitor, infliximab (p. 68), was encouraging. Systemic steroids are not indicated.

## Parapsoriasis and premycotic eruption

Parapsoriasis is a contentious term, which many would like to drop. We still find it useful clinically for lesions that look a little like psoriasis but

**Fig. 6.9** A bizarre eruption: its persistence and variable colour suggested a prelymphomatous eruption. Biopsy confirmed this.

which scale subtly rather than grossly, and which persist despite antipsoriasis treatment. It is worth trying to distinguish a benign type of parapsoriasis from a 'premycotic' type, which is a forerunner of cutaneous T-cell lymphoma (mycosis fungoides) (Fig. 6.9) – although they can look alike early in their development. Clonality of infiltrating lymphocytes suggests that these lesions are mycosis fungoides right from the start. Many prefer to call this form of parapsoriais 'patch stage cutaneous T-cell lymphoma', particularly if there is lymphocyte clonality in the patches and plaques (p. 319).

## Cause

The cause is otherwise unknown.

## Presentation

Pink scaly well-marginated plaques appear, typically on the buttocks, breasts, abdomen or flexural skin. Often they are large and irregularly shaped, and develop asymmetrically. The clinical features that distinguish the small-plaque (benign) and large-plaque (premycotic/prelymphomatous) types are given in Table 6.3. Perhaps the most important point is the presence of poikiloderma (atrophy, telangiectasia and reticulate pigmentation) in the latter type. Both conditions are stubborn in their response to topical treatment, although often responding temporarily to PUVA. Itching is variable.

**Table 6.3** Distinguishing features of parapsoriasis and premycotic/prelymphomatous eruptions.

| Parapsoriasis (benign type) | Premycotic/prelymphomatous eruptions |
| --- | --- |
| Smaller plaques | Larger |
| Yellowish | Not yellow – pink, or slightly violet, or brown |
| Sometimes finger-shaped lesions | Asymmetrical with bizarre outline running around the trunk |
| No atrophy | Atrophy ± poikiloderma |
| Responds to UVB | Responds better to PUVA |
| Remains benign although rarely clears | May progress to a cutaneous T-cell lymphoma |

## Complications

Patients with suspected premycotic/prelympho-matous eruptions should be followed up carefully, even though a cutaneous T-cell lymphoma may not develop for years. If poikiloderma or indura-tion develops, the diagnosis of a cutaneous T-cell lymphoma becomes likely.

## Differential diagnosis

This includes psoriasis, tinea and nummular (discoid) eczema. In contrast to psoriasis and pityriasis rosea, the lesions of parapsoriasis, characteristically, are asymmetrical. Topical steroids can cause atrophy and confusion.

## Investigations

Several biopsies should be taken if a premycotic eruption is suspected, if possible from thick or atrophic untreated areas. These may suggest an early cutaneous T-cell lymphoma, with bizarre mono-nuclear cells both in the dermis and in microscopic abscesses within the epidermis. Polymerase chain reaction (PCR), single-stranded conformational polymorphism or Southern blot analysis can deter-mine clonality of the T cells within the lymphoid infiltrate of mycosis fungoides based on rearrange-ments of the T-cell receptor genes (p. 23). The use of these techniques and of immunophenotyping helps to differentiate benign parapsoriasis from premycotic/prelymphomatous eruptions. Staging studies rarely disclose lymphoma of nodes or internal organs at this stage, but it may be worth feeling for lymphadenopathy and hepatosplenomegaly.

In the same spirit, some experts advocate baseline tomography, chest x-ray, blood counts and liver biochemistry.

## Treatment

Treatment is controversial. Less aggressive treat-ments are used for the benign type of parapsoriasis. Usually, moderately potent steroids or ultraviolet radiation bring some resolution, but lesions tend to recur when these are stopped. For premycotic/ prelymphomatous eruptions, treatment with PUVA (p. 66) or with topical nitrogen mustard paints is advocated by some, although it is not clear that this slows down or prevents the development of a subsequent cutaneous T-cell lymphoma.

## Pityriasis lichenoides

Pityriasis lichenoides is uncommon. It occurs in two forms (both latin mouthfuls) at each end of a spectrum that, more often than not, includes patients with overlapping features.

**1** *Pityriasis lichenoides et varioliformis acuta* This acute type is characterized by crops of papules that become necrotic and leave scars like those of chickenpox. They rarely affect the face and the rash, which lasts much longer than chickenpox, is usually scattered on the trunk and limbs.

**2** *Pityriasis lichenoides chronica* The numerous small circular scaly macules and papules of the chronic type are easy to confuse with guttate psoriasis (p. 57). However, their scaling is distinctive in that single silver-grey scales (mica scales) surmount the lesions. The rash usually grumbles on for months or, rarely, years.

## Treatment

Long-term antibiotics (tetracycline or erythromycin) have their advocates and UVB radiation can reduce the number of lesions. Spontaneous resolution occurs eventually.

## Other papulosquamous diseases

Discoid lupus erythematosus is typically papulosquamous; it is discussed with subacute cutaneous lupus erythematosus in Chapter 10. Fungus infections are nummular and scaly and can appear papulosquamous or eczematous; they are dealt with in Chapter 16. Seborrhoeic and nummular discoid eczema are discussed in Chapter 7. Secondary syphilis is discussed in Chapter 16.

## Erythroderma/exfoliative dermatitis

Sometimes the whole skin becomes red and scaly (see Fig. 5.13). The disorders that can cause this are listed in Table 6.4. The best clue to the underlying cause is a history of a previous skin disease. Sometimes the histology is helpful but often it is non-specific. 'Erythroderma' is the term used when the skin is red with little or no scaling, while the

**Table 6.4** Some causes of erythroderma/exfoliative dermatitis.

Psoriasis
Pityriasis rubra pilaris
Ichthyosiform erythroderma
Pemphigus erythematosus
Contact, atopic or seborrhoeic eczema
Reiter's syndrome
Lymphoma (including the Sézary syndrome)
Drug eruptions
Crusted (Norwegian) scabies

term 'exfoliative dermatitis' is preferred if scaling predominates. In dark skin the presence of pigment may mask the erythema, giving a purplish hue.

Most patients have lymphadenopathy, and many have hepatomegaly as well. If the condition becomes chronic, tightness of the facial skin leads to ectropion, scalp and body hair may be lost, and the nails become thickened and may be shed too. Temperature regulation is impaired and heat loss through the skin usually makes the patient feel cold and shiver. Oedema, high output cardiac failure, tachycardia, anaemia, failure to sweat and dehydration can occur. Treatment is that of the underlying condition.

> **Learning points**
>
> The dangers of erythroderma are the following
> - Poor temperature regulation
> - High-output cardiac failure
> - Protein deficiency

## Further reading

Bhattacharya M, Kaur I & Kumar B. (2000) Lichen planus: a clinical and epidemiological study. *Journal of Dermatology* **27**, 576–582.

Clayton BD, Jorrizzo JL & Hitchcock MG. (1997) Adult pityriasis rubra pilaris: a 10-year case series. *Journal of the American Academy of Dermatology* **36**, 959–964.

Cribier B, Frances C & Chosidow O. (1998) Treatment of lichen planus. An evidence-based medicine analysis of efficacy. *Archives of Dermatology* **135**, 1420–1421.

Gonzalez LM, Allen R, Janniger CK & Schwartz RA. (2005) Pityriasis rosea: an important papulosquamous disorder. *International Journal of Dermatology* **44**, 757–764.

Scarisbrick JJ. (2006) Staging and management of cutaneous T cell lymphoma. *Clinical and Experimental Dermatology* **31**, 181–186.

# **7** Eczema and dermatitis

The disorders grouped under this heading are the most common skin conditions seen by family doctors, and make up some 20% of all new patients referred to our clinics.

The eczemas are a disparate group of diseases, but unified by the presence of itch and, in the acute stages, of oedema (spongiosis) in the epidermis. In early disease the stratum corneum remains intact, so the eczema appears as a red, smooth, oedematous plaque. With worsening disease the oedema becomes more severe, tense blisters appear on the plaques or they may weep plasma. If less severe or if the eczema becomes chronic, scaling and epithelial disruption occur, giving chronic eczemas a characteristic appearance. All these are phases of the reaction pattern known as 'eczema'.

## Terminology

The word 'eczema' comes from the Greek for 'boiling' – a reference to the tiny vesicles (bubbles) that are often seen in the early acute stages of the disorder, but less often in its later chronic stages. 'Dermatitis' means inflammation of the skin and is therefore, strictly speaking, a broader term than eczema – which is just one of several possible types of skin inflammation.

> **Learning point**
>
> 'When I use a word it means just what I choose it to mean' said Humpty Dumpty. Choose to make the words eczema and dermatitis mean the same to you

To further complicate matters, the classification of eczemas is a messy legacy from a time when little was known about the subject. Some are given names based on aetiology (e.g. irritant contact dermatitis and venous eczema). Others are based on the appearance of lesions (e.g. discoid eczema and hyperkeratotic eczema), while still others are classified by site (e.g. flexural eczema and hand eczema) or age (e.g. infantile eczema and senile eczema). These classifications invite overlap. However, until the causes of all eczemas are clear, both students and dermatologists are stuck with the time-honoured, yet muddled, nomenclature that we use here (Table 7.1).

A rational subdivision of dermatitis into exogenous (or contact) and endogenous (or constitutional) types has recently been formalized by the World Allergy Organization into the classification shown in Table 7.2. This has not yet caught on, but if it does we will be happy to use it in our next edition.

## Pathogenesis

Eczema has many causes, but the pathogenesis follows some common pathways (Fig. 7.1). One hallmark is the activated keratinocyte. It metabolizes rapidly and this is associated with increased

**Table 7.1** Eczema: a working classification.

*Mainly caused by exogenous (contact) factors*
Irritant
Allergic
Photodermatitis (Chapter 18)

*Other types of eczema*
Atopic
Seborrhoeic
Discoid (nummular)
Pompholyx
Gravitational (venous, stasis)
Asteatotic
Neurodermatitis
Juvenile plantar dermatosis
Napkin (diaper) dermatitis

**Table 7.2** Dermatitis: World Allergy Organization classification.

*Eczema*
Atopic
Non-atopic

*Contact dermatitis*
Allergic
Non-allergic (irritant)

*Other types of dermatitis*
e.g. nummular, photosensitive, seborrhoeic

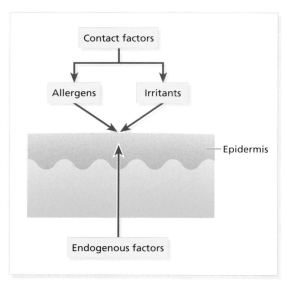

**Fig. 7.1** The causes of eczema.

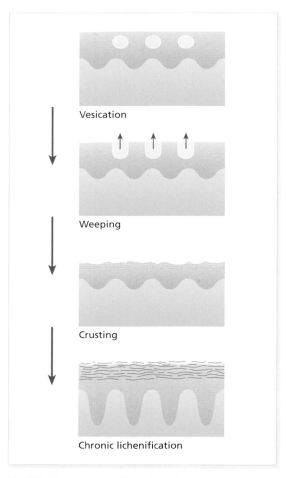

**Fig. 7.2** The sequence of histological events in eczema.

proliferation of basal cells and secretion of various cytokines. The epidermis contains large amounts of interleukin 1 (IL-1). This is released whenever the epidermis is damaged (e.g. by trauma, chemical irritation, and a type IV cell-mediated immune reaction; p. 30). IL-8 acts as a chemotactic factor for neutrophils. It is not surprising that neutrophil infiltration (exocytosis) of the epidermis is characteristic of most eczemas. γ-Interferon stimulates lymphocytes to perpetuate the perivascular lymphocytic infiltrate commonly observed in eczemas of all types. Hyperproliferation causes the epidermis to thicken (acanthosis) and to scale. Cytokines cause oedema, blistering and weeping, and especially itching.

## Histology (Fig. 7.2)

The clinical appearance of the different stages of eczema mirrors their histology. In the acute stage, oedema in the epidermis (spongiosis) progresses to the formation of intra-epidermal vesicles, which may coalesce into larger blisters or rupture. The chronic stages of eczema show less spongiosis and vesication but more thickening of the prickle cell layer (acanthosis) and horny layers (hyperkeratosis and parakeratosis). These changes are accompanied by a variable degree of vasodilatation and infiltration with lymphocytes.

**Fig. 7.4** Acute vesicular contact eczema of the hand.

**Fig. 7.3** Typical features of eczema with excoriations, fissuring, weeping/wetness and crusting.

**Fig. 7.5** Vesicular and crusted contact eczema of the face (cosmetic allergy).

## Clinical appearance

The different types of eczema have their own distinguishing marks, and these will be dealt with later; most share certain general features, which it is convenient to consider here. The absence of a sharp margin is a particularly important feature that separates eczema from most papulosquamous eruptions. Other distinguishing features are epithelial disruption (Fig. 7.3), shown by coalescing vesicles, bullae and oedematous papules on pink plaques, and a tendency for intense itching.

### Acute eczema

Acute eczema (Figs 7.4 and 7.5) is recognized by its:
- weeping and crusting;
- blistering – usually with vesicles but, in fierce cases, with large blisters;
- redness, papules and swelling – usually with an ill-defined border; and
- scaling.

### Chronic eczema

Chronic eczema may show all of the above changes but in general is:
- less vesicular and exudative;
- more scaly, pigmented and thickened;
- more likely to show lichenification (Fig. 7.6) – a dry leathery thickened state, with increased skin markings, secondary to repeated scratching or rubbing; and
- more likely to fissure.

**Fig. 7.6** Lichenification of the wrists – note also the increased skin markings on the palms ('atopic palms').

> **Learning points**
>
> - Eczema is like jazz; it is hard to define – but it should be easy to recognize if you bear in mind the physical signs listed above
> - If it does not itch, it is probably not eczema

## Complications

Heavy bacterial colonization is common in all types of eczema but overt infection is most troublesome in the seborrhoeic, nummular and atopic types. Local superimposed allergic reactions to medicaments can provoke dissemination, especially in gravitational eczema.

All severe forms of eczema have a huge effect on the quality of life. An itchy sleepless child can wreck family life. Eczema can interfere with work, sporting activities and sex lives. Jobs can be lost through it.

## Differential diagnosis

This falls into two halves. First, eczema has to be separated from other skin conditions that look like it. Table 7.3 plots a way through this maze. Always remember that eczemas are scaly, with poorly defined margins. They also exhibit features of epidermal disruption such as weeping, crust, excoriation, fissures and yellow scale (because of plasma coating the scale). Papulosquamous dermatoses, such as psoriasis or lichen planus, are sharply defined and show no signs of epidermal disruption.

Occasionally, a biopsy is helpful in confirming a diagnosis of eczema, but it will not determine the cause or type. Once the diagnosis of eczema becomes solid, look for clinical pointers towards an external cause. This determines both the need for investigations and the best line of treatment. Sometimes, an eruption will follow one of the well-known patterns of eczema, such as the way atopic eczema picks out the skin behind the knees, and a diagnosis can then be made readily enough. Often, however, this is not the case, and the history then becomes especially important.

A contact element is likely if:
- there is obvious contact with known irritants or allergens;
- the eruption clears when the patient goes on holiday, or at the weekends;
- the eczema is asymmetrical, or has a linear or rectilinear configuration; or
- the rash picks out the eyelids, external ear canals, hands and feet, the skin around stasis ulcers, or the perianal skin.

> **Learning point**
>
> Time spent thinking about contact factors may well help even those patients with the most blatantly 'constitutional' types of eczema

## Investigations

Each pattern of eczema needs a different line of inquiry.

### Exogenous eczema

Here the main decision is whether or not to undertake patch testing (p. 41) to confirm allergic contact dermatitis and to identify the allergens responsible for it. In patch testing, standardized non-irritating concentrations of common allergens are applied to the normal skin of the back. If the patient is allergic to the allergen, eczema will develop at the site of contact after 48–96 h. Patch testing with irritants is of no value in any type of eczema, but testing with suitably diluted allergens is essential in suspected allergic contact eczema. The technique is not easy. Its problems include separating irritant from allergic patch test reactions, and picking the right allergens to test. If legal issues depend on the results, testing should be carried out by a dermatologist who

**Table 7.3** Is the rash eczematous?

Atypical physical signs? Could
be eczema but consider other
erythematosquamous eruptions

Sharply marginated, strong colour, very scaly? Points of elbows and knees involved? — Yes → Likely to be psoriasis (Chapter 5) → Can be confused with seborrhoeic eczema and neurodermatitis on the scalp, with seborrhoeic eczema in the flexures, and discoid eczema on the limbs. Look for confirmatory nail and joint changes. Ask about family history

No

Itchy social contacts? Face spared? Burrows found? Genitals and nipples affected? — Yes → This is scabies (p. 262) → Ensure all contacts are treated adequately – whether itchy or not

No

Mouth lesions? Violaceous tinge? Shiny flat-topped papules? — Yes → Could be lichen planus (p. 72) → Also consider lichenoid drug eruptions

No

Annular lesions with active scaly edges? — Yes → Probably a fungal infection (Chapter 16) → More likely if the rash affects the groin, or is asymmetrical, perhaps affecting the palm of one hand only; and not doing well with topical steroids. Look at scales, cleared with potassium hydroxide, under a microscope or send scrapings to mycology laboratory. Check for contact with animals and for thickened toe nails

No

Localized to palms and soles? Obvious pustules? — Yes → Probably palmoplantar pustulosis (p. 58) → Expect poor response to most topical treatments

No

Unusually swollen; on the face? — Yes → Consider angioedema (p. 10) or erysipelas (p. 225) or allergic contact dermatitis (p. 86) → Needs rapid treatment with antihistamines and systemic steroids or antibiotics

No

Consider dermatitis herpetiformis, the various pityriases (rosea, versicolor and rubra pilaris) and drug eruptions (Chapter 25)

will have the standard equipment and a suitable selection of properly standardized allergens (see Fig. 3.8). Patch testing can be used to confirm a suspected allergy or, by the use of a battery of common sensitizers, to discover unsuspected allergies, which then have to be assessed in the light of the history and the clinical picture. A visit to the home or workplace may help with this.

Photopatch testing is more specialized and facilities are only available in a few centres. A chemical is applied to the skin for 24 h and then the site is irradiated with a suberythemal dose of ultraviolet irradiation; the patches are inspected for an eczematous reaction 48 h later.

## Other types of eczema

The only indication for patch testing here is when an added contact allergic element is suspected. This is most common in gravitational eczema; neomycin, framycetin, lanolin or preservative allergy can perpetuate the condition and even trigger dissemination.

Ironically, rubber gloves, so often used to protect eczematous hands, can themselves sensitize.

The role of prick testing in atopic eczema is discussed on p. 94.

The presence of a raised level of immunoglobulin E (IgE) antibodies is necessary to make a diagnosis of atopic eczema under the new World Allergy Organization criteria (Table 7.2). If the patient also has asthma or allergic rhinitis, the test results may be misleading even though they do tend to indicate an atopic state. Total and specific IgE antibodies are measured by a radio-allergosorbent test. Prick and RAST testing give similar results but many now prefer the more expensive RAST test as it carries no risk of anaphylaxis, is easier to perform and is less time consuming. Although not all children with eczema have elevated IgE levels, those who do are more likely to have eczema persisting into adult life, and are also more likely to develop asthma.

If the eczema is worsening despite treatment, or if there is much crusting, heavy bacterial colonization may be present. Opinions vary about the value of cultures for bacteria and *Candida*, but antibiotic treatment may be helpful. Scrapings for microscopical examination (p. 40) and culture for fungus will rule out tinea if there is clinical doubt – as in some cases of discoid eczema.

Finally, malabsorption should be considered in otherwise unexplained widespread pigmented atypical patterns of endogenous eczema.

## Treatment

### Acute weeping eczema

This does best with rest and liquid applications. Non-steroidal preparations are helpful and the techniques used will vary with the facilities available and the site of the lesions. In general practice, a simple and convenient way of dealing with weeping eczema of the hands or feet is to use thrice daily 10-min soaks in a cool 0.65% aluminium acetate solution (Formulary 1, p. 382) – saline or even tap water will do almost as well – each soaking being followed by a smear of a corticosteroid cream or lotion and the application of a non-stick dressing or cotton gloves. One reason for dropping the dilute potassium

permanganate solution that was once so popular is because it stains the skin and nails brown.

Wider areas on the trunk respond well to corticosteroid creams and lotions. However, traditional remedies such as exposure and frequent applications of calamine lotion, and the use of half-strength magenta paint for the flexures are also effective.

An experienced doctor or nurse can teach patients how to use wet dressings, and supervise this. The aluminium acetate solution, saline or water can be applied on cotton gauze, under a polythene covering, and changed twice daily. Details of wet wrap techniques are given below. Rest at home will also help.

### *Wet wrap dressings*

This is a labour-intensive but highly effective technique, of value in the treatment of troublesome atopic eczema in children. After a bath, a corticosteroid is applied to the skin and then covered with two layers of tubular dressing – the inner layer already soaked in warm water, the outer layer being applied dry. Cotton pyjamas or a T-shirt can be used to cover these, and the dressings can then be left in place for several hours. The corticosteroid may be one that is rapidly metabolized after systemic absorption such as a beclometasone diproprionate ointment diluted to 0.025% (available only in the UK). Alternatives include 1 or 2.5% hydrocortisone cream for children and 0.025 or 0.1% triamcinolone cream for adults. The bandages can be washed and reused. The evaporation of fluid from the bandages cools the skin and provides rapid relief of itching. With improvement, the frequency of the dressings can be cut down and a moisturizer can be substituted for the corticosteroid. Parents can be taught the technique by a trained nurse, who must follow up treatment closely. Parents easily learn how to modify the technique to suit the needs of their own child. Side-effects seem to be minimal.

### Subacute eczema

Steroid lotions or creams are the mainstay of treatment; their strength is determined by the severity of the attack. Yellow crusting and yellow scales suggest impetigo, and *Staphylococcus aureus* can be routinely isolated from most lesions. In high numbers, these bacteria can themselves aggravate eczemas or slow healing. Vioform, bacitracin, fusidic acid,mupirocin or neomycin (Formulary 1, p. 385) can be incorporated into the application if an infective element is present, but watch out for sensitization to neomycin, especially when treating gravitational eczema.

## Chronic eczema

This responds best to steroids in an ointment base, but is also often helped by non-steroid applications such as ichthammol and zinc cream or paste. Calcineurin inhibitors such as tacrolimus and pimecrolimus work well, although they lack the potency of strong topical corticosteroids.

The strength of the steroid is important (Fig. 7.7). Nothing stronger than 0.5 or 1% hydrocortisone ointment should be used on the face or in infancy. Even in adults one should be reluctant to prescribe more than 200 g/week of a mildly potent steroid, 50 g/week of a moderately potent or 30 g/week of a potent one for long periods. Very potent topical steroids should not be used long-term.

Bacterial superinfection may need systemic antibiotics but can often be controlled by the incorporation of antibiotics (e.g. fusidic acid, mupirocin, neomycin or chlortetracycline) or antiseptics (e.g. Vioform) into the steroid formulation. Many proprietary mixtures of this type are available in the UK. Chronic localized hyperkeratotic eczema of the palms or soles can be helped by salicylic acid (1–6% in emulsifying ointment) or stabilized urea preparations (Formulary 1, p. 381).

## Systemic treatment

Short courses of systemic steroids may occasionally be justified in extremely acute and severe eczema, particularly when the cause is known and already eliminated (e.g. allergic contact dermatitis from a plant such as poison ivy). However, prolonged systemic steroid treatment should be avoided in chronic cases, particularly in atopic eczema. Hydroxyzine, doxepin, trimeprazine and other antihistamines (Formulary 2, p. 398) may help at night. Systemic antibiotics may be needed in widespread bacterial superinfection. *Staphylococcus aureus* routinely colonizes all weeping eczemas, and most dry ones as well. Simply isolating it does not automatically prompt a prescription for an antibiotic, although if the density of organisms is high, usually manifest as extensive crusting, then systemic antibiotics can help.

## Common patterns of eczema

### Irritant contact dermatitis

This accounts for more than 80% of all cases of contact dermatitis, and for the vast majority of industrial cases. However, it can also occur in children (e.g. as a reaction to a bubble bath, play dough or lip-licking) (Fig. 7.8).

### *Cause*

Strong irritants elicit an acute reaction after brief contact and the diagnosis is then usually obvious.

**Fig. 7.7** Stretch marks following the use of too potent topical steroids to the groin.

**Fig. 7.8** Licking the lips as a nervous habit has caused this characteristic pattern of dry fissured irritant eczema.

**Fig. 7.9** Typical chronic hand eczema – irritants have played a part here.

Prolonged exposure, sometimes over years, is needed for weak irritants to cause dermatitis, usually of the hands and forearms (Fig. 7.9). Detergents, alkalis, solvents, cutting oils and abrasive dusts are common culprits. There is a wide range of susceptibility; those with very dry or fair skins are especially vulnerable. Past or present atopic dermatitis doubles the risk of irritant hand eczema developing.

### Course

The need to continue at work, or with housework, often stops the skin regaining its normal barrier function. Even under ideal circumstances this may take several months. All too often, therefore, irritant eczema, probably reversible in the early stages, becomes chronic.

### Complications

The condition may lead to loss of work.

### Differential diagnosis

It is often hard to differentiate irritant from allergic contact dermatitis, and from atopic eczema of the hands – the more so as atopic patients are especially prone to develop irritant eczema.

### Investigations

Patch testing with irritants is not helpful and may be misleading but patch testing to a battery of common allergens (Table 7.4) is worthwhile if an allergic element is suspected. Even if the results are negative, patch testing is not a waste of time and provides a valuable opportunity to educate patients about their condition.

### Treatment

Management is based upon avoidance of the irritants responsible for the condition, but often this is not possible and the best that can be achieved is reduced exposure by the use of protective gloves and clothing. The factory doctor or nurse can often advise here. Washing facilities at work should be good. Barrier creams seldom help established cases, and dirty hands should not be cleaned with harsh solvents.

Prevention is better than cure because, once started, irritant eczema can persist long after contact with offending substances has ceased, despite the vigorous use of emollients and topical corticosteroids. Vulnerable people should be advised to avoid jobs that carry an especially heavy exposure to skin irritants (see Table 7.5). If the right person can be placed in the right job, fewer trainee hairdressers and mechanics will find out the hard way that their skins are easily irritated. Moderately potent topical corticosteroids and emollients are valuable, but are secondary to the avoidance of irritants and protective measures.

## Allergic contact dermatitis

### Cause

The mechanism is that of delayed (type IV) hypersensitivity, which is dealt with in detail on p. 30. It has the following features.
- Previous contact is needed to induce allergy.
- It is specific to one chemical and its close relatives.
- After allergy has been established, all areas of skin will react to the allergen.
- Sensitization persists indefinitely.
- Desensitization is seldom possible.

## Allergens

In an ideal world, allergens would be replaced by less harmful substances, and some attempts are already being made to achieve this. A whole new industry has arisen around the need for predictive patch testing before new substances or cosmetics are let out into the community. Similarly, chrome allergy is less of a problem now in enlightened countries that insist on adding ferrous sulphate to cement to reduce its water-soluble chromate content. However, contact allergens will never be abolished completely and family doctors still need to know about the most common ones and where to find them (Table 7.4). It is not possible to guess which substances are likely to sensitize just by looking at their formulae. In fact, most allergens are relatively simple chemicals that have to bind

**Table 7.4** The allergens in our battery and what they mean.

| Allergen | Common sources | Comments |
| --- | --- | --- |
| *Metals* | | |
| The classic metal allergy for men is still to chrome, present in cement. In the past, more women than men have been allergic to nickel but the current fashion for men to have their ears and other parts of their body pierced is changing this | | |
| Chrome | Cement; chromium-plating processes; anti-rust paints; tattoos (green) and some leathers. Sensitization follows contact with chrome salts rather than chromium metal | A common problem for building site workers. In Scandinavia putting iron sulphate into cement has been shown to reduce its allergenicity by making the chrome salts insoluble |
| Nickel | Nickel-plated objects, especially cheap jewellery. Remember jean studs | The best way of becoming sensitive is to pierce your ears. Nickel is being taken out of some good costume jewellery. Stainless steel is relatively safe |
| Cobalt | A contaminant of nickel and occurs with it | Eruption similar to that of nickel allergy. The main allergen for those with metal on metal arthroplasties |
| *Cosmetics* | | |
| Despite attempts to design 'hypoallergenic' cosmetics, allergic reactions are still seen. The most common culprits are fragrances, followed by preservatives, dyes and lanolin | | |
| Fragrance mix | An infinite variety of cosmetics, sprays and toiletries | Any perfume will contain many ingredients. This convenient mix picks up some 80% of perfume allergies. Some perfume-allergic subjects also react to balsam of Peru, tars or colophony |
| Balsam of Peru | Used in some scented cosmetics. Also in some spices and suppositories (e.g. Anusol) | May indicate allergy to perfumes also. Can cross-react with colophony, orange peel, cinnamon and benzyl benzoate |
| Paraphenylene diamine (PPD) | Dark dyes for hair and clothing | Few heed the manufacturer's warning to patch test themselves before dyeing their hair. May cross-react with other chemicals containing the 'para' group (e.g. some local anaesthetics, sulphonamides or para-aminobenzoic acid, in some sunscreens) |
| Wool alcohols | Anything with lanolin in it | Common cause of reactions to cosmetics and topical medicaments. The newer purified lanolins cause fewer problems |
| Cetosteryl alcohol | Emollient, and base for many cosmetics | Taking over now as a vehicle from lanolin |

**Table 7.4** (*cont'd*)

| Allergen | Common sources | Comments |
|---|---|---|
| *Preservatives and biocides* No one likes rancid cosmetics or smelly cutting oils. Biocides are hidden in many materials to stop this sort of thing from happening | | |
| Formaldehyde | Used as a preservative in some shampoos and cosmetics. Also in pathology laboratories and white shoes | Many pathologists are allergic to it. Quaternium 15 (see below) releases formaldehyde as do some formaldehyde resins |
| Parabens-mix | Preservatives in a wide variety of creams and lotions, both medical and cosmetic | Common cause of allergy in those who react to a number of seemingly unrelated creams |
| Chlorocresol | Common preservative | Cross-reacts with chloroxylenol – a popular antiseptic |
| Kathon | Preservative in many cosmetics, shampoos, soaps and sunscreens | Also found in some odd places such as moist toilet papers, and washing-up liquids |
| Quaternium 15 | Preservative in many topical medicaments and cosmetics | Releases formaldehyde and may cross-react with it |
| Imidazolidinyl urea | Common ingredient of moisturizers and cosmetics | Cosmetic allergy |
| Other biocides | In glues, paints, cutting oils, etc. | Responsible for some cases of occupational dermatitis |
| *Medicaments* These may share allergens, such as preservatives and lanolin, with cosmetics (see above). In addition the active ingredients can sensitize, especially when applied long term to venous ulcers, pruritus ani, eczema or otitis externa | | |
| Neomycin | Popular topical antibiotic. Safe in short bursts (e.g. for impetigo and cuts) | Common sensitizer in those with leg ulcers. Simply swapping to another antibiotic may not always help as neomycin cross-reacts with framycetin and gentamicin |
| Quinoline mix | Used as an antiseptic in creams, often in combination with a corticosteroid | Its aliases include Vioform and chinoform |
| Ethylenediamine dihydrochloride | Stabilizer in some topical steroid mixtures (e.g. Mycolog and the alleged active ingredient in fat removal creams). A component in aminophylline. A hardener for epoxy resin | Cross-reacts with some antihistamines (e.g. hydroxyzine) |
| Benzocaine | A local anaesthetic which lurks in some topical applications (e.g. for piles and sunburn) | Dermatologists seldom recommend using these preparations – they have seen too many reactions |
| Tixocortol pivalate | Topical steroid | A marker for allergy to various topical steroids. Hydrocortisone allergy exists. Think of this when steroid applications seem to be making things worse |
| Budesonide | Topical steroid | Testing with both tixocortol pivalate and budesonide will detect 95% of topical steroid allergies |

**Table 7.4** (*cont'd*)

| Allergen | Common sources | Comments |
| --- | --- | --- |

*Rubber*
Rubber itself is often not the problem but it has to be converted from soft latex (p. 106) to usable rubber by adding vulcanizers to make it harder, accelerators to speed up vulcanization, and antioxidants to stop it perishing in the air. These additives are allergens

| Allergen | Common sources | Comments |
| --- | --- | --- |
| Mercapto-mix | Chemicals used to harden rubber | Diagnosis is often obvious, sometimes less so. Remember shoe soles, rubber bands and golf club grips |
| Thiuram-mix | Another set of rubber accelerators | Common culprit in rubber glove allergy |
| Black rubber mix | All black heavy-duty rubber (e.g. tyres, rubber boots, squash balls) | These are paraphenylene diamine derivatives, cross-reacting with PPD dyes (see above) |
| Carba mix | Mainly in rubber gloves | Patch testing with rubber chemicals occasionally sensitizes patients to them |

*Plants*
In the USA, the Rhus family (poison ivy and poison oak) are important allergens; in Europe, *Primula obconica* holds pride of place. Both cause severe reactions with streaky erythema and blistering. The Rhus antigen is such a potent sensitizer that patch testing with it is unwise. Other reaction patterns include a lichenified dermatitis of exposed areas from chrysanthemums, and a fingertip dermatitis from tulip bulbs

| Allergen | Common sources | Comments |
| --- | --- | --- |
| Primin | Allergen in *Primula obconica* | More reliable than patch testing to *Primula* leaves |
| Sesquiterpene lactone mix | Compositae plant allergy | Picks up chrysanth allergy. Flying pollen affects exposed parts and reactions can look like light sensitivity |

*Resins*
Common sensitizers such as epoxy resins can cause trouble both at home, as adhesives, and in industry

| Allergen | Common sources | Comments |
| --- | --- | --- |
| Epoxy resin | Common in 'two-component' adhesive mixtures (e.g. Araldite). Also used in electrical and plastics industries | 'Cured' resin does not sensitize. A few become allergic to the added hardener rather than to the resin itself |
| Paratertiary butylphenol formaldehyde resin | Used as an adhesive (e.g. in shoes, wrist watch straps, prostheses, hobbies) | Cross-reacts with formaldehyde. Depigmentation has been recorded |
| Colophony | Naturally occurring and found in pine sawdust. Used as an adhesive in sticking plasters and bandages. Also found in various varnishes, paper and rosin | The usual cause of sticking plaster allergy; also of dermatitis of the hands of violinists who handle rosin |

to protein to become 'complete' antigens. Their ability to sensitize varies – from substances that can do so after a single exposure (e.g. poison ivy) to those that need prolonged exposure (e.g. chrome – bricklayers take an average of 10 years to become allergic to it).

### Presentation and clinical course

The original site of the eruption gives a clue to the likely allergen but secondary spread may later obscure this. Easily recognizable patterns exist. Nickel allergy, for example, gives rise to eczema

**Fig. 7.10** Contact eczema caused by allergy to nickel in a jean stud.

under jewellery, bra clips and jean studs (Fig. 7.10). The lax skin of the eyelids and genitalia is especially likely to become oedematous. Possible allergens are numerous and to spot the less common ones in the environment needs specialist knowledge. Table 7.4 lists some common allergens and their distribution.

Allergic contact dermatitis should be suspected if:
**1** certain areas are involved (e.g. the eyelids, external auditory meati, hands [Fig. 7.11] or feet, and around gravitational ulcers);
**2** there is known contact with the allergens mentioned in Table 7.4; or
**3** the individual's work carries a high risk (e.g. hairdressing, working in a flower shop, or dentistry).

**Fig. 7.11** Dry fissured eczema of the fingertips caused by handling garlic.

### Investigations

Questioning should cover both occupational and domestic exposure to allergens. The indications for patch testing have already been discussed on p. 41. Techniques are constantly improving and dermatologists will have access to a battery of common allergens, suitably diluted in a bland vehicle. These are applied in aluminium cups held in position on the skin for 2 or 3 days by tape. Patch testing will often start with a standard series (battery) of allergens whose selection is based on local experience. Table 7.4 shows the battery we use and how it helps us with the most common types of contact allergy. This picks up some 80% of reactions. Extra series of relevant allergens will be used for problems such as hand eczema, leg ulcers and suspected cosmetic allergy, and for those in jobs like dentistry or hairdressing, which carry unusual risks. Some allergies are more common than others: in most centres, nickel tops the list, with a positive reaction in some 15% of those tested; fragrance allergy usually comes second. It is important to remember that positive reactions are not necessarily relevant to the patient's current skin problem; some are simply 'immunological scars' left behind by previous unrelated problems.

### Treatment

Topical corticosteroids give temporary relief, but far more important is avoidance of the relevant allergen. Reducing exposure is usually not enough; active steps have to be taken to avoid the allergen completely. Job changes are sometimes needed to achieve this. Even then, other factors may come into play (e.g. some believe that reactions to nickel can be kept going by nickel in the diet, released from cans or steel saucepans, as changes in diet and cooking utensils may rarely be helpful).

## Occupational dermatitis

The size of this problem has been underestimated in the past but, in both the UK and the USA, dermatitis is the second most common occupational disorder – second only to musculoskeletal injuries. In the UK, it is most common in younger women (Fig. 7.12), and

**Fig. 7.12** Assembly workers in an electronic factory – potential victims of industrial dermatitis.

**Table 7.5** Occupations with the highest rates of contact dermatitis in the UK.

| Men | Women |
| --- | --- |
| Chemical plant workers | Hairdressers |
| Machine tool setters and operatives | Biological scientists and laboratory workers |
| Coach and spray painters | Nurses |
| Metal workers | Catering workers |

then is often associated with wet work. The incidence in men rises with age, and in older workers it is often caused by contact with cutting oils. Table 7.5 lists the types of work particularly associated with high rates of contact dermatitis in the UK. The hands are affected in 80–90% of cases. Often several factors (constitutional, irritant and allergic) have combined to cause this, and a change of job does not always lead to a cure, particularly in long-established cases. In one large series, hand dermatitis was most common in caterers, metal workers, hairdressers, health care workers and mechanics.

## Atopic eczema

The word 'atopy' comes from the Greek (*a-topos* meaning 'without a place'). It was introduced by Coca and Cooke in 1923 and refers to the lack of a niche in the medical classifications then in use for the grouping of asthma, hay fever and eczema. Atopy is a state in which an exuberant production of IgE occurs as a response to common environmental allergens. Atopic subjects may, or may not, develop one or more of the atopic diseases such as asthma, hay fever, eczema and food allergies, and the prevalence of atopy has been steadily rising.

The prevalence of atopic eczema varies around the world from around 2% in parts of the developing world to 20% in children in western Europe, Australia and the USA. This prevalence has risen over the last 20 years, but now appears to be stabilizing. The reasons for this rise are not yet clear, but cannot be because of a change in the genetic pool in the population. Several environmental factors have been shown to reduce the risk of developing atopic disease. These include having many older siblings, growing up on a farm, having childhood measles and gut infections. The 'hygiene hypothesis' unites these, blaming the early use of antibiotics and a reduced exposure to orofaecal and other infections for preventing normal immunological maturation and shifting the circulating T lymphocytes of children destined to develop allergies from a Th1 to a Th2 response. However, this theory of a simple Th1–Th2 imbalance fails to explain the simultaneous rise in Th1-mediated diseases such as diabetes and inflammatory bowel disease. More recently it has been suggested that failure to develop regulatory T cells, which also develop as part of the response to infection, may explain the rise in incidence of allergic and autoimmune disease.

One promising but still experimental way of tackling these problems has emerged recently, involving the use of probiotics, which are cultures of potentially beneficial live gut commensal bacteria. Perinatal administration of a Gram-positive probiotic (*Lactobacillus* GG) to infants at risk of atopic disease significantly reduces the incidence of eczema for up to 4 years. Unfortunately, no such benefit is seen following administration to older children or adults.

### Inheritance

A strong genetic component is obvious, although affected children can be born to clinically normal parents. The concordance rates for atopic eczema in monozygotic and dizygotic twins are around 80%

and 22%, respectively, and atopic diseases tend to run true to type within each family. In some, most of the affected members will have eczema; in others, respiratory allergy will predominate. There is also a tendency for atopic diseases to be inherited more often from the mother than the father, and if both parents have atopic eczema, a child has a 75% chance of developing the disease. Environmental factors too are important and, not surprisingly, a simple genetic explanation has not yet been found in all patients.

Many patients are heterozygous or homozygous for a mutation of the filaggrin gene. New insights have come from the finding that a 50% reduction or complete absence of a critical structural protein in the skin due to highly prevalent genetic mutations is a major genetic factor in eczema development. Loss of function mutations in the filaggrin gene causes ichthyosis vulgaris (p. 47) but is also strongly predictive for atopic eczema. In European populations, about 10% of individuals carry mutations that completely deactivate one copy of the filaggrin gene; 1 in 400 make no filaggrin whatsoever. However, in a cohort of Irish paediatric cases of atopic eczema, more than 50% carried one or more filaggrin-deactivating mutations. There was also a very strong association with eczema-associated asthma. This is the most significant genetic factor yet identified in atopy and points to a skin barrier defect being an early initiating event or even a prerequisite for development of the disease.

Probably the inheritance of atopic eczema requires genes that predispose to the state of atopy itself, and others that determine whether it is asthma, eczema or hay fever that occurs. Genome-wide scans in different populations have suggested various linkages with atopic eczema but there has been a disappointing lack of overlap between findings in these studies, perhaps because of lack of a consistent phenotype and definition of atopic eczema. Evidence for linkage has been shown in at least two independent studies in regions on chromosomes 3q, 3p, 17q and 18q. Using the alternative candidate gene approach, changes in three genes have consistently been associated with atopic eczema. These are the genes for the Th2 cytokines IL-13, IL-4 receptor α in the cytokine gene cluster on chromosome 5q31-33 and *SPINK5*, the gene linked to Netherton's syndrome. In genome scans, several areas of overlap have been reported with psoriasis susceptibility loci, and there is an evolving understanding that eczema may not be primarily an allergic disorder with IgE-mediated sensitization and Th2-tilted immune dysregulation as major characteristics, but depends on aberrant genes controlling epidermal differentiation and skin defence.

### Presentation and course

Seventy-five per cent of cases of atopic eczema begin before the age of 6 months, and 80–90% before the age of 5 years. It affects at least 3% of infants, but the onset may be delayed until childhood or adult life. Some 60–70% of children with atopic eczema will clear by their early teens, although subsequent relapses are possible. The distribution and character of the lesions vary with age (Fig. 7.13) but a general dryness of the skin may persist throughout life.

● In infancy, atopic eczema tends to be vesicular and weeping. It often starts on the face (Fig. 7.14) with a non-specific distribution elsewhere, commonly sparing the napkin (diaper) area.

● In childhood, the eczema becomes leathery, dry and excoriated, affecting mainly the elbow and knee flexures (Fig. 7.15), wrists and ankles. A stubborn 'reverse' pattern affecting the extensor aspects of the limbs is also recognized.

● In adults, the distribution is as in childhood with a marked tendency towards lichenification and a more widespread but low-grade involvement of the trunk, face and hands. White dermographism (Fig. 7.16) is often striking, but not diagnostic of atopic eczema.

The cardinal feature of atopic eczema is itching, and scratching may account for most of the clinical picture. Affected children may sleep poorly, be hyperactive and sometimes manipulative, using the state of their eczema to get what they want from their parents. Luckily, the condition remits spontaneously before the age of 10 years in at least two-thirds of affected children, although it may come back at times of stress. Eczema and asthma may seesaw, so that while one improves the other may get worse.

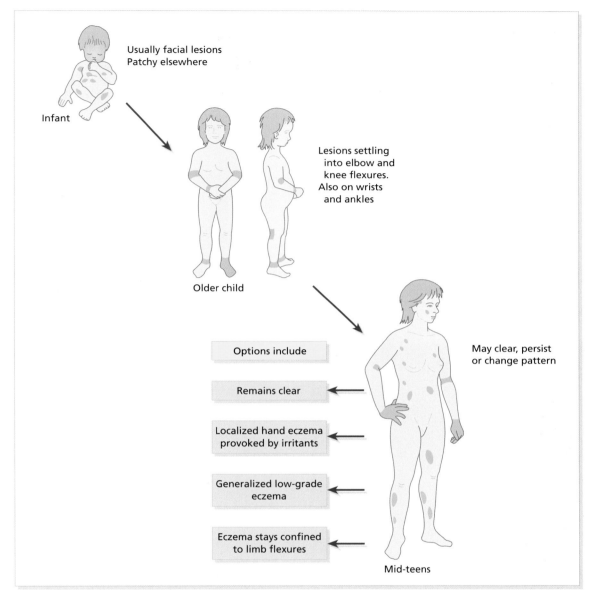

**Usually facial lesions
Patchy elsewhere**

Infant

**Lesions settling
into elbow and
knee flexures.
Also on wrists
and ankles**

Older child

Options include

Remains clear

Localized hand eczema
provoked by irritants

Generalized low-grade
eczema

Eczema stays confined
to limb flexures

May clear, persist
or change pattern

Mid-teens

**Fig. 7.13** The pattern of atopic eczema varies with age. It may clear at any stage.

## Diagnostic criteria

Diagnostic criteria shown to be accurate in hospital and community settings, and used for epidemiological research worldwide, are shown in Table 7.6.

## Complications

Overt bacterial infection is troublesome in many patients with atopic eczema (Fig. 7.17). They are also especially prone to viral infections, most dangerously

**Fig. 7.14** Atopic eczema in a child: worse around the eyes due to rubbing.

**Fig. 7.16** Trivial scratching has led to striking white dermographism.

**Table 7.6** Clinical diagnosis criteria for atopic eczema.

*Must have*:
A chronically itchy skin (or report of scratching or rubbing in a child)

*Plus three or more of the following*:
History of itchiness in skin creases such as folds of the elbows, behind the knees, fronts of ankles or around the neck (or the cheeks in children under 4 years)
History of asthma or hay fever (or history of atopic disease in a first-degree relative in children under 4 years)
General dry skin in the past year
Visible flexural eczema (or eczema affecting the cheeks or forehead and outer limbs in children under 4 years)
Onset in the first 2 years of life (not always diagnostic in children under 4 years)

**Fig. 7.15** Chronic excoriated atopic eczema behind the knees.

with widespread herpes simplex (eczema herpeticum; Fig. 7.18), but also with molluscum contagiosum and warts. Growth hormone levels rise during deep sleep (stages 3 and 4), but these stages may not be reached during the disturbed sleep of children with severe atopic eczema and as a consequence they may grow poorly. The absorption of topical steroids can contribute to this too.

## Investigations

Prick testing (see Fig. 3.10) demonstrates immediate-type hypersensitivity and is helpful in the investigation of asthma and hay fever. However, the value of prick testing in atopic eczema remains controversial. Often the finding of multiple positive reactions, and a high IgE level, does little more than support a

**Fig. 7.17** Facial eczema in a young boy worsening recently. Crusting on the cheeks and upper lip points to possible bacterial superinfection.

**Fig. 7.18** Infected facial eczema – herpes simplex was isolated.

doubtful clinical diagnosis. Treatment of eczema is the same whether atopic (IgE positive) or non-atopic.

### Treatment

Management here is complex and should include the following.

● Explanation, reassurance and encouragement. Educating patients and parents has been shown to improve long-term outcome. Many benefit from an introduction to the National Eczema Society in the UK or the National Eczema Association for Science and Education or the Inflammatory Skin Institute in the USA.

● The avoidance of exacerbating factors such as irritants (e.g. woollen clothing next to the skin) and later of careers such as hairdressing and engineering, which would inevitably lead to much exposure to irritants. Also avoid extremes of temperature, and contact with soaps and detergents.

● The judicious use of topical steroids and other applications as for other types of chronic eczema (p. 84; Table 7.7). A technique useful for extensive and troublesome eczema, particularly in children, is that of 'wet wrap' dressings (p. 84). A nurse who is expert in applying such dressings is an asset to any practice (Fig. 7.19).

Tacrolimus (Formulary 1, p. 387) is a macrolide immunosuppressant produced by a streptomycete. It is used systemically in kidney, liver and heart transplantation and is now available as an ointment for topical use in eczema unresponsive to conventional therapy. The 0.1% ointment is equivalent in strength to a moderate or potent topical corticosteroid but without the potential to cause skin atrophy. Long-term safety data are not yet available, and the drug is probably best used for treatment

**Table 7.7** Principles of treatment with topical corticosteroids.

Use the weakest steroid that controls the eczema effectively
Review their use regularly; check for local and systemic side-effects
In primary care, avoid using potent and very potent steroids for children with atopic eczema
Be wary of repeat prescriptions

**Fig. 7.19** Protective tubular gauze dressings being applied over a topical steroid ointment.

**Table 7.8** Winning ways with emollients.

Make sure they are applied when the skin is moist
Prescribe plenty (at least 500 g/week for the whole skin of an adult and 250 g/week for the whole skin of a child) and ensure they are used at least 3–4 times a day
For maximal effect, combine the use of creams, ointments, bath oils and emollient soap substitutes

of resistant eczema on sensitive sites, such as the face, or in patients requiring constant use of topical steroids. Local infection might be troublesome and concerns remain about the development of skin cancer or lymphoma in the long term. Patients should be advised to avoid excessive exposure to sunlight or UV lamps while using tacrolimus.

Pimecrolimus (Formulary 1, p. 387) is another topical immunosuppressant and a derivative of askamycin, but is less effective than potent topical corticosteroids. Its benefits over mild corticosteroids such as 1% hydrocortisone in the treatment of mild eczema remain unclear, and there are as yet no suitable trials comparing these agents.

● The regular use of bland emollients, either directly to the skin or in the form of oils to be used in the bath. Some of these can also be used as soap substitutes. A list of suitable preparations is given in Formulary 1 (p. 381). Some rules governing the use of emollients are given in Table 7.8.
● Those with an associated ichthyosis should generally use ointments rather than creams.
● The scratch–itch cycle can often be interrupted by occlusive bandaging (e.g. with a 1% ichthammol paste bandage). Nails should be kept short.
● Sedative antihistamines (e.g. trimeprazine or hydroxyzine; Formulary 2, p. 398) are of value if sleep is interrupted, but histamine release is not the main cause of the itching, so the newer non-sedative antihistamines help less than might be expected.
● Acute flares are often induced by the surface

proliferation of staphylococci, even without frank sepsis. A month's course of a systemic antibiotic (e.g. erythromycin) may then be helpful.
● Allergen avoidance: prick tests confirm that most patients with atopic eczema have immediate hypersensitivity responses to allergens in the faeces of house dust mites. Sometimes, but not always, measures to reduce contact with these allergens help eczema. These measures should include encasing the mattress in a dustproof bag, washing the duvets and pillows every 3 months at a temperature greater than 55°C, and thorough and regular vacuuming in the bedroom, where carpets should preferably be avoided.
● Do not keep pets to which there is obvious allergy.
● The role of diet in atopic eczema is even more debatable, and treatments based on changing the diet of patients are often disappointing. Similarly, it is not certain that the avoidance of dietary allergens (e.g. cow's milk and eggs) by a pregnant or lactating woman lessens the risk of her baby developing eczema. It may still be wise to breastfeed children at special risk for 6 months.

---

**Learning point**

Do not encourage cranky dieting for atopic eczema: it causes anxiety and seldom if ever does much good

---

● Routine inoculations are permissible during quiet phases of the eczema. However, children who are allergic to eggs should not be inoculated against measles, influenza and yellow fever.
● Those with active herpes simplex infections should be avoided to cut the risk of developing eczema herpeticum.
● In stubborn cases, UVB, UVA-1 (340–400 nm) or even PUVA therapy may be useful.
● Ciclosporin: severe and unresponsive cases may be helped by short courses under specialist

supervision (Formulary 2, p. 399). Short (6 week) courses may induce long-term remission in adults, but in children continuous therapy is usually needed.

• Azathioprine (Formulary 2, p. 399): patients with moderate to severe eczema can benefit from this purine analogue. Relatively common polymorphisms in the gene coding for thiopurinemethyltransferase (TPMT) lead to low or absent levels of this azathioprine metabolizing enzyme. TPMT levels must thus be checked before starting azathioprine to determine in whom the drug must be avoided because of absent activity, and in whom lower doses should be given because of low activity. Mycophenolate mofetil may be used as an alternative to Azathioprine, but trial data of this are limited.

• Chinese herbal remedies: properly conducted trials have given promising results but difficulties remain. The active ingredients within these complex mixtures of herbs have still not been identified. We have some hope for the future but currently do not prescribe these treatments for our patients.

## Seborrhoeic eczema

### *Presentation and course*

The term covers at least three common patterns of eczema, mainly affecting hairy areas, and often showing characteristic greasy yellowish scales. These patterns may merge together (Fig. 7.20).

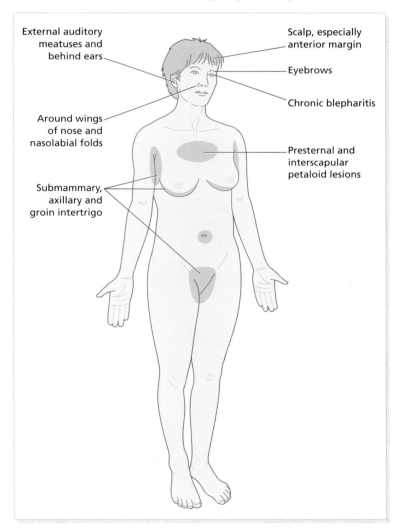

**Fig. 7.20** Areas most often affected by seborrhoeic eczema.

**Fig. 7.21** Dry scaly seborrhoeic eczema of the ear.

1 A red scaly or exudative eruption of the scalp, ears (Fig. 7.21), face (Fig. 7.22) and eyebrows. May be associated with chronic blepharitis and otitis externa.
2 Dry scaly 'petaloid' lesions of the presternal

**Fig. 7.22** Active seborrhoeic eczema of the face.

**Fig. 7.23** Typical presternal patch of seborrhoeic eczema.

(Fig. 7.23) and interscapular areas. There may also be extensive follicular papules or pustules on the trunk (seborrhoeic folliculitis or pityrosporum folliculitis).
3 Intertriginous lesions of the armpits, umbilicus or groins, or under spectacles or hearing aids.

### Cause

This condition is not obviously related to seborrhoea. It may run in some families, often affecting those with a tendency to dandruff. The success of treatments directed against yeasts has suggested that overgrowth of the pityrosporum yeast skin commensals plays an important part in the development of seborrhoeic eczema. This fits well with the fact that seborrhoeic eczema is often an early sign of AIDS, and that it responds to anti-yeast agents such as topical ketoconazole shampoo or cream.

Seborrhoeic eczema may affect infants (Fig. 7.24)

**Fig. 7.24** Infantile seborrhoeic eczema.

but is most common in adult males. In infants it clears quickly but in adults its course is unpredictable and may be chronic or recurrent. Some particularly severe cases have occurred in patients with AIDS (p. 246; Fig. 16.35).

### Complications

May be associated with furunculosis. In the intertriginous type, superadded *Candida* infection is common.

### Investigations

None are usually needed, but bear possible HIV infection and Parkinson's disease in mind.

### Treatment

Therapy is suppressive rather than curative and patients should be told this. Topical imidazoles (Formulary 1, p. 388) are perhaps the first line of treatment. Two per cent sulphur and 2% salicylic acid in aqueous cream is often helpful and avoids the problem of topical steroids. It may be used on the scalp overnight and removed by a medicated shampoo, which may contain ketoconazole, tar, salicylic acid, sulphur, zinc or selenium sulphide (Formulary 1, p. 382). For intertriginous lesions a weak steroid – antiseptic or steroid – antifungal combination (Formulary 1, p. 386) is often effective. For severe and unresponsive cases a short course of oral itraconazole may be helpful.

## Discoid (nummular) eczema

### Cause

No cause has been established but chronic stress is often present. A reaction to bacterial antigens has been suspected as the lesions often yield staphylococci on culture, and as steroid–antiseptic or steroid–antibiotic mixtures do better than either separately.

### Presentation and course

This common pattern of endogenous eczema classically affects the limbs of middle-aged males. The

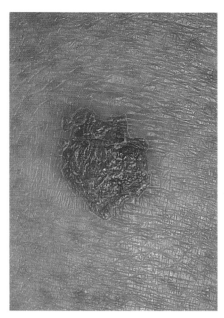

**Fig. 7.25** Vesicular and weeping patch of discoid eczema.

lesions are multiple, coin-shaped, vesicular or crusted, highly itchy plaques (Fig. 7.25), usually less than 5 cm across. The condition tends to persist for many months, and recurrences often appear at the site of previous plaques.

### Investigations

None are usually needed.

### Treatment

With topical steroid–antiseptic or steroid–antibiotic combinations (see above).

## Pompholyx

### Cause

The cause is usually unknown, but pompholyx is sometimes provoked by heat or emotional upsets. In subjects allergic to nickel, small amounts of nickel in food may trigger pompholyx. The vesicles are not plugged sweat ducts, and the term 'dyshidrotic eczema' should now be dropped.

**Fig. 7.26** Pompholyx vesicles along the side of a finger.

### Presentation and course

In this tiresome and sometimes very unpleasant form of eczema, recurrent bouts of vesicles or larger blisters appear on the palms, fingers (Fig. 7.26) and/or the soles of adults. Bouts lasting a few weeks recur at irregular intervals. Secondary infection and lymphangitis are a recurrent problem for some patients.

### Investigations

None are usually needed; sometimes a pompholyx-like eruption of the hands can follow acute tinea pedis (an 'ide reaction'). If this is suspected, scrapings or blister roofs, not from the hand lesions but from those on the feet, should be sent for mycological examination. Swabs from infected vesicles should be cultured for bacterial pathogens.

### Treatment

As for acute eczema of the hands and feet (p. 84). Appropriate antibiotics should be given for bacterial infections. Aluminium acetate or potassium permanganate soaks, followed by applications of a very potent corticosteroid cream, are often helpful.

## Gravitational (stasis) eczema

### Cause

Poor circulation, often but not always accompanied by obvious venous insufficiency.

**Fig. 7.27** Chronic gravitational eczema, perhaps with a superimposed contact dermatitis from a local medication.

### Presentation and course

A chronic patchy eczematous condition of the lower legs, sometimes accompanied by varicose veins, oedema and haemosiderin deposition (Fig. 7.27). When severe it may spread to the other leg or even become generalized.

### Complications

Patients often become sensitized to local antibiotic applications or to the preservatives in medicated bandages. The natural course and excoriations may lead to ulcer formation.

### Treatment

This should include the elimination of oedema by elevation, pressure bandages or diuretics. A moderately potent topical steroid may be helpful, but stronger ones are best avoided. Bland applications (e.g. Lassar's paste or zinc cream BNF, or medicated bandages; Formulary 1, p. 391) are useful but gravitational eczema is liable to persist, despite surgery to the underlying veins.

**Fig. 7.28** Asteatotic eczema with network of fine fissures in the stratum corneum.

## Asteatotic eczema

### Cause

Many who develop asteatotic eczema in old age will always have had a dry skin and a tendency to chap. Other contributory factors include the removal of surface lipids by over-washing, the low humidity of winter and central heating, the use of diuretics and hypothyroidism.

### Presentation and course

Often unrecognized, this common and itchy pattern of eczema occurs usually on the legs of elderly patients. Against a background of dry skin, a network of fine red superficial fissures creates a 'crazy paving' appearance (Fig. 7.28).

### Investigations

None are usually needed. Very extensive cases may be part of malabsorption syndromes, zinc deficiency or internal malignancy.

### Treatment

Can be cleared by the use of a mild or moderately potent topical steroid in a greasy base, and aqueous cream as a soap substitute for the area. Baths should be restricted until clearance. Thereafter, daily use of unmedicated emollients (Formulary 1, p. 381) usually prevents recurrence.

## Localized neurodermatitis (lichen simplex)

### Cause

The skin is damaged as a result of repeated rubbing or scratching, as a habit or in response to stress, but there is no underlying skin disorder.

### Presentation and course

Usually occurs as a single, fixed, itchy, lichenified plaque (Fig. 7.29). Favourite areas are the nape of the neck in women, the legs in men and the anogenital area in both sexes. Lesions may resolve with treatment but tend to recur either in the same place or elsewhere.

### Investigations

None are usually needed.

### Treatment

Potent topical steroids or occlusive bandaging, where feasible, help to break the scratch–itch cycle. Tranquillizers are often disappointing.

**Fig. 7.29** It is often hard to tell palmar lichen simplex from hyperkeratotic fissured eczema, as shown here.

**Fig. 7.30** The shiny skin and fissures of juvenile plantar dermatosis.

## Juvenile plantar dermatosis (Fig. 7.30)

### Cause

This condition is thought to be related to the impermeability of modern socks and shoe linings with subsequent sweat gland blockage, and so has been called the 'toxic sock syndrome'! Some feel the condition is a manifestation of atopy.

### Presentation and course

The skin of the weight-bearing areas of the feet, particularly the forefeet and undersides of the toes, becomes dry and shiny with deep painful fissures that make walking difficult. The toe webs are spared. Onset can be at any time after shoes are first worn, and even if untreated the condition clears in the early teens.

### Investigations

Much time has been wasted in patch testing and scraping for fungus.

### Treatment

The child should use a commercially available cork insole in all shoes, and wear cotton or wool socks. An emollient such as emulsifying ointment or 1% ichthammol paste, or an emollient containing lactic acid, is as good as a topical steroid.

## Napkin (diaper) dermatitis

### Cause

The most common type of napkin eruption is irritant in origin, and is aggravated by the use of waterproof plastic pants. The mixture of faecal enzymes and ammonia produced by urea-splitting bacteria, if allowed to remain in prolonged contact with the skin, leads to a severe reaction. The overgrowth of yeasts is another aggravating factor. The introduction of modern disposable napkins has helped to reduce the number of cases sent to our clinics.

### Presentation

The moist, often glazed and sore erythema affects the napkin area generally (Fig. 7.31), with the exception of the skin folds, which tend to be spared.

### Complications

Superinfection with *Candida albicans* is common, and this may lead to small erythematous papules

**Fig. 7.31** Irritant napkin erythema with a hint of sparing of the skin folds.

or vesicopustules appearing around the periphery of the main eruption.

### Differential diagnosis

The sparing of the folds helps to separate this condition from infantile seborrhoeic eczema and candidiasis.

### Treatment

It is never easy to keep this area clean and dry, but this is the basis of all treatment. Theoretically, the child should be allowed to be free of napkins as much as possible but this may lead to a messy nightmare. On both sides of the Atlantic disposable nappies (diapers) have largely replaced washable ones. The superabsorbent type is best and should be changed regularly, especially in the middle of the night. When towelling napkins are used they should be washed thoroughly and changed frequently. The area should be cleaned at each nappy change with aqueous cream and water. Protective ointments (e.g.

---

**Learning points**

- Do not accept 'eczema' as an adequate diagnosis: treatment hinges on establishing its cause and type
- Keep fluorinated steroids off the face of adults and off the skin of infants
- Monitor repeat prescriptions of topical steroids, keeping an eye on the amount used and their potency
- Do not promise that atopic eczema will be clear by any particular age: guesses are always wrong and the patients lose faith

---

zinc and castor oil ointment) or silicone protective ointments are often useful (Formulary 1, p. 382), as are topical imidazole preparations that stop yeast growth. Potent steroids should be avoided but combinations of hydrocortisone with antifungals or antiseptics (Formulary 1, p. 386) are often useful.

### Further reading

Ashcroft DM, Dimmock P, Garside R, Stein K & Williams HC. (2005) Efficacy and tolerability of topical pimecrolimus and tacrolimus in the treatment of atopic dermatitis: meta-analysis of randomised controlled trials. *British Medical Journal* **330**, 516–522.

Bieber T & Leung DYM. (2002) *Atopic Dermatitis*. Marcel Dekker, New York.

Brown S & Reynolds NJ. (2006) Atopic and non-atopic eczema. *British Medical Journal* **332**, 584–588.

Flohr C, Johansson SG, Wahlgren CF & Williams H. (2004) How atopic is atopic dermatitis? *Journal of Allergy and Clinical Immunology* **114**, 150–158.

Hanifin J & Saurat J-H. (2001) Understanding atopic dermatitis: pathophysiology and etiology. *Journal of the American Academy of Dermatology* **45** (Supplement), S67–68.

Hoffjan S & Epplen JT. (2005) The genetics of atopic dermatitis: recent findings and future options. *Journal of Molecular Medicine* **83**, 682–692.

Irvine AD. (2007) Fleshing out filaggrin phenotypes. *Journal of Investigative Dermatology*; **127**: 504–7.

Kanerva L, Elsner P, Wahlberg JE & Maibach HI. (2000) *Handbook of Occupational Dermatology*. Springer, Berlin.

Rycroft RJG, Menne T, Frosch P & Lepoittevin J-P. (2001) *Textbook of Contact Dermatitis*, 3rd edn. Springer, Berlin.

# 8 Reactive erythemas and vasculitis

Blood vessels can be affected by a variety of insults, both exogenous and endogenous. When this occurs, the epidermis remains unaffected, but the skin becomes red or pink and often oedematous. This is a reactive erythema. If the blood vessels are damaged more severely – as in vasculitis – purpura or larger areas of haemorrhage mask the erythematous colour.

## Urticaria (hives, 'nettle-rash')

Urticaria is a common reaction pattern in which pink, itchy or 'burning' swellings (wheals) can occur anywhere on the body. Individual wheals do not last longer than 24 h, but new ones may continue to appear for days, months or even years. Traditionally, urticaria is divided into acute and chronic forms, based on the duration of the disease rather than of individual wheals. Urticaria that persists for more than 6 weeks is classified as chronic. Most patients with chronic urticaria, other than those with an obvious physical cause, have what is often known as 'ordinary urticaria'.

### Cause

The signs and symptoms of urticaria are caused by mast cell degranulation, with release of histamine (Fig. 8.1). The mechanisms underlying this may be different but the end result, increased capillary permeability leading to transient leakage of fluid into the surrounding tissue and development of a wheal, is the same (Fig. 8.1). For example, up to half of those patients with chronic urticaria have circulating antibodies directed against the high affinity

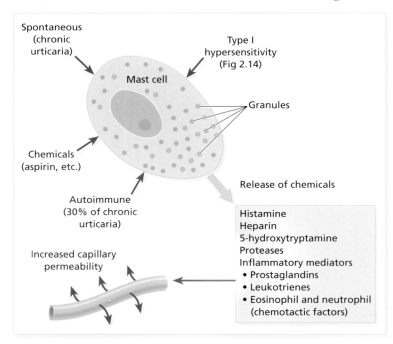

Spontaneous (chronic urticaria)

Type I hypersensitivity (Fig 2.14)

Mast cell

Granules

Chemicals (aspirin, etc.)

Autoimmune (30% of chronic urticaria)

Increased capillary permeability

Release of chemicals

Histamine
Heparin
5-hydroxytryptamine
Proteases
Inflammatory mediators
• Prostaglandins
• Leukotrienes
• Eosinophil and neutrophil (chemotactic factors)

**Fig. 8.1** Ways in which a mast cell can be degranulated and the ensuing reaction.

**Table 8.1** The main types of urticaria.

Physical
    cold
    solar
    heat
    cholinergic
    dermographism (immediate pressure urticaria)
    delayed pressure
Hypersensitivity
Autoimmune
Pharmacological
Contact

immunoglobulin E (IgE) receptor on mast cells whereas the reaction in others in this group may be caused by immediate IgE-mediated hypersensitivity (see Fig. 2.14), direct degranulation by a chemical or trauma, or complement activation.

## Classification

The various types of urticaria are listed in Table 8.1. They can often be identified by a careful history; laboratory tests are less useful. The duration of the wheals is an important pointer. Contact and physical urticarias, with the exception of delayed pressure urticaria, start shortly after the stimulus and go within an hour. Individual wheals of other forms resolve within 24 h.

## Physical urticarias

### Cold urticaria

Patients develop wheals in areas exposed to cold (e.g. on the face when cycling or freezing in a cold wind).

A useful test in the clinic is to reproduce the reaction by holding an ice cube, in a thin plastic bag to avoid wetting, against forearm skin. A few cases are associated with the presence of cryoglobulins, cold agglutinins or cryofibrinogens.

### Solar urticaria

Wheals occur within minutes of sun exposure. Some patients with solar urticaria have erythropoietic protoporphyria (p. 328); most have an IgE-mediated urticarial reaction to sunlight.

### Heat urticaria

In this condition wheals arise in areas after contact with hot objects or solutions.

### Cholinergic urticaria

Anxiety, heat, sexual excitement or strenuous exercise elicits this characteristic response. The vessels over-react to acetylcholine liberated from sympathetic nerves in the skin. Transient 2–5 mm follicular macules or papules resemble a blush or viral exanthem (Fig. 8.2). Some patients develop blotchy patches on their necks.

### Aquagenic urticaria

This resembles cholinergic urticaria and is precipitated by contact with water, irrespective of its temperature.

### Dermographism (Fig. 8.3)

This is the most common type of physical urticaria, the skin mast cells releasing extra histamine after rubbing or scratching. The linear wheals are therefore an exaggerated triple response of Lewis. They can readily be reproduced by rubbing the skin of the back lightly at different pressures, or by scratching the back with a fingernail or blunt object.

### Delayed pressure urticaria

Sustained pressure causes oedema of the underlying skin and subcutaneous tissue 3–6 h later. The

**Fig. 8.2** Typical small transient wheals of cholinergic urticaria – in this case triggered by exercise.

**Fig. 8.3** Dermographism: a frenzy of scratching by an already dermographic individual led to this dramatic appearance.

swelling may last up to 48 h and kinins or prostaglandins, rather than histamine, probably mediate it. It occurs particularly on the feet after walking, on the hands after clapping and on the buttocks after sitting. It can be disabling for manual labourers.

## Other types of urticaria

### Hypersensitivity urticaria

This common form of urticaria is caused by hypersensitivity, often an IgE-mediated (type I) allergic reaction (Chapter 2). Allergens may be encountered in 10 different ways (the 10 I's listed in Table 8.2).

**Table 8.2** The 10 I's of antigen encounter in hypersensitive urticaria.

| |
| --- |
| Ingestion |
| Inhalation |
| Instillation |
| Injection |
| Insertion |
| Insect bites |
| Infestations |
| Infection |
| Infusion |
| Inunction (contact) |

### Autoimmune urticaria

Some patients with chronic urticaria have an autoimmune disease with IgG antibodies to IgE or to FcIgE receptors on mast cells. Here the autoantibody acts as antigen to trigger mast cell degranulation.

### Pharmacological urticaria

This occurs when drugs cause mast cells to release histamine in a non-allergic manner (e.g. aspirin, non-steroidal anti-inflammatory drugs [NSAIDs], angiotensin-converting enzyme [ACE] inhibitors and morphine).

### Contact urticaria

This may be IgE mediated or caused by a pharmacological effect. The allergen is delivered to the mast cell from the skin surface rather than from the blood. Wheals occur most often around the mouth. Foods and food additives are the most common culprits but drugs, animal saliva, caterpillars, insect repellents and plants may cause the reaction. Recently, latex allergy has become a significant public health concern.

### Latex allergy

Possible reactions to the natural rubber latex of the *Hevea brasiliensis* tree include irritant dermatitis, contact allergic dermatitis (Chapter 7) and type I allergy (Chapter 2). Reactions associated with the latter include hypersensitivity urticaria (both by contact and by inhalation), hay fever, asthma, anaphylaxis and, rarely, death.

Medical latex gloves became universally popular after precautions were introduced to protect against HIV and hepatitis B infections. The demand for the gloves increased and this led to alterations in their manufacture and to a flood of high allergen gloves on the market. Cornstarch powder in these gloves bound to the latex proteins so that the allergen became airborne when the gloves were put on. Individuals at increased risk of latex allergy include health care workers, those undergoing multiple surgical procedures (e.g. spina bifida patients) and workers in mechanical, catering and electronic trades. Around 1–6% of the general population is believed to be sensitized to latex.

Latex reactions should be treated on their own merits (for urticaria see p. 109; for anaphylaxis see Fig. 25.5; for dermatitis see Chapter 7). Prevention of latex allergy is equally important. Non-latex (e.g. vinyl) gloves should be worn by those not handling infectious material (e.g. caterers) and, if latex gloves are chosen for those handling infectious material, then powder-free low allergen ones should be used.

## Presentation

Most types of urticaria share the sudden appearance of pink itchy wheals, which can come up anywhere on the skin surface (Figs 8.4 and 8.5). Each lasts for less than a day, and most disappear within a few hours. Lesions may enlarge rapidly and some resolve centrally to take up an annular shape. In an acute anaphylactic reaction, wheals may cover most of the skin surface. In contrast, in chronic urticaria only a few wheals may develop each day.

Angioedema is a variant of urticaria that primarily affects the subcutaneous tissues, so that the swelling is less demarcated and less red than an

**Fig. 8.4** A classic wheal.

**Fig. 8.5** Severe and acute urticaria caused by penicillin allergy.

**Fig. 8.6** Angioedema of the upper lip.

urticarial wheal. Angioedema most commonly occurs at junctions between skin and mucous membranes (e.g. peri-orbital, peri-oral and genital; Fig. 8.6). It may be associated with swelling of the tongue and laryngeal mucosa. It sometimes accompanies chronic urticaria and its causes may be the same.

## Course

The course of an urticarial reaction depends on its cause. If the urticaria is allergic, it will continue until the allergen is removed, tolerated or metabolized. Most such patients clear up within a day or two, even if the allergen is not identified. Urticaria may recur if the allergen is met again. At the other end of the scale, only half of patients attending hospital clinics with chronic urticaria and angioedema will be clear 5 years later. Those with urticarial lesions alone do better, half being clear after 6 months.

## Complications

Urticaria is normally uncomplicated, although its itch may be enough to interfere with sleep or daily activities and to lead to depression. In acute anaphylactic reactions, oedema of the larynx may lead to asphyxiation, and oedema of the tracheo-bronchial tree to asthma.

## Differential diagnosis

There are two aspects to the differential diagnosis of urticaria. The first is to tell urticaria from other eruptions that are not urticaria at all. The second is

**Fig. 8.7** A massive urticarial reaction to a wasp sting.

to define the type of urticaria (Table 8.1). Insect bites or stings (Fig. 8.7) and infestations commonly elicit urticarial responses, but these may have a central punctum and individual lesions may last longer than 24 h. Erythema multiforme can mimic an annular urticaria. A form of vasculitis (urticarial vasculitis; p. 114) may resemble urticaria, but individual lesions last for longer than 24 h, blanch incompletely and may leave bruising in their wake. Some bullous diseases (e.g. dermatitis herpetiformis, bullous pemphigoid and pemphigoid gestationis) begin as urticarial papules or plaques, but later bullae make the diagnosis obvious. In these patients, individual lesions last longer than 24 h, providing an additional tip-off for further studies (Chapter 9). On the face, erysipelas can be distinguished from angioedema by its sharp margin, redder colour and accompanying pyrexia. Hereditary angioedema (p. 110) must be distinguished from the angioedema accompanying urticaria as their treatments are completely different.

## Investigations

The investigations will depend upon the presentation and type of urticaria. Many of the physical urticarias can be reproduced by appropriate physical tests. It is important to remember that antihistamines should be stopped for at least 3 days before these are undertaken.

Almost invariably, more is learned from the history than from the laboratory. The history should include details of the events surrounding the onset of the eruption. A review of systems may uncover evidence of an underlying disease. Careful attention should be paid to drugs, remembering that self-prescribed

ones can also cause urticaria. Over-the-counter medications (e.g. aspirin and herbal remedies) and medications given by other routes (Table 8.2) can produce wheals.

If a patient has ordinary urticaria and its cause is not obvious, investigations are often deferred until it has persisted for a few weeks or months, and are based on the history. If no clues are found in the history, investigations can be confined to a complete blood count and erythrocyte sedimentation rate (ESR). An eosinophilia should lead to the exclusion of bullous and parasitic disease, and a raised ESR might suggest urticarial vasculitis or a systemic cause. If the urticaria continues for 2–3 months, the patient may be referred to a dermatologist for further evaluation. In general, the focus of such investigations will be on internal disorders associated with urticaria (Table 8.3) and on external allergens (Table 8.4). Patients frequently suspect a food allergy, but this is rarely found in chronic urticaria. Prick tests are unhelpful, although many patients with chronic urticaria are sure that their problems could be solved by intensive 'allergy tests', and ask repeatedly for them. Even after extensive evaluation and environmental change, the cause cannot always be found.

**Table 8.3** Some endogenous causes of urticaria.

Infection
    Viral (e.g. hepatitis, infectious mononucleosis, HIV infection during seroconversion)
    Bacterial
    Mycoplasma
Intestinal parasites
Connective tissue disorders
Hypereosinophilic syndrome (unexplained eosinophilia with multiple internal organ involvement, especially cardiac)
Hyperthyroidism
Cancer
Lymphomas

**Table 8.4** Some exogenous causes of urticaria.

Drugs, both topical and systemic
Preservatives in lotions (especially sorbic acid)
Foods and food additives
Bites
Inhalants
Pollens
Insect venoms
Animal dander

## Treatment

The ideal is to find a cause and then to eliminate it. In addition, aspirin – in any form – should be banned. The treatment for each type of urticaria is outlined in Table 8.5. In general, antihistamines are the mainstays of symptomatic treatment. Cetirizine 10 mg/day and loratadine 10 mg/day, both with half-lives of around 12 h, are useful. If necessary, these can be supplemented with shorter acting antihistamines (e.g. hydroxyzine 10–25 mg up to every 6 h; Formulary 2, p. 398, or acrivastine 8 mg three times daily). Alternatively, they can be combined with a longer acting antihistamine (e.g. chlorphenamine [chlorpheniramine] maleate 12 mg sustained-release tablets every 12 h) so that peaks and troughs are blunted, and histamine activity is blocked throughout the night. If the eruption is not controlled, the dose of hydroxyzine can often be increased and still tolerated. H2-blocking antihistamines (e.g. cimetidine) may add a slight benefit if used in conjunction with an H1 histamine antagonist. Chlorphenamine or diphenhydramine are often used during pregnancy because of their long record of safety, but cetirizine, loratadine and mizolastine should be avoided. Sympathomimetic agents can help urticaria, although the effects of adrenaline (epinephrine) are short lived. Pseudoephedrine (30 or 60 mg every 4 h) or terbutaline (2.5 mg every 8 h) can sometimes be useful adjuncts.

A tapering course of systemic corticosteroids may be used, but only when the cause is known and there are no contraindications, and certainly not as a panacea to control chronic urticaria or urticaria of unknown cause. Low doses of ciclosporin may be used for particularly severe cases. For the treatment of anaphylaxis see p. 362.

### Learning points

- The treatment of choice is to find the cause and eliminate it
- You can learn more about the cause from the history than from tests
- Most patients with hives clear up quickly even if the cause is not obvious
- Use antihistamines in relatively high doses
- Avoid aspirins and systemic steroids in chronic urticaria
- Do not promise patients that all will be solved by allergy tests
- Take respiratory tract blockage seriously

**Table 8.5** Some types of urticaria and their management.

| Type | Treatment |
| --- | --- |
| Cold urticaria | Avoid cold |
| | Protective clothing |
| | Antihistamines |
| Solar urticaria | Avoid sun exposure |
| | Protective clothing |
| | Sunscreens and sun blocks |
| | Beta-carotene |
| | Antihistamines |
| Cholinergic urticaria | Avoid heat |
| | Minimize anxiety |
| | Avoid excessive exercise |
| | Anticholinergics |
| | Antihistamines |
| | Tranquillizers |
| Dermographism | Avoid trauma |
| | Antihistamines |
| Hereditary angioedema | Avoid trauma |
| | Attenuated androgenic steroids as prophylaxis |
| | Tracheotomy may be necessary |
| Hypersensitivity urticarias | Remove cause |
| | Antihistamines (H1 + H2) |
| | Sympathomimetics |
| | Systemic steroids (rarely justified) |
| | Avoid aspirin-containing drugs |

## Hereditary angioedema

Recurrent attacks of abdominal pain and vomiting, or massive oedema of soft tissues, which may involve the larynx, characterize this autosomal dominant condition. Urticaria does not accompany the tissue swellings. Tooth extraction, cheek biting and other forms of trauma may precipitate an attack. A deficiency of an inhibitor to C1 esterase allows complement consumption to go unchecked so that vasoactive mediators are generated. To confirm the diagnosis, plasma complement C4 levels should be checked, and if low, functional serum C1 esterase inhibitor level measured.

This type of angioedema is controlled with maintenance anabolic steroids, and replacement C1 esterase inhibitor concentrate for acute episodes. Mechanical trauma should be avoided. Trachyotomy may be necessary in an acute attack.

## Erythema multiforme

### Cause

In erythema multiforme, the patient has usually reacted to an infection, often herpes simplex, or to a drug, but other factors have occasionally been implicated (Table 8.6).

### Presentation

The symptoms of an upper respiratory tract infection may precede the eruption. Typically, annular non-scaling plaques appear on the palms, soles,

**Table 8.6** Some causes of erythema multiforme.

Viral infections, especially:
  herpes simplex
  hepatitis A, B and C
  mycoplasma
  orf
Bacterial infections
Fungal infections
  coccidioidomycosis
Parasitic infestations
Drugs
Pregnancy
Malignancy, or its treatment with radiotherapy
Idiopathic

**Fig. 8.8** Erythema multiforme: bullous and target lesions occurring in a favourite site.

forearms and legs. They may be slightly more purple than the wheals of ordinary urticaria. Individual lesions enlarge but clear centrally. A new lesion may begin at the same site as the original one, so that the two concentric plaques look like a target (Fig. 8.8). Some lesions blister. The Stevens–Johnson syndrome is a severe variant of erythema multiforme associated with fever and mucous membrane lesions. The oral mucosa, lips and bulbar conjunctivae are most commonly affected, but the nares, penis, vagina, pharynx, larynx and tracheo-bronchial tree may also be involved (Fig. 8.9). This merges with toxic epidermal necrolysis (p. 127), where the whole skin is affected.

### Course

Crops of new lesions appear for 1–2 weeks, or until the responsible drug or other factor has been eliminated. Individual lesions last several days, and this differentiates them from the more fleeting lesions of an annular urticaria. The site of resolved lesions is marked transiently by grey or brown patches, particularly in pigmented individuals. A recurrent

**Fig. 8.9** Stevens–Johnson type of erythema multiforme. The eyelids were also severely involved.

variant of erythema multiforme exists, characterized by repeated attacks; this merges with a rare form in which lesions continue to develop over a prolonged period, even for years.

## Complications

There are usually no complications. However, severe lesions in the tracheo-bronchial tree of patients with Stevens–Johnson syndrome can lead to asphyxia, and ulcers of the bulbar conjunctiva to blindness. Corneal ulcers, anterior uveitis and panophthalmitis may also occur. Genital ulcers can cause urinary retention, phimosis or vaginal stricture after they heal.

## Differential diagnosis

Erythema multiforme can mimic the annular variant of urticaria as described above. However, target lesions are pathognomonic of erythema multiforme. Its acral distribution, the way individual lesions last for more than 24 h, their purple colour and the involvement of mucous membranes all help to identify erythema multiforme. Other bullous disorders may enter the differential diagnosis (Chapter 9). Rings of granuloma annulare (p. 325) take weeks or months to develop.

## Investigations

The histology of erythema multiforme is distinctive. Its main features are epidermal necrosis and dermal changes, consisting of endothelial swelling, a mixed lymphohistiocytic perivascular infiltrate and papillary dermal oedema. The abnormalities may be predominantly epidermal or dermal, or a combination of both; they probably depend on the age of the lesion biopsied.

Most investigations are directed towards identifying a cause. A careful history helps rule out a drug reaction. A polymerase chain reaction (PCR) test, Tzanck smear (p. 41) or culture of suspicious prodromal vesicles may identify a precipitating herpes simplex infection, which usually is almost healed by the time the erythema multiforme erupts. A chest X-ray and serological tests should identify mycoplasmal pneumonia. A search for other infectious agents, neoplasia, endocrine causes or collagen disease is sometimes necessary, especially when the course is prolonged or recurrent. About 50% of cases have no demonstrable provoking factor.

## Treatment

The best treatment for erythema multiforme is to identify and remove its cause. In mild cases, only symptomatic treatment is needed and this includes the use of antihistamines.

The Stevens–Johnson syndrome, however, may demand immediate consultation between dermatologists and specialists in other fields such as ophthalmology, urology and infectious diseases, depending on the particular case. This is because affected mucous membranes may scar, and affected skin may slough. Intravenous infusions of human $\gamma$-globulin seem to be worthwhile. The use of systemic steroids to abort the Stevens–Johnson syndrome is debatable, but many believe that a short course (e.g. prednisolone 80 mg/day in divided doses in an adult) helps. However, the dose should be tapered rapidly or stopped because prolonged treatment in the Stevens–Johnson syndrome has been linked, controversially, with a high complication rate. They probably should not be used at all for patients with full-blown toxic epidermal necrolysis (p. 127). Ciclosporin may be a better choice if infection, as a cause or an effect, is ruled out. Good nursing care with attention to the mouth and eyes is essential. The prevention of secondary infection, maintenance of a patent airway, good nutrition, and proper fluid and electrolyte balance are important.

Herpes simplex infections should be suspected in recurrent or continuous erythema multiforme of otherwise unknown cause. Treatment with oral valaciclovir 500 mg once or twice daily or famciclovir 250 mg once or twice daily (Formulary 2, p. 397) may prevent attacks, both of herpes simplex and of the recurrent erythema multiforme that follows it.

---

**Learning points**

- Look for target lesions and involvement of the palms
- Herpes simplex infection is the most common provoking factor of recurrent erythema multiforme, but do not forget drugs
- Stevens–Johnson syndrome calls for fast action and a team approach to therapy

---

## Erythema nodosum

Erythema nodosum is an inflammation of the subcutaneous fat (a panniculitis). It is an immunological reaction, elicited by various bacterial, viral and fungal infections, malignant disorders, drugs and by a variety of other causes (Table 8.7).

### Presentation

The characteristic lesion is a tender red nodule developing alone or in groups on the legs and forearms or, rarely, on other areas such as the thighs, face, breasts or other areas where there is fat (Fig. 8.10). Some patients also have painful joints and fever.

**Table 8.7** Some causes of erythema nodosum.

| |
| --- |
| Infections |
|   Bacteria (e.g. streptococci, tuberculosis, brucellosis, leprosy, yersinia) |
|   Viruses |
|   Mycoplasma |
|   Rickettsia |
|   Chlamydia |
|   Fungi (especially coccidioidomycosis) |
| Drugs (e.g. sulphonamides, oral contraceptive agents) |
| Systemic disease (e.g. sarcoidosis, ulcerative colitis, Crohn's disease, Behçet's disease) |
| Pregnancy |

**Fig. 8.10** Erythema nodosum: large painful dusky plaques on the shins. Always investigate this important reaction pattern (see text).

### Course

Lesions usually resolve in 6–8 weeks. In the interim, lesions may enlarge and new ones may occur at other sites. Like other reactive erythemas, erythema nodosum may persist if its cause is not removed. Persisting erythema nodosum is sometimes called nodular vasculitis.

### Complications

The nodules may be so tender that walking is difficult. Erythema nodosum leprosum occurs when lepromatous leprosy patients establish cell-mediated immunity to *Mycobacterium leprae*. These patients have severe malaise, arthralgia and fever.

### Differential diagnosis

The differential diagnosis of a single tender red nodule is extensive and includes trauma, infection (early cellulitis or abscess) and phlebitis.

When lesions are multiple or bilateral, infection becomes less likely unless the lesions are developing in a sporotrichoid manner (p. 233). Other causes of a nodular panniculitis, which may appear like erythema nodosum, include panniculitis from pancreatitis, cold, trauma, the injection of drugs or other foreign substances, withdrawal from systemic steroids, lupus erythematosus, superficial migratory thrombophlebitis, polyarteritis nodosa and a deficiency of $\alpha_1$-antitrypsin.

## Investigations

Erythema nodosum demands a careful history, physical examination, a chest X-ray, throat culture for *Streptococcus*, a Mantoux test and an antistreptolysin-O (ASO) titre. Serological testing for deep fungal infections such as coccidioidomycosis should be obtained, at least in endemic areas. If the results are normal, and there are no symptoms or physical findings to suggest other causes, extensive investigations can be deferred because the disease will usually resolve.

## Treatment

The ideal treatment for erythema nodosum is to identify and eliminate its cause if possible. For example, if culture or an ASO test confirms a streptococcal infection, a suitable antibiotic should be recommended. Bed rest and leg elevation are also an important part of treatment. NSAIDs such as aspirin, indometacin or ibuprofen may be helpful. Systemic steroids are usually not needed. For reasons that are not clear, potassium iodide in a dosage of 400–900 mg/day can help, but should not be used for longer than 6 months.

## Acute febrile neutrophilic dermatosis (Sweet's syndrome)

Red, indurated, often painful plaques (Fig. 21.2), nodules or tumours erupt suddenly and dramatically, sometimes being associated with fever, malaise, myalgias and ocular signs. Coalescence of areas of more and less acute inflammation may lead to curious irregularities of the surface resembling a mountain range. Neutrophils gather in the dermis and subcutaneous fat to cause this, and in peripheral blood counts these cells are frequently elevated. The ESR is often raised and involvement of other organs

can occur. Acute myelocytic leukaemia is one cause. Other malignancies, infections, inflammatory bowel disease, pregnancy, treatments with granulocyte–macrophage colony-stimulating factor (GM-CSF) and Behçet's disease are among other associated causes. Sometimes, a precipitating cause cannot be found. The differential diagnosis is large, the list of causes is long, the disease may be severe and treatments can be tricky. Refer these patients to a dermatologist.

## Vasculitis

Whereas the reactive erythemas are associated with some inflammation around superficial or deep blood vessels, the term vasculitis is reserved for those showing inflammation within the vessel wall, with endothelial cell swelling, necrosis or fibrinoid change. The clinical manifestations depend upon the size of the blood vessel affected.

## Leucocytoclastic (small vessel) vasculitis (allergic or hypersensitivity vasculitis, anaphylactoid purpura)

### Cause

Immune complexes may lodge in the walls of blood vessels, activate complement and attract polymorphonuclear leucocytes (Fig. 8.11). Enzymes released from these can degrade the vessel wall. Antigens in these immune complexes include drugs, autoantigens and infectious agents such as bacteria.

### Presentation

The most common presentation of vasculitis is painful palpable purpura (Fig. 8.12). Crops of 3–6 mm purpuric papules arise in dependent areas (the forearms and legs in ambulatory patients, or on the buttocks and flanks in bedridden ones; Fig. 8.13). Some have a small livid or black centre, caused by necrosis of the tissue overlying the affected blood vessel.

Henoch–Schönlein purpura is a small-vessel vasculitis associated with palpable purpura, arthritis and abdominal pain, and is often preceded by an upper respiratory tract infection. Children are most commonly affected.

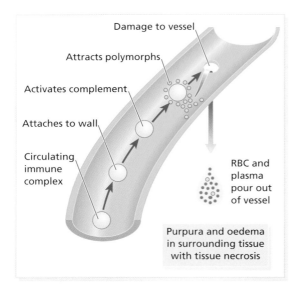

**Fig. 8.11** Pathogenesis of vasculitis.

**Fig. 8.12** The three P's of small-vessel vasculitis.

**Fig. 8.13** The palpable purpuric lesions of small-vessel vasculitis.

**Fig. 8.14** Urticarial vasculitis: a combination of urticaria and bruising.

Urticarial vasculitis is a small-vessel vasculitis characterized by urticaria-like lesions which last for longer than 24 h, sometimes leaving bruising and then pigmentation (haemosiderin) at the site of previous lesions (Fig. 8.14). There may be foci of purpura in the wheals, low serum complement levels, elevated erythrocyte sedimentation rates and sometimes angioedema. General features include malaise and arthralgia.

## Course

The course of the vasculitis varies with its cause, its extent, the size of blood vessel affected and the involvement of other organs.

## Complications

Vasculitis may simply be cutaneous; alternatively, it may be systemic and then other organs will be damaged, including the kidney, central nervous system, gastrointestinal tract and lungs.

### Differential diagnosis

Small-vessel vasculitis has to be separated from other causes of purpura (p. 159) such as abnormalities of the clotting system and sepsis (with or without vasculitis). Vasculitic purpuras are raised (palpable). Occasionally, the vasculitis may look like urticaria if its purpuric element is not marked. Blanching such an urticarial papule with a glass slide (diascopy) may reveal subtle residual purpura.

### Investigations

Investigations should be directed toward identifying the cause and detecting internal involvement. Questioning may indicate infections; myalgias, abdominal pain, claudication, mental confusion and mononeuritis may indicate systemic involvement. A physical examination, chest X-ray, ESR and biochemical tests monitoring the function of various organs are indicated. However, the most important test is urine analysis, checking for proteinuria and haematuria, because vasculitis can affect the kidney subtly and so lead to renal insufficiency.

Skin biopsy will confirm the diagnosis of small-vessel vasculitis. The finding of circulating immune complexes, or a lowered level of total complement (CH50) or C4, will implicate immune complexes as its cause. Tests for paraproteins, hepatitis viruses, cryoglobulins, rheumatoid factor and antinuclear antibodies may also be needed.

Direct immunofluorescence can be used to identify immune complexes in blood vessel walls, but is seldom performed because of false positive and false negative results, as inflammation may destroy the complexes in a true vasculitis and induce non-specific deposition in other diseases. Henoch–Schönlein vasculitis is confirmed if IgA deposits are found in the blood vessels of a patient with the clinical triad of palpable purpura, arthritis and abdominal pain.

### Treatment

The treatment of choice is to identify the cause and eliminate it. In addition, antihistamines and bed rest sometimes help. Colchicine 0.6 mg twice daily or dapsone 100 mg/day may be worth a trial, but require monitoring for side-effects (Formulary 2, p. 405). Patients whose vasculitis is damaging the kidneys or other internal organs may need systemic corticosteroids or immunosuppressive agents such as cyclophosphamide.

> **Learning point**
>
> Leucocytoclastic vasculitis of the skin may indicate that the kidneys are being damaged. Be sure to check the urine

## Polyarteritis nodosa

### Cause

This necrotizing vasculitis of large arteries causes skin nodules, infarctive ulcers and peripheral gangrene. Immune complexes may initiate this vasculitis, and sometimes contain hepatitis B or C virus or antigen. Other known causes are adulterated drugs, B-cell lymphomas and immunotherapy.

### Presentation

Tender subcutaneous nodules appear along the line of arteries. The skin over them may ulcerate or develop stellate patches of purpura and necrosis. Splinter haemorrhages and a peculiar net-like vascular pattern (livedo reticularis) aid the clinical diagnosis. The disorder may be of the skin only (cutaneous polyarteritis nodosa), or also affect the kidneys, gut, heart muscle, nerves and joints (Fig. 8.15). Patients may be febrile, lose weight and feel pain in the muscles, joints or abdomen. Some develop peripheral neuropathy, hypertension and ischaemic heart disease. Renal involvement, with or without hypertension, is common.

### Course

Untreated, systemic polyarteritis nodosa becomes chronic. Death, often from renal disease, is common, even in treated patients.

### Differential diagnosis

Embolism, panniculitis and infarctions can cause a similar clinical picture. Wegener's granulomatosis,

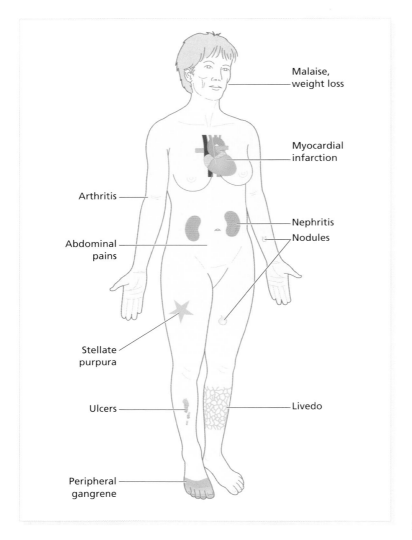

Malaise, weight loss

Myocardial infarction

Arthritis

Nephritis

Nodules

Abdominal pains

Stellate purpura

Ulcers

Livedo

Peripheral gangrene

**Fig. 8.15** Clinical features of polyarteritis nodosa.

allergic granulomatosis, temporal arteritis, and the vasculitis that accompanies systemic lupus erythematosus and rheumatoid arthritis should be considered. Occasionally, pyoderma gangrenosum can mimic polyarteritis nodosa.

## Investigations

The laboratory findings are non-specific. An elevated ESR, neutrophil count, and γ-globulin level are common. Investigations for cryoglobulins, rheumatoid factor, antinuclear antibody, antineutrophil cytoplasmic antibodies, hepatitis C antibodies and hepatitis B surface antigen are worthwhile, as are checks for disease in the kidneys, heart, liver and gut. Low levels of complement C4 suggest active disease. The use of a biopsy to confirm the diagnosis of large-vessel vasculitis is not always easy as the arterial involvement may be segmental, and surgery itself difficult. Histological confirmation is most likely when biopsies are from a fresh lesion. Affected vessels show aneurysmal dilatation or necrosis, fibrinoid changes in their walls, and an intense neutrophilic infiltrate around and even in the vessel wall.

## Treatment

Systemic steroids and cyclophosphamide improve the chances of survival. Low-dose systemic steroids alone or methotrexate are usually sufficient for the purely cutaneous form.

## Wegener's granulomatosis

In this granulomatous vasculitis of unknown cause, fever, weight loss and fatigue accompany naso-respiratory symptoms such as rhinitis, hearing loss or sinusitis. Only half of the patients have skin lesions, usually symmetrical ulcers or papules on the extremities. Other organs can be affected, including the eye, joints, heart, nerves, lung and kidney. Antineutrophil antibodies are present in most cases and are a useful but non-specific diagnostic marker. Cyclophosphamide is the treatment of choice, used alone or with systemic steroids.

## Further reading

Carlson JA, Ng BT & Chen KR. (2005) Cutaneous vasculitis update: diagnostic criteria, classification, epidemiology, etiology, pathogenesis, evaluation and prognosis. *American Journal of Dermatopathology* **27**, 504–528.

Carlson JA, Cavaliere LF & Grant-Kels JM. (2006) Cutaneous vasculitis: diagnosis and management. *Clinics in Dermatology* **24**, 414–429.

Cousin F, Philips K, Favier B, Bienvenu J & Nicolas JF. (2001) Drug-induced urticaria. *European Journal of Dermatology* **11**, 181–187.

Cuellar ML & Espinoza LR. (2000) Laboratory testing in the evaluation and diagnosis of vasculitis. *Current Rheumatology Reports* **2**, 417–422.

Dibbern DA. (2006) Urticaria: selected highlights and recent advances. *Medical Clinics of North America* **90**, 187–209.

Grattan C, Powell S & Humphreys F. (2001) Management and diagnostic guidelines for urticaria and angio-oedema. *British Journal of Dermatology* **144**, 708–714.

Greaves MW. (2005) Antihistamines in dermatology. *Skin Pharmacology and Physiology* **18**, 220–209.

Joint Task Force on Practice Parameters (2000) The diagnosis and management of urticaria: a practice parameter. I. Acute urticaria/angioedema. II. Chronic urticaria/angioedema. *Annals of Allergy, Asthma and Immunology* **85**, 521–544.

Kaplan AP & Greaves MW. (2005) Angioedema. *Journal of the American Academy of Dermatology* **53**, 373–388.

Russell JP & Gibson LE. (2006) Primary cutaneous small vessel vasculitis: approach to diagnosis and treatment. *International Journal of Dermatology* **45**, 3–13.

Schachner LA. (2000) Erythema multiforme. *Pediatric Dermatology* **17**, 75–83.

Sunderkotter C & Sindrilaru A. (2006) Clinical classification of vasculitis. *European Journal of Dermatology* **16**, 114–124.

# 9 Bullous diseases

Vesicles and bullae are accumulations of fluid within or under the epidermis. They have many causes, and a correct clinical diagnosis must be based on a close study of the physical signs.

The appearance of a blister is determined by the level at which it forms. Subepidermal blisters occur between the dermis and the epidermis. Their roofs are relatively thick and so they tend to be tense and intact. They may contain blood. Intra-epidermal blisters appear within the prickle cell layer of the epidermis, and so have thin roofs and rupture easily to leave an oozing denuded surface. This tendency is even more marked with subcorneal blisters, which form just beneath the stratum corneum at the outermost edge of the viable epidermis, and therefore have even thinner roofs.

Sometimes the morphology or distribution of a bullous eruption gives the diagnosis away, as in herpes simplex or zoster. Sometimes the history helps too, as in cold or thermal injury, or in an acute contact dermatitis. When the cause is not obvious, a biopsy should be taken to show the level in the skin at which the blister has arisen. A list of differential diagnoses, based on the level at which blisters form, is given in Fig. 9.1.

The bulk of this chapter is taken up by the three most important immunobullous disorders – pemphigus, pemphigoid and dermatitis herpetiformis (Table 9.1) – and by the group of inherited bullous disorders known as epidermolysis bullosa. Our understanding of both groups has advanced in parallel, as several of the skin components targeted by autoantibodies in the immunobullous disorders are the same as those inherited in an abnormal form in epidermolysis bullosa.

## Bullous disorders of immunological origin

Many chronic bullous diseases are caused directly or indirectly with antibodies binding to normal tissue antigens. In the pemphigus family, these are cadherins holding keratinocytes of the epidermis together. In the pemphigoid family, antigens are constitutents of the dermal–epidermal junction that anchor the epidermis to the dermis. In dermatitis herpetiformis, the antigen is a transglutaminase.

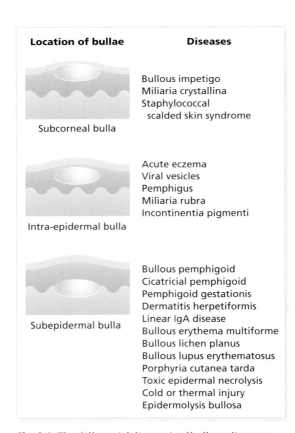

| Location of bullae | Diseases |
|---|---|
| Subcorneal bulla | Bullous impetigo<br>Miliaria crystallina<br>Staphylococcal scalded skin syndrome |
| Intra-epidermal bulla | Acute eczema<br>Viral vesicles<br>Pemphigus<br>Miliaria rubra<br>Incontinentia pigmenti |
| Subepidermal bulla | Bullous pemphigoid<br>Cicatricial pemphigoid<br>Pemphigoid gestationis<br>Dermatitis herpetiformis<br>Linear IgA disease<br>Bullous erythema multiforme<br>Bullous lichen planus<br>Bullous lupus erythematosus<br>Porphyria cutanea tarda<br>Toxic epidermal necrolysis<br>Cold or thermal injury<br>Epidermolysis bullosa |

**Fig. 9.1** The differential diagnosis of bullous diseases based on the histological location of the blister.

**Table 9.1** Distinguishing features of the three main immunobullous diseases.

| | Age | Site of blisters | General health | Blisters in mouth | Nature of blisters | Circulating antibodies | Fixed antibodies | Treatment |
|---|---|---|---|---|---|---|---|---|
| Pemphigus | Middle age | Trunk, flexures and scalp | Poor | Common | Superficial and flaccid | IgG to intercellular adhesion proteins | IgG in intercellular space | Steroids Immunosuppressives |
| Bullous pemphigoid | Old | Often flexural | Good | Rare | Tense and blood-filled | IgG to basement membrane region | IgG at basement membrane | Steroids Immunosuppressives |
| Dermatitis herpetiformis | Primarily adults | Elbows, knees, upper back, buttocks | Itchy | Rare | Small, excoriated and grouped | IgG to endomysium and transglutaminase | IgA granular deposits in papillary dermis | Gluten-free diet Dapsone Sulfapyridine |

## The pemphigus family

Pemphigus is severe and potentially life-threatening. There are two main types. The most common is pemphigus vulgaris, which accounts for at least three-quarters of all cases, and for most of the deaths. Pemphigus vegetans is a rare variant of pemphigus vulgaris. The other important type of pemphigus, superficial pemphigus, also has two variants: the generalized foliaceus type and localized erythematosus type. A few drugs, led by penicillamine, can trigger a pemphigus-like reaction, but auto-antibodies are then seldom found. Finally, a rare type of pemphigus (paraneoplastic pemphigus) with severe mucosal erosions arrises in association with a neoplasm such as thymoma, Castleman's tumour or lymphoma.

### Cause

All types of pemphigus are autoimmune diseases in which pathogenic immunoglobulin G (IgG) antibodies bind to antigens within the epidermis. The main antigens are desmoglein 3 (in pemphigus vulgaris) and desmoglein 1 (in superficial pemphigus). Both are cell-adhesion molecules of the cadherin family (see Table 2.5), found in desmosomes. The antigen–antibody reaction interferes with adhesion, causing the keratinocytes to fall apart (acantholysis). Pemphigus vulgaris is particularly common in Ashkenazi Jews and people of Mediterranean or Indian origin. There is linkage between it and certain HLA class II alleles.

### Presentation

Pemphigus vulgaris is characterized by flaccid blisters of the skin (Fig. 9.2) and mouth (Fig. 9.3). The blisters rupture easily to leave widespread painful erosions. Most patients develop the mouth lesions first. Shearing stresses on normal skin can cause new erosions to form (a positive Nikolsky sign). In the vegetans variant (Fig. 9.4), heaped-up cauliflower-like weeping areas are present in the groin and body folds. The blisters in pemphigus foliaceus are so superficial, and rupture so easily, that the clinical picture is dominated more by weeping and crusting erosions than by blisters. In the

**Fig. 9.2** Pemphigus vulgaris: widespread erosions that have followed blisters.

**Fig. 9.3** Painful sloughy mouth ulcers in pemphigus vulgaris.

rarer pemphigus erythematosus, the facial lesions are often pink, rough and scaly.

### Course

The course of all forms of pemphigus is prolonged, even with treatment, and the mortality rate of pemphigus vulgaris is still at least 15%. Most patients have a terrible time with weight gain and other side-effects from systemic corticosteroids and from

**Fig. 9.4** Pemphigus vegetans in the axilla, some intact blisters can be seen.

the lesions, which resist healing. About one-third of patients with pemphigus vulgaris will go into complete remission within 3 years. Superficial pemphigus is less severe. With modern treatments, most patients with pemphigus can live relatively normal lives, with occasional exacerbations.

## Complications

Complications are inevitable with the high doses of steroids and immunosuppressive drugs that are needed to control the condition. Indeed, side-effects of treatment are now the leading cause of death. Infections of all types are common. The large areas of denudation may become infected and smelly, and severe oral ulcers make eating painful.

## Differential diagnosis

Widespread erosions may suggest a pyoderma, impetigo, epidermolysis bullosa or ecthyma. Mouth ulcers can be mistaken for aphthae, Behçet's disease or a herpes simplex infection. Scalp erosions suggest bacterial or fungal infections.

## Investigations

Biopsy shows that the vesicles are intra-epidermal, with rounded keratinocytes floating freely within the blister cavity (acantholysis). Direct immuno-fluorescence (p. 45) of adjacent normal skin shows intercellular epidermal deposits of IgG and C3 (Fig. 9.5). The serum from a patient with pemphigus contains antibodies that bind to the desmogleins in the desmosomes of normal epidermis, so that indirect immunofluorescence (p. 45) or enzyme-linked immunosorbent assays (ELISA) can also be used to confirm the diagnosis. The titre of these antibodies correlates loosely with clinical activity and may guide changes in the dosage of systemic steroids.

## Treatment

Because of the dangers of pemphigus vulgaris, and the difficulty in controlling it, patients should be treated by dermatologists. Resistant and severe cases need very high doses of systemic steroids, such as 80–180 mg/day prednisolone (Formulary 2, p. 401). These 'industrial doses' work because prednisolone up-regulates the expression of desmoglein molecules on the surfaces of keratinocytes, in addition to other effects above and beyond their anti-inflammatory ones. The dose is reduced only when new blisters stop appearing. Immunosuppressive agents, such as azathioprine, gold salts or cyclophosphamide and, recently, mycophenylate mofetil, are often used as steroid-sparing agents. New and promising approaches include plasmapheresis and administration of intravenous immunoglobulin. Rituximab is a humanized murine monoclonal antibody to CD20 that may knock out B cells, pre-B cells and antibody production. Dapsone may sometimes be helpful, especially to allow healing. After control has been achieved, prolonged maintenance therapy and regular follow-up will be needed. In superficial pemphigus, smaller doses of systemic corticosteroids are usually needed, and the use of topical corticosteroids may also help.

> **Learning point**
>
> Pemphigus is more attacking than pemphigoid and needs higher doses of steroids to control it

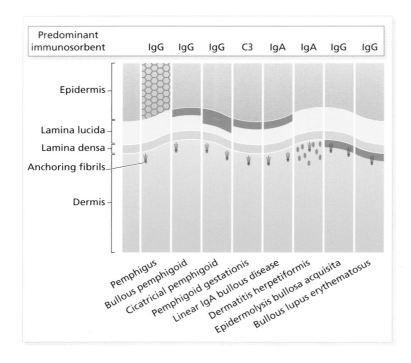

**Fig. 9.5** Immunofluorescence (red) in bullous diseases.

## Other causes of subcorneal and intra-epidermal blistering

### Bullous impetigo (p. 222)

This is a common cause of blistering in children. The bullae erupt suddenly, are flaccid, often contain pus and are frequently grouped or located in body folds. Bullous impetigo is caused by *Staphylococcus aureus*.

### Scalded skin syndrome (p. 224)

A toxin (exfoliatin) elaborated by some strains of *S. aureus* makes the skin painful and red; later it peels like a scald. The staphylococcus is usually hidden (e.g. conjunctiva, throat, wound, furuncle). The toxin causes dyshesion of desmoglein I, the same cadherin injured in pemphigus foliaceus.

### Miliaria crystallina (p. 175)

Here sweat accumulates under the stratum corneum leading to the development of multitudes of uniformly spaced vesicles without underlying redness. Often this occurs after a fever or heavy exertion. The vesicles look like droplets of water lying on the surface, but the skin is dry to the touch. The disorder is self-limiting and needs no treatment.

### Subcorneal pustular dermatosis

As its name implies, the lesions are small groups of pustules rather than vesicles. However, the pustules pout out of the skin in a way that suggests they were once vesicles (like the vesico-pustules of chickenpox). Oral dapsone (Formulary 2, p. 405) usually suppresses it. Many patients have IgA antibodies to intercellular epithelial antigens.

### Acute dermatitis (Chapter 7)

Severe acute eczema, especially of the contact allergic type, can be bullous. Plants such as poison ivy, poison oak or primula are common causes. The varied size of the vesicles, their close grouping, their asymmetry, their odd configurations (e.g. linear, square, rectilinear), their intense itch and a history of contact with plants are helpful guides to the diagnosis.

### Pompholyx (p. 99)

In pompholyx, highly itchy small eczematous

vesicles occur along the sides of the fingers, and sometimes also on the palms and soles. Some call it 'dyshidrotic eczema', but the vesicles are not related to sweating or sweat ducts. The disorder is very common, but its cause is not known.

## Viral infections (Chapter 16)

Some viruses create blisters in the skin by destroying epithelial cells. The vesicles of herpes simplex and zoster are the most common examples.

## Transient acantholytic dermatosis (Grover's disease)

Itchy vesicles appear on the sun-damaged skin of the trunk, usually of middle-aged males. The cause is not known and the condition can be persistent-despite its name.

# Subepidermal immunobullous disorders

These can be hard to separate on clinical grounds and only the two most important, pemphigoid and dermatitis herpetiformis, are described in detail here. Several others are mentioned briefly.

## The pemphigoid family

Pemphigoid is an autoimmune disease. Serum from about 70% of patients contains antibodies that bind *in vitro* to normal skin at the basement membrane zone. However, their titre does not correlate with clinical disease activity. The IgG antibodies bind to two main antigens: most commonly to BP230 (which anchors keratin intermediate filaments to the hemidesmosome; p. 18), and less often to BP180 (a transmembrane molecule with one end within the hemidesmosome and the other bound to the lamina lucida). Complement is then activated (p. 18), starting an inflammatory cascade. Eosinophils often participate in the process, causing the epidermis to separate from the dermis.

### Presentation

Pemphigoid is a chronic, usually itchy, blistering disease, mainly affecting the elderly. Usually no

**Fig. 9.6** Blisters of pemphigoid arise as tense yellow bullae, often on a pink, urticated base.

precipitating factors can be found, but rarely ultraviolet light or radiation therapy seems to play a part. The skin often erupts with smooth, itching red plaques in which tense vesicles and bullae form (Fig. 9.6). Occasionally they arise from normal skin. The flexures are often affected; the mucous membranes usually are not. The Nikolsky test is negative. Denudation occurs only over small areas as blisters rupture, so the disorder would not be fatal were it not for its propensity to affect elderly people who may be already in poor health; factors carrying a high risk include old age, the need for high steroid dosage and low serum albumin levels.

### Course

Pemphigoid is usually self-limiting and treatment can often be stopped after 1–2 years.

### Complications

Untreated, the disease causes much discomfort and loss of fluid from ruptured bullae. Systemic steroids and immunosuppressive agents carry their usual complications if used long term (Formulary 2, p. 401 and p. 399, respectively).

### Differential diagnosis

Most of the time, a clinical diagnosis proves correct.

**Fig. 9.7** Indirect immunofluorescence using serum from a patient with pemphigoid, showing basement zone immunofluorescence.

Pemphigoid may look like other bullous diseases, especially epidermolysis bullosa acquisita, bullous lupus erythematosus, dermatitis herpetiformis, pemphigoid gestationis, bullous erythema multiforme and linear IgA bullous disease. Immunofluorescence helps to separate it from these (Fig. 9.5).

### Investigations

A subepidermal blister is often filled with eosinophils. Direct immunofluorescence shows a linear band of IgG and C3 along the basement membrane zone. Indirect immunofluorescence, using serum from the patient, identifies IgG antibodies that react with the basement membrane zone in some 70% of patients (Fig. 9.7). Most patients have peripheral blood eosinophilia.

### Treatment

Mild pemphigoid can sometimes be controlled by the use of potent topical steroids alone. However, in the acute phase, prednisolone or prednisone (Formulary 2, p. 401) at a dosage of 40–60 mg/day is usually needed to control the eruption – although starting doses of over 0.75 mg/kg/day give no additional benefit. The dosage is reduced as soon as possible, and patients end up on a low maintenance regimen of systemic steroids, taken on alternate days until treatment is stopped. Immunosuppressive agents such as azathioprine may also be required. For unknown reasons, tetracyclines and niacinamide help some patients.

> **Learning points**
>
> - Death is uncommon and the disease is self-limiting
> - Some elderly people have fatal side-effects from their systemic steroids. Reduce the dosage as soon as possible

### Pemphigoid gestationis (herpes gestationis)

This is pemphigoid occurring in pregnancy, or in the presence of a hydatidiform mole or a choriocarcinoma. Certain paternally derived histocompatability antigens carried by the fetus might provoke an autoimmune response in some mothers. As in pemphigoid, most patients have linear deposits of C3 along the basement membrane zone (Fig. 9.5), although IgG is detected less often. The condition usually remits after the birth but may return in future pregnancies. It is not caused by a herpes virus: the name herpes gestationis should be discarded now so that the disease is not confused with herpes genitalis. Treatment is with systemic steroids. Oral contraceptives should be avoided, because their hormones may precipitate the disease.

### Cicatricial pemphigoid (Fig. 9.8)

Like pemphigoid itself, cicatricial pemphigoid is an autoimmune skin disease showing IgG and C3 deposition at the basement membrane zone (Fig. 9.5). The antigens are often as in pemphigoid, but other antigens at the dermal–epidermal junction are sometimes targeted such as laminin 5 (in anchoring filaments). The condition differs from pemphigoid

**Fig. 9.8** Long-standing cicatricial pemphigoid. Adhesions are now forming between the upper and lower eyelids.

in that its blisters and ulcers occur mainly on mucous membranes such as the conjunctivae, the mouth and genital tract. Bullae on the skin itself are uncommon. Lesions heal with scarring; around the eyes this may cause blindness, especially when the palpebral conjunctivae are affected (Fig. 9.8). The condition tends to persist and treatment is relatively ineffective, although very potent local steroids, dapsone, systemic steroids and immunosuppressive agents are usually tried. Good eye hygiene and the removal of ingrowing eyelashes are important.

### Linear IgA bullous disease

This is clinically similar to pemphigoid, but affects children as well as adults. Blisters arise on urticarial plaques, and are more often grouped, and on extensor surfaces, than is the case with pemphigoid. The so-called 'string of pearls sign', seen in some affected children, is the presence of blistering around the rim of polycyclic urticarial plaques. The conjunctivae may be involved. Linear IgA bullous disease is, as its name implies, associated with linear deposits of IgA and C3 at the basement membrane zone (Fig. 9.5). IgG is sometimes also found. The disorder responds well to oral dapsone (Formulary 2, p. 405).

### Acquired epidermolysis bullosa

This can also look like pemphigoid, but has two important extra features: many of the blisters arise in response to trauma on otherwise normal skin; and milia are a feature of healing lesions. The target of the autoantibodies is type VII collagen in anchoring fibrils (Fig. 9.5). The antigen lies on the dermal side of the lamina densa, in contrast to the pemphigoid antigens, which lie on the epidermal side – a difference that can be demonstrated by immunofluorescence after the basement membrane is split at the lamina densa by incubating skin in a saline solution (the 'salt-split' technique). The condition responds poorly to systemic corticosteroids or immunosuppressive agents.

## Dermatitis herpetiformis

Dermatitis herpetiformis is a very itchy chronic subepidermal vesicular disease, in which the vesicles erupt in groups as in herpes simplex – hence the name 'herpetiformis'.

### Cause

Gluten-sensitive enteropathy (sprue, adult coeliac disease), demonstrable by small bowel biopsy, is always present, but most patients do not suffer from diarrhoea, constipation or malnutrition as the enteropathy is mild, patchy and involves only the proximal small intestine. A range of antibodies can be detected in serum, notably directed against tissue transglutaminase, reticulin, gliadin and endomysium – a component of smooth muscle. In a minority of patients with gluten-sensitive enteropathy, IgA antibodies against tissue transglutaminase cross-react with antigens of epidermal transglutaminase leading to granular deposits of IgA and then C3 in the superficial dermis under the basement membrane zone (Fig. 9.5). These induce a neutrophil-rich inflammation, which separates the epidermis from the dermis. The IgA deposits in skin clear slowly after the introduction of a gluten-free diet. There is a strong association with certain human leucocyte antigen (HLA) types, particularly HLA-DR3 and HLA-DQw2.

### Presentation

The extremely itchy, grouped vesicles (Fig. 9.9) and urticated papules develop particularly over the elbows (Fig. 9.10) and knees, buttocks and shoulders. They are often broken by scratching before they reach any size. A typical patient therefore shows only grouped excoriations. Sometimes a secondary eczematous dermatitis develops from fierce scratching. Thus, the name 'dermatitis' comes from scratching, and 'herpetiformis' comes from grouping of vesicles and crusts.

### Course

The condition typically lasts for decades unless patients avoid gluten entirely.

### Complications

The complications of gluten-sensitive enteropathy

**Fig. 9.9** The typical small tense grouped itchy blisters of dermatitis herpetiformis.

**Fig. 9.10** The itchy blisters of dermatitis herpetiformis favour the points of the elbows and knees, where they are quickly destroyed by scratching.

include diarrhoea, abdominal pain, anaemia and, rarely, malabsorption. Small bowel lymphomas have been reported, and the use of a gluten-free diet may reduce this risk. There is a proven association with other autoimmune diseases, most commonly of the thyroid.

### Differential diagnosis

The disorder masquerades as scabies, an excoriated eczema, insect bites or neurodermatitis.

### Investigations

If a vesicle can be biopsied before it is scratched away, the histology will be that of a subepidermal blister, with neutrophils packing the adjacent dermal papillae. Direct immunofluorescence of uninvolved skin shows granular deposits of IgA, and usually C3, in the dermal papillae and superficial dermis (Fig. 9.5). Serum antibody tests for anti-endomysial antibodies or tissue transglutaminase can help diagnose the enteropathy. Small bowel biopsy is no longer recommended as routine because the changes are often patchy and serum tests are more sensitive. Tests for malabsorption are seldom needed.

### Treatment

The disorder responds to a gluten-free diet, which should be supervised by a dietitian. Adherence to this can be monitored using the titre of antibodies to anti-endomysial antigens or to tissue transglutaminase, which fall if gluten is strictly avoided. The bowel changes revert quickly to normal but IgA deposits remain longer in the skin, so the skin disease can drag on for many months. Because of this, and because a gluten-free diet is hard to follow and enjoy, some patients prefer to combine the diet with dapsone (Formulary 2, p. 405) or sulfapyridine at the start, although both can cause severe rashes, haemolytic anaemia (especially in those with glucose-6-phosphate dehydrogenase deficiency), leucopenia, thrombocytopenia, methaemoglobinaemia and peripheral neuropathy. Regular blood checks are therefore necessary.

**Learning points**

- Biopsy non-involved skin to demonstrate the diagnostic granular deposits of IgA in the dermal papillae
- The gluten enteropathy of dermatitis herpetiformis seldom causes frank malabsorption
- Dapsone works quickly and a gluten-free diet only very slowly. Combine the two at the start and slowly reduce the dapsone

## Other causes of subepidermal blisters

### Porphyria cutanea tarda (p. 328)

Flaccid bullae and erosions occur on the backs of the hands and on other areas exposed to sunlight.

### Blisters in diabetes and renal disease

A few diabetics develop unexplained blisters on their legs or feet. The backs of the hands of patients with chronic renal failure may show changes rather like those of porphyria cutanea tarda (pseudoporphyria). Furosemide (frusemide) can contribute to blister formation.

### Bullous lupus erythematosus

Vesicles and bullae may be seen in severe active systemic lupus erythematosus (p. 132). This disorder is uncommon and carries a high risk of kidney disease. Non-cutaneous manifestations of systemic lupus erythematosus do not respond to dapsone; however, the bullae do.

### Bullous erythema multiforme

Bullous erythema multiforme in the form of the Stevens–Johnson syndrome is discussed in Chapter 8.

### Toxic epidermal necrolysis (Lyell's disease)

#### Cause

Toxic epidermal necrolysis is usually a drug reaction, most commonly to sulphonamides, lamo-

**Fig. 9.11** The burn-like appearance of toxic epidermal necrolysis.

trigine, barbiturates, carbamazepine or allopurinol (Chapter 25), but can also be a manifestation of graft-vs.-host disease and there is an increased incidence in patients with AIDs. Sometimes it is unexplained.

#### Presentation

The skin becomes red and intensely painful, and then begins to come off in sheets like a scald. This leaves an eroded painful glistening surface (Fig. 9.11). Nikolsky's sign is positive (p. 120). The mucous membranes may be affected, including the mouth, eyes, and even the bronchial tree.

#### Course

The condition usually clears if the patient lives and if the offending drug is stopped. New epidermis grows out from hair follicles so that skin grafts are not usually needed. The disorder may come back if the drug is taken again.

#### Complications

Toxic epidermal necrolysis is a skin emergency and can be fatal. Infection, and the loss of fluids and electrolytes, are life-threatening, and the painful denuded skin surfaces make life a misery. Corneal scarring may remain when the acute episode has settled.

## Differential diagnosis

The epidermolysis of the staphylococcal scalded skin syndrome (p. 224) looks like toxic epidermal necrolysis clinically, but only the stratum corneum is lost. Whereas toxic epidermal necrolysis affects adults, the staphylococcal scalded skin syndrome is seen in infancy or early childhood. Histology differentiates the two. Pemphigus may also look similar, but starts more slowly and is more localized. Severe graft-vs.-host reactions can also cause this syndrome. Some believe that toxic epidermal necrolysis can evolve from Stevens–Johnson syndrome because some patients have the clinical features of both.

## Investigations

Biopsy helps to confirm the diagnosis. The split is subepidermal in toxic epidermal necrolysis, and the entire epidermis may be necrotic. A frozen section provides a quick answer if there is genuine difficulty in separating toxic epidermal necrolysis from the scalded skin syndrome where the split is subcorneal (p. 224). There are no tests to tell which drug, if any, caused the disease.

## Treatment

If toxic epidermal necrolysis is caused by a drug, this must be stopped (Chapter 25); otherwise, treatment relies mainly on symptomatic management. Intensive nursing care and medical support are needed, including the use of central venous lines, intravenous fluids and electrolytes. Many patients are treated in units designed to deal with extensive thermal burns. Air suspension beds increase comfort. The weight of opinion has turned against the use of systemic corticosteroids. Intravenous IgG seems more promising and ciclosporin treatment has been associated with a decreased mortality rates. Plasmapheresis may remove triggering drugs, or inflammatory mediators.

> **Learning points**
>
> - The skin is programmed to die. Treatments may not stop it
> - This is an emergency. Death is common
> - Refer the patient to a unit that treats thermal burns

## Epidermolysis bullosa (also known as the mechanobullous disorders)

There are many types of epidermolysis bullosa: the five main ones are listed in Table 9.2. All are characterized by an inherited tendency to develop blisters after minimal trauma, although at different levels in the skin (Fig. 9.12). The more severe types have a catastrophic impact on the lives of patients. Acquired epidermolysis bullosa is not inherited and was discussed earlier in this chapter.

### Simple epidermolysis bullosa

Several subtypes are recognized, of which the most common are the Weber–Cockayne (mainly affecting the hands and feet) and the Dowling–Meara

**Table 9.2** Simplified classification of epidermolysis bullosa.

| Type | Mode of inheritance | Level of split | Mutations in |
|---|---|---|---|
| Simple epidermolysis bullosa | Usually autosomal dominant | Intra-epidermal | Keratins 5 and 14 |
| Junctional epidermolysis bullosa (epidermolysis bullosa letalis) | Autosomal recessive | Lamina lucida | Components of the hemidesmosome-anchoring filaments (e.g. laminins, integrins and bullous pemphigoid 180 molecule) |
| Dystrophic epidermolysis bullosa | Autosomal dominant | Beneath lamina densa | Type VII collagen |
| Dystrophic epidermolysis bullosa | Autosomal recessive | Beneath lamina densa | Type VII collagen |
| Acquired epidermolysis bullosa | Not inherited | Dermal side of lamina densa | Nil |

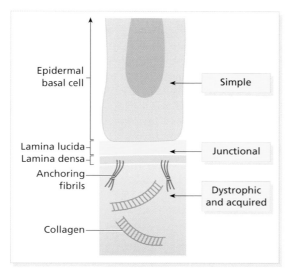

**Fig. 9.12** Levels of blister formation in epidermolysis bullosa at the dermo-epidermal junction.

**Fig. 9.13** Junctional epidermolysis bullosa: minor trauma has caused large blisters and erosions which will heal slowly or not at all.

(featuring herpetiform blisters on the trunk) types. Most are inherited as autosomal dominant conditions and are caused by abnormalities in genes responsible for production of the paired keratins (K5 and K14) expressed in basal keratinocytes (see Fig. 2.4). Linkage studies show that the genetic defects responsible for the most common types of simple epidermolysis bullosa lie on chromosomes 17 and 12.

Blisters form within or just above the basal cell layers of the epidermis and so tend to heal without scarring. Involvement of nails and mucosae is frequent but subtle. The problems are made worse by sweating and ill-fitting shoes. Blistering can be minimized by avoiding trauma, wearing soft well-fitting shoes and using foot powder. Large blisters should be pricked with a sterile needle and dressed. Their roofs should not be removed. Local antibiotics may be needed.

## Junctional epidermolysis bullosa

The separation occurs in the lamina lucida of the basement membrane, usually following mutations in the genes responsible for laminin formation (p. 19; see Fig. 2.9). This rare and often lethal condition is evident at birth. The newborn child has large raw areas and flaccid blisters, which are slow to

heal (Fig. 9.13). The perioral and perianal skin is usually involved, as are the nails and oral mucous membrane. There is no effective systemic treatment. Hopes for the future include adding the normal gene to epidermal stem cells, and then layering these onto the denuded skin.

## Dystrophic epidermolysis bullosa

There are many subtypes, all of which probably result from abnormalities of collagen VII, the major structural component of anchoring fibrils.

## Autosomal dominant dystrophic epidermolysis bullosa

In this type blisters appear in late infancy. They are most common on friction sites (e.g. the knees, elbows and fingers), healing with scarring and milia formation. The nails may be deformed or even lost. The mouth is not affected. The only treatment is to avoid trauma and to dress the blistered areas.

## Autosomal recessive dystrophic epidermolysis bullosa

In this tragic form of epidermolysis bullosa, blisters start in infancy. They are subepidermal and may be filled with blood. They heal with scarring, which can be so severe that the nails are lost and webs form between the digits (Fig. 9.14). The hands and feet may become useless balls, having lost all fingers

**Fig. 9.14** Autosomal recessive dystrophic epidermolysis bullosa: note large blood-filled blister. Scarring has led to fixed deformity of the fingers and loss of nails.

and toes. The teeth, mouth and upper part of the oesophagus are all affected; oesophageal strictures may form. Squamous cell carcinomas of the skin are a late complication. Treatment is unsatisfactory. Phenytoin, which reduces the raised dermal collagenase levels found in this variant, and systemic steroids are disappointing. It is especially important to minimize trauma, maintain nutrition, prevent contractures and web formation between the digits, and combat anaemia and secondary infection. Referral to centres with expertise in management of these patients is strongly recommended.

## Further reading

Chavez TA, Mortimer MJ, Hall AP & Hutchinson PE. (2005) Toxic epidermal necrolysis: current evidence, practical management, and future directions. *British Journal of Dermatology* **153**, 241–253.

Cotell S, Robinson ND & Chan LS. (2000) Autoimmune blistering skin disease. *American Journal of Emergency Medicine* **18**, 288–299.

Fassihi H, Wong T, Wessagowit V, McGrath JA & Mellerio JE. (2006) Target proteins in inherited and acquired blistering skin disorders. *Clinical and Experimental Dermatology* **31**, 252–259.

Fleming TE & Korman NJ. (2000) Cicatricial pemphigoid. *Journal of the American Academy of Dermatology* **43**, 571–591.

Harman KE, Albert S & Black MM. (2003) Guidelines for the management of pemphigus vulgaris. *British Journal of Dermatology* **149**, 926–937.

Nousari HC & Anhalt GJ. (1999) Pemphigus and bullous pemphigoid. *Lancet* **354**, 667–672.

Schmidt E & Zillikens D. (2000) Autoimmune and inherited subepidermal blistering diseases: advances in the clinic and the laboratory. *Advances in Dermatology* **16**, 113–157.

Wojnarowska F, Kirtschig G, Highet AS, Venning VA & Khumalo NP. (2002) Guidelines for the management of bullous pemphigoid. *British Journal of Dermatology* **147**, 214–221.

# **10** Connective tissue disorders

The cardinal feature of these conditions is inflammation in the connective tissues which leads to dermal atrophy or sclerosis, to arthritis and sometimes to abnormalities in other organs. In addition, antibodies form against normal tissues and cellular components; these disorders are therefore classed as autoimmune. Many have difficulty in remembering which antibody features in which condition; Table 10.1 should help here.

The main connective tissue disorders present as a spectrum ranging from the benign cutaneous variants to severe multisystem diseases (Table 10.2).

## Lupus erythematosus

Lupus erythematosus (LE) is a good example of such a spectrum, ranging from the purely cutaneous type (discoid LE), through patterns associated with some internal problems (disseminated discoid LE and subacute cutaneous LE), to a severe multisystem disease (systemic lupus erythematosus, SLE; Table 10.2).

### Systemic lupus erythematosus

#### *Cause*

This is unknown, but hereditary factors, such as complement deficiency and certain HLA types, increase susceptibility. Exposure to sunlight and artificial ultraviolet radiation (UVR) may precipitate the disease or lead to flare-ups, probably by exposing

**Table 10.1** Some important associations with non-organ-specific antibodies.

| Disease | Autoantibody | Frequency (%) |
|---|---|---|
| Systemic lupus erythematosus | Double-stranded DNA | 50–70 |
| | Sm antigens (U1, U2, etc.) | 15–30 |
| | Phospholipid | 10–20 |
| Drug-induced lupus | Nuclear histones | Common |
| Subacute cutaneous lupus | SS-A(Ro) | 50–70 |
| | SS-B(La) | 20–30 |
| Dermatomyositis | Jo-1 | 20–30 |
| | Mi-2 | (5–10) |
| Systemic sclerosis | SCL-70 (topoisomerase 1) | 20–30 |
| CREST syndrome | Centromere | 20–30 |
| Mixed connective tissue disease | U1-RNP | 100 |
| Lichen sclerosis | Extracellular matrix protein 1 | Uncertain |

**Table 10.2** Classification of connective tissue disease.

| Localized disease | Intermediate type | Aggressive multisystem disease |
|---|---|---|
| Discoid lupus erythematosus | Subacute lupus erythematosus | Systemic lupus erythematosus |
| | Juvenile dermatomyositis | Adult dermatomyositis |
| Morphoea | Limited scleroderma | Systemic sclerosis |

**Fig. 10.1** In systemic lupus erythematosus (SLE) (left) the eruption is often just an erythema, sometimes transient, but occupying most of the 'butterfly' area. In discoid LE (right) the fixed scaling and scarring plaques may occur in the butterfly area (dotted line), but can occur outside it too.

previously hidden nuclear or cytoplasmic antigens to which autoantibodies are formed. Such auto-antibodies to DNA, nuclear proteins and other normal antigens are typical of LE, and immune complexes formed from these are deposited in the tissues or found in the serum. Some drugs, such as hydralazine and procainamide, trigger SLE in a dose-dependent way, whereas others, including oral contraceptives, anticonvulsants, minocycline, etanercept and captopril, precipitate the disease just occasionally.

### Presentation

Typically, but not always, the onset is acute. SLE is an uncommon disorder, affecting women more often than men (in a ratio of about 8 : 1). The classic rash of acute SLE is an erythema of the cheeks and nose in the rough shape of a butterfly (Figs 10.1 and 10.2), with facial swelling. Blisters occur rarely, and when they do they signify very active systemic disease. Some patients develop widespread discoid or annular papulosquamous plaques very like those of discoid LE; others, about 20% of patients, have no skin disease at any stage.

Other dermatological features include periungual telangiectasia (Fig. 10.7), erythema over the digits, hair fall (especially at the frontal margin of the scalp) and photosensitivity. Ulcers may occur on the palate, tongue or buccal mucosa.

### Course

The skin changes may be transient, continuous or recurrent; they correlate well with the activity of the systemic disease. Acute SLE may be associated with fever, arthritis, nephritis, polyarteritis, pleurisy, pneumonitis, pericarditis, myocarditis and

**Fig. 10.2** Erythema in the butterfly area, suggestive of systemic lupus erythematosus.

involvement of the central nervous system. Internal involvement can be fatal, but about three-quarters of patients survive for 15 years. Renal involvement suggests a poorer prognosis.

## Complications

The skin disease may cause scarring or hyperpigmentation, but the main dangers lie with damage to other organs and the side-effects of treatment, especially systemic steroids.

## Differential diagnosis

SLE is a great imitator. Its malar rash can be confused with sunburn, polymorphic light eruption (p. 273) and rosacea (p. 170), but is more livid in colour and swollen in texture. The discoid lesions are distinctive, but are also seen in discoid LE and in subacute cutaneous LE. Occasionally, they look like psoriasis or lichen planus (p. 72). The hair fall suggests telogen effluvium (p. 184). Plaques on the scalp may cause a scarring alopecia. SLE should be suspected when a characteristic rash is combined with fever, malaise and internal disease (Table 10.3).

## Investigations

Conduct a full physical examination, looking for internal disease. Biopsy of skin lesions is worthwhile because the pathology and immunopathology are distinctive. There is usually some thinning of the epidermis, liquefaction degeneration of epidermal

**Table 10.3** Criteria for the diagnosis of systemic lupus erythematosus (must have at least four).

Malar rash
Discoid plaques
Photosensitivity
Mouth ulcers
Arthritis
Serositis
Renal disorder
Neurological disorder
Haematological disorder
Immunological disorder
Antinuclear antibodies

basal cells, and a mild perivascular mononuclear cell infiltrate. Direct immunofluorescence is helpful: IgG, IgM, IgA and C3 are found individually or together in a band-like or granular pattern at the dermo-epidermal junction of involved skin and often uninvolved skin as well. Relevant laboratory tests are listed in Table 10.4.

## Treatment

Systemic steroids are the mainstay of treatment, with bed rest needed during exacerbations. Large doses of prednisolone (Formulary 2, p. 401) are often needed to achieve control, as assessed by symptoms, signs, erythrocyte sedimentation rate (ESR), total complement level and tests of organ function. The dosage is then reduced to the smallest that suppresses the disease. Immunosuppressive agents, such as azathioprine (Formulary 2, p. 399),

**Table 10.4** Investigations in systemic lupus erythematosus.

| Test | Usual findings |
| --- | --- |
| Skin biopsy | Degeneration of basal cells, epidermal thinning, inflammation around appendages |
| Skin immunofluorescence | Fibrillar or granular deposits of IgG, IgM, IgA and/or C3 alone in basement membrane zone |
| Haematology | Anaemia, raised ESR, thrombocytopenia, decreased white cell count |
| Immunology | Antinuclear antibody, antibodies to double-stranded DNA, false positive tests for syphilis, low total complement level, lupus anticoagulant factor |
| Urine analysis | Proteinuria or haematuria, often with casts if kidneys involved |
| Tests for function of other organs | As indicated by history but always test kidney and liver function |

ESR, erythrocyte sedimentation rate.

cyclophosphamide and other support drugs (e.g. antihypertensive therapy or anticonvulsants) may also be needed. Antimalarial drugs may help some patients with marked photosensitivity, as may sunscreens. Intermittent intravenous infusions of γ globulin show promise. Long-term and regular follow-up is necessary.

## Subacute cutaneous lupus erythematosus

This is less severe than acute SLE. Sometimes only the skin is affected but about half of patients also have marked systemic disease. While the aetiology is not fully understood, clues have been given by experiments *in vivo*. Autoantibodies to SSA(Ro) are particularly common in subacute cutaneous lupus erythematosus (SCLE), and blebs containing SSA(Ro) and other intracellular antigens form on the nuclear surface of irradiated keratinocytes. SSA(Ro) autoantibodies can activate complement. Antibody-dependent cellular cytotoxicity and autoantibody binding to SSA(Ro) are enhanced by oestradiol, perhaps accounting for the increased prevalence of SCLE in women.

### Presentation

Patients with SCLE are often photosensitive. The skin lesions are sharply marginated psoriasiform plaques, sometimes annular, lying on the forehead, nose, cheeks, chest, hands and sun-exposed surfaces of the arms and forearms. They tend to be symmetrical and are hard to tell from discoid LE, or SLE with widespread discoid lesions.

### Course

As in SLE, the course is prolonged. The skin lesions are slow to clear but, in contrast to discoid LE, do so with little or no scarring.

### Complications

Systemic disease is frequent, but not usually serious. SSA(Ro) can cross the placenta and children born to mothers who have, or have had, this condition are liable to neonatal LE with transient annular skin lesions and permanent heart block.

### Differential diagnosis

The morphology is characteristic, but lesions can be mistaken for psoriasis or widespread discoid LE. Annular lesions may resemble tinea corporis (p. 249) or figurate erythemas (p. 147).

### Investigations

Patients with SCLE should be evaluated in the same way as those with acute SLE, although deposits of immunoglobulins in the skin and antinuclear antibodies in serum are present less often. Many have antibodies to the cytoplasmic antigen SS-A(Ro) and SS-B(La).

### Treatment

SCLE does better with antimalarials, such as hydroxychloroquine (Formulary 2, p. 405), than acute SLE. Moderate potency topical corticosteroid creams help, and oral retinoids (Formulary 2, p. 401) are also effective in some cases. Systemic steroids may be needed too, especially if there are signs of internal disease.

## Discoid lupus erythematosus

This is the most common form of LE. Patients with discoid LE may have one or two plaques only, or many in several areas. The cause is also unknown but UVR is one factor.

### Presentation

Plaques show erythema, scaling, follicular plugging (like a nutmeg grater), scarring and atrophy, telangiectasia, hypopigmentation and a peripheral zone of hyperpigmentation. They are well demarcated and lie mostly on sun-exposed skin of the scalp, face and ears (Figs 10.1 and 10.3). In one variant (chilblain LE) dusky lesions appear on the fingers and toes.

### Course

The disease may spread relentlessly, but in about half of the cases the disease goes into remission over the course of several years. Scarring is common and

**Fig. 10.4** Discoid lupus erythematosus of the scalp leading to permanent hair loss. Note the marked follicular plugging.

**Fig. 10.3** Red scaly fixed plaques of discoid lupus erythematosus. This degree of scaling is not uncommon in the active stage. Follicular plugging is seen on the nose.

hair may be lost permanently if there is scarring in the scalp (Fig. 10.4). Whiteness remains after the inflammation has cleared, and hypopigmentation is common in dark-skinned people. Discoid LE rarely progresses to SLE.

### Differential diagnosis

Psoriasis is hard to tell from discoid LE when its plaques first arise but psoriasis has larger, thicker scales, and later it is usually symmetrical and affects different sites from those of discoid LE. Discoid LE is common on the face and ears, and on sun-exposed areas, whereas psoriasis favours the elbows, knees,

scalp and sacrum. Discoid LE is far more prone than psoriasis to scar and cause hair loss.

### Investigations

Most patients with discoid LE remain well. However, screening for SLE and internal disease is still worthwhile. A skin biopsy is most helpful if taken from an untreated plaque where appendages are still present (Fig. 10.5). Direct immunofluorescence shows deposits of IgG, IgM, IgA and C3 at the basement membrane zone. Biopsies for direct immunofluorescence are best taken from older untreated plaques. Blood tests are usually normal but occasionally serum contains antinuclear antibodies (Table 10.5).

### Treatment

Discoid LE needs potent or very potent topical corticosteroids (Formulary 1, p. 385). In this condition, it is justifiable to use them on the face, as the risk of scarring is worse than that of atrophy.

**Table 10.5** Some factors distinguishing the different types of lupus erythematosus (LE).

|  | Antinuclear antibodies | Sun sensitivity | Internal organ involvement |
|---|---|---|---|
| Systemic LE | Often against DNA ++++ | +++ | ++ |
| Subacute LE | Often against SSA + | ++++ | + |
| Discoid LE | ± | + | − |

SSA,

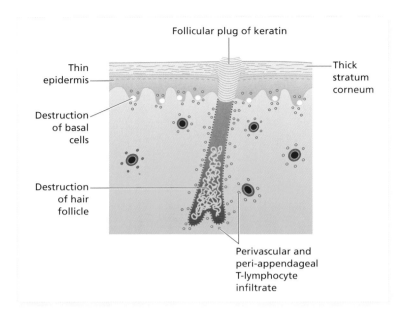

Follicular plug of keratin

Thin epidermis

Thick stratum corneum

Destruction of basal cells

Destruction of hair follicle

Perivascular and peri-appendageal T-lymphocyte infiltrate

**Fig. 10.5** The histology of discoid lupus erythematosus.

Topical steroids should be applied twice daily until inflammation disappears or side-effects develop (e.g. atrophy); weaker preparations can then be used for maintenance. If discoid LE does not respond to this, intralesional injections of triamcinolone (2.5 or 10 mg/mL) may help. Stubborn and widespread lesions often do well with oral antimalarials such as hydroxychloroquine (Formulary 2, p. 405), but rarely these cause irreversible eye damage. The eyes should therefore be tested before and at intervals during treatment. Sun avoidance and screens are also important. Oral retinoids (Formulary 2, p. 401) and thalidomide have proved helpful in stubborn cases but a specialist with experience of their use should prescribe these controlled treatments and supervise management.

### Tumid lupus erythematosus

This is a dermal form of discoid LE. The epidermis remains smooth although the blood vessels and adnexae are surrounded by a lymphocytic infiltrate very similar to that seen in discoid LE. The lesions are smooth, tumid, round, violaceous plaques, usually on the face. Treatment is with oral antimalarials. Jessner's lymphocytic infiltration is viewed by some as a photosensitive form of tumid LE.

## Dermatomyositis

Dermatomyositis is a subset of polymyositis with distinctive skin changes. There are adult and juvenile types (Table 10.2). The cause is unknown but an auto-immune mechanism seems likely. Autoantibodies to striated muscle are found. When starting after the age of 40 years, dermatomyositis may signal an internal malignancy. Presumably, the epitopes of some tumour antigens are so similar to those of muscle antigens that immune reactions directed against the tumour cross-react with muscle cells and initiate the disease in a few adults with internal malignancy. Serological evidence for acute toxoplasmosis in poly-myositis/dermatomyositis was found in one series.

### Presentation

The skin signs are characteristic. Typical patients have a faint lilac discoloration around their eyes (sometimes called 'heliotrope' because of the colour of the flower). This is associated with malar erythema and oedema (Fig. 10.6) and, sometimes, less striking erythema of the neck and presternal area (shawl sign). Most patients also develop lilac, slightly atrophic papules over the knuckles of their fingers (Gottron's papules, Fig. 10.7), streaks of erythema over the

**Fig. 10.6** Acute dermatomyositis: oedematous purple face with erythema on presternal area. Severe progressive muscle weakness, but no underlying tumour was found.

**Fig. 10.7** Erythema and telangiectasia of the nail folds are important clues to systemic connective tissue disorders. This patient has dermatomyositis. Note Gottron's papules over the knuckles.

extensor tendons of the hand, periungual telangiectasia and ragged cuticles (Fig. 10.7). The skin signs usually appear at the same time as the muscle symptoms but occasionally appear months or even years earlier. Sometimes the skin signs appear in isolation. Many, but not all, patients have weakness of proximal muscles. Climbing stairs, getting up from chairs and combing the hair become difficult.

## Course

In children the disorder is often self-limiting, but in adults it may be prolonged and progressive. Raynaud's phenomenon, arthralgia, dysphagia and calcinosis may follow. The rash may become scaly and, rarely, itchy; eventually that on the light-exposed areas and overlying involved muscles develops poikiloderma (p. 288). Features of mixed connective disease may develop (p. 142). The presence of calcinosis suggests a good prognosis.

## Complications

Myositis may lead to permanent weakness and immobility, and inflammation to contractures or cutaneous calcinosis. Some die from progressive and severe myopathy.

## Differential diagnosis

Other connective tissue disorders may look similar, particularly mixed connective tissue disease (p. 142) and SLE. In LE, the finger lesions favour the skin between the knuckles whereas in dermatomyositis the knuckles are preferred. Toxoplasmosis may cause a dermatomyositis-like syndrome. Myopathy can be a side-effect of systemic steroids, so weakness is not always caused by the disease itself.

## Investigations

Thirty to 40% of adults over the age of 40 years with dermatomyositis also have an underlying malignancy. Their dermatomyositis coincides with the onset of the tumour and may improve if it is removed. Adult dermatomyositis or polymyositis therefore requires a search for such an underlying malignancy. In women, the ovaries are a favourite hiding place. The levels of muscle enzymes such as aldolase and creatinine phosphokinase (CPK) are often elevated. Electromyography (EMG) detects muscle abnormalities, and biopsy of an affected muscle shows inflammation and destruction. Surprisingly, the ESR is often normal and antinuclear antibodies may not be detected. The presence of Jo-1 antibodies in plasma suggests high risk for myositis, arthritis and interstitial lung disease. Toxoplasmosis should be excluded by serology.

## Treatment

Systemic steroids, often in high doses (e.g. 60 mg/day prednisolone for an average adult; Formulary 2, p. 401), are the cornerstone of treatment and protect the muscles from destruction. A maintenance regimen may be needed for several years. Immunosuppressive agents, such as azathioprine (Formulary 2, p. 399) or methotrexate (Formulary 2, p. 400), also help to control the condition and to reduce the high steroid dose. Maintenance treatment is adjusted according to clinical response and CPK level. As in SLE, intravenous γ globulin infusions seem effective in stubborn cases. Long-term and regular follow-up is necessary.

> **Learning point**
>
> Hunt for internal malignancy in the middle aged and elderly, but not in juvenile cases

## Scleroderma

Dermatologists tend to think of scleroderma (excessive fibrosis in the skin) as a differential diagnosis rather than as a disease. Table 10.6 lists the differential diagnoses.

**Table 10.6**  Differential diagnosis of scleroderma.

*Systemic*
Diffuse scleroderma (systemic sclerosis)
Limited scleroderma
Diabetic sclerodactyly
Chronic graft-vs.-host reaction
Chronic vibration exposure
Phenylketonuria
Porphyria cutanea tarda
Chemicals (polyvinylchloride monomers)
Drugs (bleomycin, pentazocine, taxanes)
Amyloidosis
Nephrogenic sclerosing dermopathy
Progeria
Werner's syndrome
Scleroderma carcinoid syndrome scleroderma

*Localized*
Lichen sclerosus
Morphoea
Morphoea profunda
Fasciitis with eosinophilia
Pansclerotic morphoea
Linear morphoea
*En coup de sabre*
Injections (silicone, paraffin, vitamin K)
*Borrelia burgdorferi* infections (Europe & Asia)
Trauma
Radiation therapy

**Table 10.7**  Skin signs of systemic sclerosis.

Raynaud's phenomenon (95%)
Sclerosis (especially hands and fingers)
Diffuse darkening (hyperpigmentation)
Pinched nose
Mask-like face
Decreased oral aperture
Square mat telangiectasias
Thin lips
Prominent periungual capillaries
Nail abnormalities (pterygium)
Calcinosis cutis
Painful digital ulcers

## Diffuse scleroderma (systemic sclerosis, generalized scleroderma, diffuse sclerosis)

In this disorder the skin becomes hard as connective tissues thicken (Table 10.7). The disease has vascular, inflammatory and fibrotic elements. Early in the condition, T-helper cells dominate the inflammatory infiltrate in the dermis and cause fibroblasts to proliferate and produce more hyaluronic acid and type I collagen (p. 20). In addition, there is intimal thickening of arterioles and arteries. These processes are not confined to the skin, but involve many other organs, including the gut, lungs, kidneys and heart, leading to their dysfunction and to death.

### Cause

The cause of systemic sclerosis is unknown but many, apparently unrelated, pieces of the complex jigsaw are now beginning to come together. A vascular phase often precedes the sclerosis. Adhesion molecules are up-regulated on endothelial cells and chemotactic cytokines synthesized. An oligoclonal CD4+ T lymphocyte and macrophage tissue infiltration follows with high levels of IL-4 and transforming growth factor β (TGF-β) being produced. Increased levels of growth factors induce fibroblasts to make collagen. TGF-α promotes synthesis of collagen and matrix proteins, decreases metalloproteinases that degrade collagen and keeps fibroblasts in an active state.

A diffuse sclerosis-like syndrome is a feature of the chronic graft-vs.-host disease after allogeneic bone marrow transplantation. This has lead to speculation that diffuse sclerosis may occur by similar mechanisms, perhaps brought about by fetus-derived lymphocytes that cross the placenta during pregnancy, reactivating in the mother later in her life.

### Presentation

Most patients have Raynaud's phenomenon (p. 149) and sclerodactyly. Their fingers become immobile, hard and shiny. Some become hyperpigmented and itchy early in their disease. Periungual telangiectasia is common.

### Course

As the disease progresses, sclerosis spreads to the face, scalp and trunk. The nose becomes beak-like, and wrinkles radiate around the mouth (Figs 10.8–10.10). Most have abnormalities of the gut including dysphagia, oesophagitis, constipation, diarrhoea and malabsorption. Fibrosis of the lungs leads to dyspnoea; fibrosis of the heart and pulmonary hypertension to congestive failure. The kidneys are involved late, but this has a grave prognosis from malignant hypertension.

### Complications

Most complications are caused by the involvement of organs other than the skin, but ulcers of the fingertips and calcinosis are distressing (Fig. 10.11). Hard skin immobilizes the joints and leads to contractures.

**Fig. 10.8** Systemic sclerosis: radial furrowing around the mouth.

**Fig. 10.9** Mat-like telangiectasia seen in a patient with systemic sclerosis.

### Differential diagnosis

Other causes of Raynaud's phenomenon are given in Table 11.4. The differential diagnosis includes chilblains (p. 146) and erythromelalgia (p. 146). The sclerosis should be distinguished from that of widespread morphoea, porphyria cutanea tarda, mixed connective tissue disease, eosinophilic fasciitis, diabetic sclerodactyly and an acute arthritis with swollen fingers. Rarely, the disease is mimicked by progeria, scleromyxoedema, amyloidosis or carcinoid syndrome. A more complete differential diagnosis is given in Table 10.6. Nephrogenic sclerosing dermopathy, as the name suggests, occurs in some patients with renal disease undergoing dialysis. Its cause may be erythropoietin used to treat coexisting anaemias or gadolinium used in radiological scans. Similar syndromes have been reported following ingestion of adulterated rape-seed oil, dimerized L-tryptophan, and treatment with the antitumour agent bleomycin.

### Investigations

The diagnosis is made clinically because histological

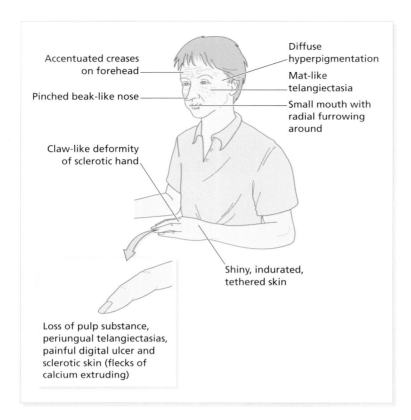

**Fig. 10.10** Signs of systemic sclerosis.

abnormalities are seldom present until the physical signs are well established. Laboratory tests should include a fluorescent antinuclear antibody test and the evaluation of the heart, kidney, lungs, joints and muscles. Barium studies are best avoided as obstruction may follow poor evacuation; other contrast media are available. X-rays of the hands, measurement of muscle enzymes and immunoglobulin levels, and a blood count, ESR and test for the scleroderma-associated antibody Scl-70 are also worthwhile.

### Treatment

This is unsatisfactory. The calcium-channel blocker nifedipine or the erectile dysfunction drug sildenafil may help Raynaud's phenomenon (p. 149). Systemic steroids, salicylates, antimalarials and long-term penicillin are used, but are not of proven value. D-penicillamine has many side-effects, especially on renal function. Physiotherapy is helpful; photopheresis is experimental. Recently, there have been promising reports of the efficacy of ultraviolet A-1 (340–400 nm) phototherapy for affected skin in systemic sclerosis. Antagonists to endothelin receptors such as bosentan reduce risks from pulmonary hypertension.

**Fig. 10.11** Loss of fingertip pulp, and extrusion of chalky material.

## Limited scleroderma

In this variant, thick skin is present only on the distal extremities and sometimes the face. A previously popular diagnosis, the CREST syndrome, is falling out of favour since it fails to suggest other non-skin elements that may be present. The mnemonic stood for Calcinosis, Raynaud's phenomenon, oEsophageal dysmotility, Sclerodactyly and Telangiectasia. Telangiectasia is periungual on the fingers and flat, mat-like or rectangular on the face. Many patients with limited scleroderma develop more diffuse skin involvement or pulmonary fibrosis after months or years. Some patients produce anti-centromere antibodies.

## Localized scleroderma

Sometimes only areas of skin become sclerotic. The differential diagnoses are listed in Table 10.6. Some people view lichen sclerosis, morphoea, morphoea profunda, eosinophilic fasciitis and pansclerotic morphoea as a spectrum of localized sclerosis based on the level of sclerosis in the skin. Overlaps occur.

## Morphoea

Morphoea is a localized form of diffuse sclerosis with pale indurated plaques on the skin but no internal sclerosis (Figs 10.12 and 10.13). Many plaques are surrounded by a violaceous halo. Its prognosis is usually good, and the fibrosis slowly clears leaving slight depression and hyperpigmentation. In pansclerotic morphoea, contractures can cause marked

**Fig. 10.13** Morphoea (*en coup de sabre* type) on the forehead. In a young child this can lead to facial hemiatrophy.

disability. A rare type may lead to arrest of growth of the underlying bones causing, for example, facial hemiatrophy or shortening of a limb. Little is known about the cause, except that Lyme borreliosis may be associated with the disease in Europe but not in the Americas. Treatments work slowly, if at all, and include topical steroids, topical calcipotriene, non-steroidal anti-inflammatory drugs (NSAIDs), psoralen with ultraviolet A (PUVA), long wavelength UVA (so-called UVA-1) or hydroxychloroquine in selected patients.

## Diffuse fasciitis with eosinophilia (eosinophilic fasciitis)

Localized areas of skin become indurated, sometimes after an upper respiratory tract infection or prolonged severe exercise. Hypergammaglobulinaemia and eosinophilia are present and a deep skin biopsy, which includes muscle, shows that the fascia overlying the muscle is thickened. Despite its common name 'eosinophilic fasciitis' and despite a profound eosinophilia in the peripheral blood, the fascia is not eosinophilic or permeated by eosinophils. The

**Fig. 10.12** Morphoea. Pale indurated plaques on the arm, showing a purplish rim.

**Fig. 10.14** Lichen sclerosus. Follicular hyperkeratosis differentiates this from morphoea.

disease responds promptly to systemic steroids; the long-term prognosis is good but disability in the short term can be severe.

## Lichen sclerosus

Many think that this condition is related to morphoea, with which it may coexist. However, its patches are non-indurated white shiny macules (Fig. 10.14), sometimes with obvious plugging in the follicular openings. Women are affected far more often than men and, although any area of skin can be involved, the classic ivory-coloured lesions often surround the vulva and anus (Fig. 13.39). Intractable itching is common in these areas and the development of vulval carcinoma is a risk. In men the condition may cause stenosis of the urethral meatus, and adhesions between the foreskin and glans of the penis (Fig. 13.38). Patients with lichen sclerosus may have antibodies to extracellular matrix protein 1.

## Mixed connective tissue disease

This is an overlap between SLE and either scleroderma or dermatomyositis.

### Presentation

As in LE, women are affected more often than men. Many develop swollen hands and sclerodactyly, and skin lesions like those of cutaneous LE may also be present. Alopecia is mild and the hair fall mimics telogen effluvium. Periungual telangiectasia and pigmentary disturbances are common. About 25% of patients have a small-vessel vasculitis with palpable purpura, leg ulcers and painful dermal nodules on the hands or elbows. Many show Raynaud's phenomenon, arthritis, serositis and myositis. Headaches, weakness, fatigue, lymph node enlargement or hoarseness occur in about one in three patients; renal and central nervous system disease are less common.

### Course

The disorder is chronic, and usually turns into either SLE or systemic sclerosis.

### Differential diagnosis

The disorder can be confused with SLE, dermatomyositis, polymyositis, systemic sclerosis and other sclerosing processes such as porphyria cutanea tarda (p. 328).

### Investigations

Patients with mixed connective tissue disease have antibodies in high titre directed against one or more extractable nuclear antigens, and in particular ribonuclear proteins. These give a speckled pattern when serum is reacted against nuclei and detected by indirect immunofluorescence. Direct immunofluorescence of involved and uninvolved skin shows IgG within the epidermal nuclei, also in a speckled pattern. Only one-third of patients have subepidermal immunoglobulin deposits in involved skin. Most have hypergammaglobulinaemia, a high ESR, oesophageal dysmotility, abnormal pulmonary function tests and a positive rheumatoid factor. Hypocomplementaemia, leucopenia, anaemia, cryoglobulinaemia and false positive biological tests for syphilis occur in a few patients.

### Treatment

Treatment depends upon which organs are involved, but systemic steroids are usually needed, in the same dosage as for SLE. Immunosuppressive agents reduce the dosage of systemic steroids, and NSAIDs help with arthralgia, myalgia and swelling of the hands.

## Other connective tissue diseases

### Rheumatoid arthritis

Most patients with rheumatoid arthritis have no skin disease, but some have tiny fingertip infarcts, purpura, ulcers, palmar or periungual erythema, or pyoderma gangrenosum. The most common skin manifestations are marble-like nodules near joints (rheumatoid nodules). These are always associated with the presence of rheumatoid factor. Some patients with rheumatoid arthritis have a vasculitis of larger blood vessels with deep 'punched out' ulcers on the legs.

### Reiter's syndrome (reactive arthritis)

Reiter's syndrome, precipitated by non-specific urethritis or dysentery, combines skin lesions, arthropathy, conjunctivitis, balanitis, mucositis and spondylitis. Arthritis is the most severe element. The skin lesions (keratoderma blennorrhagicum) are psoriasis-like red scaling plaques, often studded with vesicles and pustules, seen most often on the soles. The toes are red and swollen, and the nails thicken. Psoriasiform plaques may also occur on the penis and scrotum, with redness near the penile meatus. Sometimes nearly the whole skin may be afflicted, and Reiter's syndrome should be considered in the differential diagnosis of erythroderma. Topical steroids, systemic retinoids and systemic NSAIDs help, but many patients need methotrexate (Formulary 2, p. 400) and/or systemic steroids. There are early reports of biological agents such as those used for psoriasis being helpful (p. 403).

### Relapsing polychondritis

This process can affect any cartilage as the disorder is apparently caused by autoimmunity to type II collagen. The ears are the usual target, and often just one ear is involved at the start. The overlying skin becomes red, swollen and tender. Exacerbations and remissions may occur spontaneously. The cartilage of the nose and the tracheo-bronchial tree may be involved, so that patients develop floppy ears, a saddle nose, hoarseness, stridor and respiratory insufficiency. Aortic aneurysms are also seen. Treatment is with systemic steroids and NSAIDs. Tracheostomy may be necessary.

### Behçet's syndrome

Behçet's syndrome is discussed in Chapter 13 (p. 198).

### Polyarteritis nodosa

This is discussed in Chapter 8 (p. 115) but is considered by some to be a connective tissue disorder.

### Panniculitis

Panniculitis is an inflammation of the subcutaneous fat. It includes a number of diseases with different causes but a similar appearance; some are listed in Table 10.8.

#### *Presentation*

Most patients have tender ill-defined red nodules and indurated plaques on the lower legs, thighs and buttocks.

#### *Differential diagnosis*

Diagnosis can be tricky. Usually, the diagnosis is made from clinical suspicion linked to findings from the laboratories. If the panniculitis is unilateral, consider infection (including cellulitis), foreign bodies and phlebitis. If there is ulceration, consider lupus profundus, panniculitis-like subcutaneous T-cell lymphoma, polyarteritis and nodular vasculitis. The discharge from the ulcers associated with pancreatitis and $\alpha_1$-antitrypsin deficiency often drains

**Table 10.8** Some causes of panniculitis.

Infections, including cellulitis
Traumatic
Foreign bodies
Erythema nodosum (p. 112)
Erythema nodosum leprosum (leprosy)
Nodular vasculitis (p. 112)
Erythema induratum
Weber–Christian type
Polyarteritis nodosa (p. 115)
Associated with pancreatitis
Associated with SLE (lupus profundus)
Panniculitis-like subcutaneous T-cell lymphoma
Morphoea profunda (deep morphoea)
Cold-induced
Withdrawal of systemic steroids
Calciphylaxis
Superficial and migratory thrombophlebitis
Dermatoliposclerosis
Deficiency of $\alpha_1$-antitrypsin
Neurobiosis lipoidica
Gout
Traumatic fat necrosis
Factitial (e.g. from injection of milk)

SLE, systemic lupus erythematosus.

as an oily saponified fat. The most common bilateral panniculitis is erythema nodosum (p. 112). Calcifying panniculitis (calciphylaxis) usually occurs in the setting of haemodialysis, end-stage renal failure and secondary hyperparathyroidism. It presents acutely as livedo, stellate necrosis and eventual deep ulcerations.

### Course

This depends upon the cause. Migratory thrombophlebitis may be associated with underlying malignancy. In lupus profundus, a panniculitis is associated with discoid or systemic LE. Watch out if you suspect this, because subcutaneous T-cell lymphomas look like lupus profundus clinically and even histologically, but can cause rapid death. Causes of erythema nodosum are discussed in Chapter 8. Erythema induratum may be caused by tuberculosis. Erythema nodosum leprosum is a reactional state in leprosy (p. 230). Patients with pancreatitis may liberate enough lipase into the systemic circulation to cause cutaneous fat to liquefy

and discharge through the overlying skin. The Weber–Christian variant is associated with fever, but its cause is unknown.

### Investigations

The type of panniculitis can sometimes be identified by skin biopsy, which must include subcutaneous fat. Inflamed fat usually pulls easily off the dermis and punch biopsies are usually inadaquate. An incisional biopsy with scalpel can better provide adequate fatty tissue. When performing an incisional biopsy, ensure that there is enough extra tissue for culture for bacteria (including acid-fast organisms) and fungi. Pathologists often start by classifying panniculitis as septal (if the inflammation is mostly around the fibrous septae that separate fat lobules) or lobular (if the inflammation is primarily in the fat). They also note whether or not vascultitis is present. A complete blood count, ESR, chest X-ray, serum $\alpha_1$-antitrypsin and tests for antinuclear antibodies are often needed. Patients with pancreatitis have elevated levels of amylase and lipase, and abnormal tomography scans.

### Treatment

This depends upon the cause. Rest, elevation of affected extremities and local heat often help symptoms. NSAIDs may also bring help in the absence of specific therapy.

## Further reading

Anon. (2002) Review: systemic sclerosis: demographic, clinical, and serologic features and survival in 1,012 Italian patients. *Medicine (Baltimore)* **81**, 139–153.

Callen JP. (1998) Collagen-vascular diseases. *Medical Clinics of North America* **82**, 1217–1237.

Callen JP. (2000) Dermatomyositis. *Lancet* **355**, 53–57.

Camilleri MJ & Su WPD. (2003) Panniculitis. In: Freedberg IM, Eisen AZ, Wolff K, *et al.*, eds. *Dermatology in General Medicine*, 6th edn. McGraw-Hill, New York: 1047–1063.

Chung L, Lin J, Furst DE & Fiorentino D. (2006) Systemic and localized scleroderma. *Clinics in Dermatology* **24**, 374–392.

D'Cruz DP. (2006) Systemic lupus erythematosus. *British Medical Journal* **15**, 890–894.

Kuhn A, Lehmann P & Ruzicka T., eds. (2005) *Cutaneous Lupus Erythematosus*. Springer Verlag, Berlin.

Mimori T. (1999) Autoantibodies in connective tissue diseases: clinical significance and analysis of target autoantigens. *Internal Medicine* **7**, 523–532.

Patterson JW. (1991) Differential diagnosis of panniculitis. *Advances in Dermatology* **6**, 309–329.

# 11 Disorders of blood vessels and lymphatics

In functional diseases of the blood and lymphatic vessels, abnormalities of flow are reversible, and there is no vessel wall damage (e.g. in urticaria; discussed in Chapter 8). The diseases of structure include the many types of vasculitis; some of those with an immunological basis are also covered in Chapter 8. For convenience, disorders of the blood vessels are grouped according to the size and type of the vessels affected.

## Disorders involving small blood vessels

### Acrocyanosis

This type of 'poor circulation', often familial, is more common in females than males. The hands, feet, nose, ears and cheeks become blue–red and cold. The palms are often cold and clammy. The condition is caused by arteriolar constriction and dilatation of the subpapillary venous plexus, and by cold-induced increases in blood viscosity. The best answers are warm clothes and the avoidance of cold.

### Erythrocyanosis

This occurs in fat, often young, women. Purple–red mottled discoloration is seen over the fatty areas such as the buttocks, thighs and lower legs. Cold provokes it and causes an unpleasant burning sensation. Most young people outgrow the condition, but an area of acrocyanosis or erythrocyanosis may be the site where other disorders will settle in the future (e.g. perniosis, erythema induratum, lupus erythematosus, sarcoidosis, cutaneous tuberculosis and leprosy). Weight reduction is often recommended.

### Perniosis (chilblains)

In this common, sometimes familial, condition, inflamed purple–pink swellings appear on the fingers, toes and, rarely, ears (Fig. 11.1). They arrive with winter and are induced by cold. They are painful, and itchy or burning on rewarming. Occasionally they ulcerate. Chilblains are caused by a combination of arteriolar and venular constriction, the latter predominating on rewarming with exudation of fluid into the tissues. Warm housing and clothing help. Topical remedies rarely work, but the oral calcium-channel blocker nifedipine may be useful (p. 150). The blood pressure should be monitored at the start of treatment and at return visits. The vasodilator nicotinamide (500 mg three times daily) may be helpful alone or in addition to calcium-channel blockers. Sympathectomy may be advised in severe cases.

### Erythromelalgia

This is a rare condition in which the extremities become red, hot and painful when they or their owner are exposed to heat. The condition may be idiopathic, or caused by a myeloproliferative disease (e.g. polycythaemia rubra vera or thrombocythaemia), lupus erythematosus, rheumatoid

**Fig. 11.1** The typical purplish swellings of chilblains.

arthritis, diabetes, degenerative peripheral vascular disease or hypertension. Aspirin gives symptomatic relief. Alternatives include non-steroidal anti-inflammatory drugs (NSAIDs), beta-blockers, pentoxifylline (oxpentifylline) and the serotonin reuptake inhibitor venlafaxine.

## Erythemas

Erythema accompanies all inflammatory skin conditions, but the term 'the erythemas' is usually applied to a group of conditions with redness but without primary scaling. Such areas are seen in some bacterial and viral infections such as toxic shock syndrome and measles. Drugs are another common cause (Chapter 25). If no cause is obvious, the rash is often called a 'toxic' or 'reactive' erythema.

When erythema is associated with oedema ('urticated erythema') it becomes palpable.

### Figurate erythemas

These are chronic eruptions, made up of bizarre serpiginous and erythematous rings. In the past most carried Latin labels; happily, these eruptions are now grouped under the general term of 'figurate erythemas'. Underlying malignancy, a connective tissue disorder, a bacterial, fungal or yeast infection, worm infestation, drug sensitivity and rheumatic heart disease should be excluded, but often the cause remains obscure.

### Palmar erythema

This may be an isolated finding in a normal person or be familial. Sometimes it is seen in pregnancy, liver disease or rheumatoid arthritis. Often associated with spider telangiectases, it may be caused by increased circulating oestrogens.

## Telangiectases

This term refers to permanently dilated and visible small vessels in the skin. They appear as linear, punctate or stellate crimson–purple markings. The common causes are given in Table 11.1.

**Table 11.1** Causes of telangiectasia.

| | |
|---|---|
| *Primary telangiectasia* | |
| Hereditary haemorrhagic telangiectasia | Autosomal dominant |
| | Nose and gastrointestinal bleeds |
| | Lesions on face |
| Ataxia telangiectasia | Autosomal recessive |
| | Telangiectases develop between the ages of 3 and 5 years |
| | Cerebellar ataxia |
| | Recurrent respiratory infections |
| | Immunological abnormalities |
| Generalized essential telangiectasia | Runs benign course |
| | No other associations |
| Unilateral naevoid telangiectasia | May occur in pregnancy or in females on oral contraceptive |
| | |
| *Secondary telangiectasia* | |
| Rosacea | Associated with centrofacial erythema (erythematotelangiectatic subtype) |
| Sun-damaged skin | Sun-exposed areas, especially face and neck |
| Atrophy | Seen on exposed skin of elderly, after topical steroid applications, after X-irradiation and with poikiloderma |
| Connective tissue disorders | Always worth inspecting nail folds |
| | Mat-like on the face in systemic sclerosis |
| Prolonged vasodilatation | For example, with venous hypertension |
| Mastocytosis | Accompanying a rare and diffuse variant |
| Liver disease | Multiple spider telangiectases are common |
| Drugs | Nifedipine |
| Tumours | A tell-tale sign in nodular basal cell carcinomas |

## Spider naevi

These stellate telangiectases do look rather like spiders, with legs radiating from a central, often palpable, feeding vessel. If the diagnosis is in doubt, press on the central feeding vessel with the corner of a glass slide and the entire lesion will disappear. Spider naevi are seen frequently on the faces of normal children, and may erupt in pregnancy or be the presenting sign of liver disease, with many lesions on the upper trunk. Liver function should be checked in those with many spider naevi. The central vessel can be destroyed by electrodessication without local anaesthesia or with a pulsed dye laser (p. 379).

## Livedo reticularis

This cyanosis of the skin is net-like or marbled and caused by stasis in the capillaries furthest from their arterial supply: at the periphery of the inverted cone supplied by a dermal arteriole (see Fig. 2.1). It may be widespread or localized. 'Cutis marmorata' is the name given to the mottling of the skin seen in many normal children. It is physiological and disappears on warming, whereas true livedo reticularis remains (Fig. 11.2).

The causes of livedo reticularis are listed in Table 11.2. Livedo vasculitis and cutaneous polyarteritis are forms of vasculitis associated with livedo reticularis (Chapter 8). Localized forms suggest localized blood vessel injury (e.g. from cholesterol emboli).

**Fig. 11.2** The mottled pattern of livedo reticularis.

**Table 11.2** Causes of livedo reticularis.

*Physiological*
Cutis marmorata

*Vessel wall disease*
Atherosclerosis
Connective tissue disorders (especially polyarteritis, livedo vasculitis and systemic lupus erythematosus)
Syphilis
Tuberculosis

*Hyperviscosity states*
Polycythaemia/thrombocythaemia
Macroglobulinaemia

*Cryopathies*
Cryoglobulinaemia
Cold agglutinaemia

*Autoimmune*
Antiphospholipid syndrome

Congenital

Idiopathic

## Antiphospholipid syndrome

Some patients with an apparently idiopathic livedo reticularis develop progressive disease in their peripheral, cerebral, coronary and renal arteries. Others, usually women, have multiple arterial or venous thromboembolic episodes accompanying livedo reticularis. Recurrent spontaneous abortions and intra-uterine fetal growth retardation are also features. Prolongation of the activated partial thromboplastin time (APTT) and the presence of antiphospholipid antibodies (either anticardiolipin antibody or lupus anticoagulant, or both) help to identify this syndrome. Systemic lupus erythematosus should be excluded (Chapter 10).

## Erythema ab igne

This appearance is also determined by the underlying vascular network. Its reticulate pigmented erythema, with variable scaling, is caused by damage from long-term exposure to local heat – usually from an open fire, hot water bottle or heating pad. If on one side of the leg, it gives a clue to the side of the fire on which granny likes to sit (Fig. 11.3). The condition has become less common with the advent of central heating.

**Fig. 11.3** Erythema ab igne: this patient persisted in sitting too close to an open fire and burned herself.

**Table 11.3** Causes of flushing.

*Physiological*
Emotional
Menopausal
Exercise

*Foods*
Hot drinks
Spicy foods
Additives (monosodium glutamate)
Alcohol (especially in oriental people)

*Drugs*
Vasodilators including nicotinic acid, hydralazine
Nitrates and sildenafil
Calcium-channel blockers including nifedipine
Disulfiram or chlorpropamide + alcohol
Cholinergic agents

*Pathological*
Mastocytosis
Carcinoid tumours – with asthma and diarrhoea
Phaeochromocytoma (type producing adrenaline) – with episodic headaches (caused by transient hypertension) and palpitations
Dumping syndrome
Migraine headaches

## Flushing

This transient vasodilatation of the face may spread to the neck, upper chest and, more rarely, other parts of the body. There is no sharp distinction between flushing and blushing apart from the emotional provocation of the latter. The mechanism varies with the many causes that are listed in Table 11.3. Paroxysmal flushing ('hot flushes'), common at the menopause, is associated with the pulsatile release of luteinizing hormone from the pituitary, as a consequence of low circulating oestrogens and failure of normal negative feedback. However, luteinizing hormone itself cannot be responsible for flushing as this can occur after hypophysectomy. It is possible that menopausal flushing is mediated by central mechanisms involving encephalins. Hot flushes can usually be helped by oestrogen replacement.

Alcohol-induced flushing is most commonly seen in oriental people. Ethanol is broken down to acetaldehyde by alcohol dehydrogenase and acetaldehyde is metabolized to acetic acid by aldehyde dehydrogenase (Fig. 11.4). Acetaldehyde accumulation is in part responsible for flushing. Oriental people may have not only a high-activity variant of

**Fig. 11.4** The metabolism of ethanol.

alcohol dehydrogenase, but also defective aldehyde dehydrogenase. Disulfiram (Antabuse) and, to a lesser extent, chlorpropamide inhibit aldehyde dehydrogenase so that some individuals taking these drugs may flush.

## Arterial disease

### Raynaud's phenomenon

This is a paroxysmal pallor of the digits provoked by cold or, rarely, emotional stress. At first the top of

**Fig. 11.5** Digital gangrene. In this case caused by frostbite.

one or more fingers becomes white. On rewarming, a painful cyanosis appears and the area turns red before the hands return to their normal colour. In severe disease the fingers lose pulp substance, ulcerate or become gangrenous (Fig. 11.5). Some causes are listed in Table 11.4. Raynaud's disease, often familial, is the name given when no cause can be found. However, some patients with what seems to be Raynaud's disease will later develop a connective tissue disease, usually scleroderma.

The main treatment is to protect the vulnerable digits from cold. Warm clothing reduces the need for peripheral vasoconstriction to conserve heat. Smoking should be abandoned. Calcium-channel blockers (e.g. nifedipine 10–30 mg three times daily) are the most effective agents although they work best in patients with primary Raynaud's disease. Patients should be warned about dizziness caused by postural hypotension. Initially, it is worth giving nifedipine as a 5-mg test dose with monitoring of the blood pressure in the clinic. If this is tolerated satisfactorily the starting dosage should be 5 mg/day, increasing by 5 mg every 5 days until a therapeutic dose is achieved (e.g. 5–20 mg three times daily) or until intolerable side-effects occur. The blood pressure should be monitored before each incremental increase in the dosage. Diltiazem (30–60 mg three times daily) is less effective than nifedipine but has fewer side-effects. The systemic vasodilator inositol nicotinate may help, and a combination of low-dose acetylsalicylic acid and the antiplatelet drug dipyridamole is also worth trying.

**Table 11.4** Causes of Raynaud's phenomenon.

*Familial*
Raynaud's disease

*Connective tissue diseases*
Systemic sclerosis
Lupus erythematosus
Mixed connective tissue disease

*Arterial occlusion*
Thoracic outlet syndrome
Atherosclerosis
Endarteritis obliterans

*Repeated trauma*
Pneumatic hammer/drill operators ('vibration white finger')

*Hyperviscosity*
Polycythaemia
Macroglobulinaemia

*Cryopathies*
Cryoglobulinaemia
Cryofibrinogenaemia
Cold agglutinaemia

*Neurological disease*
Peripheral neuropathy
Syringomyelia

*Toxins*
Ergot
Vinyl-chloride

Sustained-release glycerol trinitrate patches, applied once daily, may reduce the severity and frequency of attacks and allow reduction in the dosage of calcium-channel blockers and vasodilators. Slow intravenous infusions with prostaglandin $E_1$ or prostacyclin help some severe cases.

## Polyarteritis nodosa

This is discussed in Chapter 8.

## Temporal arteritis

Here the brunt is borne by the larger vessels of the head and neck. The condition affects elderly people and may be associated with polymyalgia rheumatica. The classic site is the temporal arteries, which become tender and pulseless, in association with severe headaches. Rarely, necrotic ulcers appear on the scalp. Blindness may follow if the ophthalmic arteries are involved and, to reduce this risk, systemic steroids should be given as soon as the diagnosis has been made. In active phases the erythrocyte sedimentation rate (ESR) is high and its level can be used to guide treatment, which is often prolonged.

## Atherosclerosis

This occlusive disease, most common in developed countries, is not discussed in detail here, but involvement of the large arteries of the legs is of concern to dermatologists. It may cause intermittent claudication, nocturnal cramps, ulcers or gangrene. These may develop slowly over the years or within minutes if a thrombus forms on an atheromatous plaque. The feet are cold and pale, the skin is often atrophic, with little hair, and peripheral pulses are diminished or absent.

Investigations should include urine testing to exclude diabetes mellitus. Fasting plasma lipids (cholesterol, triglycerides and lipoproteins) should be checked in the young, especially if there is a family history of vascular disease. Doppler ultrasound measurements help to distinguish atherosclerotic from venous leg ulcers in the elderly (p. 156). Complete assessment is best carried out by a specialist in peripheral vascular disease or a vascular surgeon.

## Arterial emboli

Emboli may lodge in arteries supplying the skin and cause gangrene, ulcers or necrotic papules, depending on the size of the vessel obstructed. Causes include dislodged thrombi (usually from areas of atherosclerosis), fat emboli (after major trauma), infected emboli (e.g. gonococcal septicaemia or subacute bacterial endocarditis) and tumour emboli.

## Pressure sores (Fig. 11.6)

Sustained or repeated pressure on skin over bony prominences can cause ischaemia and pressure sores. These are common in patients over 70 years old who are confined to hospital, especially those with a fractured neck of femur. The morbidity and mortality of those with deep ulcers are high.

**Fig. 11.6** A deep pressure sore on the buttock.

### *Cause*

The skin and underlying tissues need to be continually nourished with oxygen and nutrients. Pressure prevents adequate blood flow, and if prolonged can lead to tissue death. Healthy people get neurological signals that cause them to shift position. The main factors responsible for pressure sores are:
1 prolonged immobility and recumbency (e.g. caused by a stroke, paraplegia, arthritis senility);
2 vascular disease (e.g. atherosclerosis);
3 neurological disease causing diminished sensation (e.g. in paraplegia);
4 malnutrition, severe systemic disease and general debility.

### *Clinical features*

The sore begins as an area of erythema which progresses to a superficial blister or erosion. If pressure continues, deeper damage occurs with the development of a black eschar which, when removed or shed, reveals a deep ulcer, often colonized by *Pseudomonas aeruginosa*. The skin overlying the sacrum, greater trochanter, ischial tuberosity, the heel and the lateral malleolus is especially at risk.

### Management

The following are important.

1 Prevention: by turning recumbent patients regularly and using antipressure mattresses for susceptible patients.

2 Treatment of malnutrition and the general condition.

3 Débridement. Regular cleansing with normal saline or 0.5% aqueous silver nitrate. Antibacterial preparations locally (Formulary 1, p. 388). Absorbent dressings (Formulary 1, p. 391). Hydrocolloid wafer dressings if there is no infection. Appropriate systemic antibiotic if an infection is spreading.

4 Plastic surgical reconstruction may be indicated in the young when the ulcer is clean.

## Venous disease

### Deep vein thrombosis

The common causes are listed in Table 11.5.

**Table 11.5** Some causes of deep vein thrombosis.

*Abnormalities of the vein wall*
Trauma (operations and injuries)
Chemicals (intravenous infusions)
Neighbouring infection (e.g. in leg ulcer)
Tumour (local invasion)

*Abnormalities of blood flow*
Stasis (immobility, operations, long aircraft flights, pressure, pregnancy, myocardial infarction, heart failure, incompetent valves)
Impaired venous return

*Abnormalities of clotting*
Platelets increased or sticky (thrombocythaemia, polycythaemia vera, leukaemia, trauma, splenectomy)
Decreased fibrinolysis (postoperative)
Deficiency of clotting factors (e.g. antithrombin, proteins C and S, factor V Leiden)
Alteration in clotting factors (oral contraceptive, infection, leukaemia, pregnancy, shock and haemorrhage)
Antiphospholipid antibody

*Unknown mechanisms*
Malignancy (thrombophlebitis migrans)
Smoking
Behçet's syndrome
Inflammatory bowel disease

The onset may be 'silent' or heralded by pain in the calf, often about 10 days after immobilization following surgery or a long-haul aeroplane flight, parturition or an infection. The leg becomes swollen and cyanotic distal to the thrombus. The calf may hurt when handled or if the foot is dorsiflexed (Homan's sign). Sometimes a pulmonary embolus is the first sign of a silent deep vein thrombosis.

Suitable investigations include venography, Doppler ultrasonography – which can only detect thrombi in large veins at, or above, the popliteal fossa – and $^{125}$I-fibrinogen isotope leg scanning.

Treatment is anticoagulation with heparin and later with a coumarin. The value of thrombolytic regimens has yet to be assessed properly. Prevention is important. Deep vein thrombosis after a surgical operation is less frequent now, with early postoperative mobilization, regular leg exercises, the use of elastic stockings over the operative period and prophylaxis with low-dose heparin. A mini-aspirin taken before a long flight (providing there is no contraindication), elastic stockings and leg exercises during the flight are sensible precautions.

### Thrombophlebitis

This is thrombosis in an inflamed vein. If the affected vein is varicose or superficial it will be red and feel like a tender cord. The leg may be diffusely inflamed, making a distinction from cellulitis difficult (p. 225). There may be fever, leucocytosis and a high ESR. Migratory superficial thrombophlebitis should arouse suspicion of an underlying malignancy or pancreatic disease.

Treatment is based on rest, local heat and NSAIDs. Antibiotics or anticoagulants rarely help.

### Venous hypertension, the gravitational syndrome and venous leg ulceration

Ulcers of the lower leg, secondary to venous hypertension, have an estimated prevalence of around 1%, are more common in women than in men, and account for some 85% of all leg ulcers seen in the UK and USA.

together – the perforating or communicating veins (Fig. 11.7). When the leg muscles contract, blood in the deep veins is squeezed back, against gravity, to the heart (the calf muscle pump); reflux is prevented by valves. When the muscles relax, with the help of gravity, blood from the superficial veins passes into the deep veins via the communicating vessels. If the valves in the deep and communicating veins are incompetent, the calf muscle pump now pushes blood into the superficial veins, where the pressure remains high ('venous hypertension') instead of dropping during exercise. This persisting venous hypertension enlarges the capillary bed; white cells accumulate here and are then activated (by hypoxic endothelial cells), releasing oxygen free radicals and other toxic products which cause local tissue destruction and ulceration. The increased venous pressure also forces fibrinogen and $\alpha_2$-macroglobulin out through the capillary walls; these macromolecules trap growth and repair factors so that minor traumatic wounds cannot be repaired and an ulcer develops. Patients with these changes develop lipodermatosclerosis (p. 154) and have a high serum fibrinogen and reduced blood fibrinolytic activity. The combination of pressure, shearing force (as generated by sliding down a bed), friction and moisture on this background all greatly increases the risks of developing an ulcer. Figure 11.8 shows the factors causing venous ulceration.

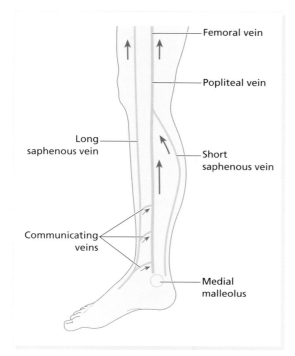

**Fig. 11.7**  The direction of blood flow in normal leg veins.

## Cause

Satisfactory venous drainage of the leg requires three sets of veins: deep veins surrounded by muscles; superficial veins; and the veins connecting these

**Fig. 11.8**  Factors causing venous leg ulceration.

## Clinical features

Venous hypertension is heralded by a feeling of heaviness in the legs and by pitting oedema. Other signs include:

1 red or bluish discoloration;
2 loss of hair;
3 brown pigmentation (mainly haemosiderin from the breakdown of extravasated red blood cells) and scattered petechiae;
4 atrophie blanche (ivory white scarring with dilated capillary loops; Fig. 11.9); and
5 induration, caused by inflammation, fibrosis and oedema of the dermis and subcutis – sometimes called 'lipodermatosclerosis'.

Ulceration is most common near the medial malleolus (Fig. 11.10). In contrast to arterial ulcers, which are usually deep and round, with a punched-out appearance, venous ulcers are often large but shallow, with prominent granulation tissue in their bases. Incompetent perforating branches (blow-outs) between the superficial and deep veins are best felt with the patient standing. Under favourable conditions the exudative phase gives way to a granulating and healing phase, signalled by a blurring of the ulcer margin, ingrowth of skin from it, and the appearance of scattered small grey epithelial islands over the base. Prolonged lipodermatosclerosis gives the leg the look and feel of an inverted champagne bottle.

## Complications

Bacterial colonisation is inevitable in a long-standing ulcer, but needs systemic antibiotics only if there is pyrexia, a purulent discharge, rapid extension or an increase in pain, cellulitis, lymphangitis or septicaemia.

Eczema (p. 100) is common around venous ulcers. Allergic contact dermatitis (p. 86) is a common complication and should be suspected if the rash worsens, itches or fails to improve with local treatment. Lanolin, parabens (a preservative) and neomycin are the most common culprits.

Malignant change can occur. If an ulcer has a hyperplastic base or a rolled edge, biopsy may be needed to rule out a squamous cell carcinoma (Fig. 11.11).

**Fig. 11.9** Irregular areas of whitish scarring and dilated capillary loops – the changes of atrophie blanche.

**Fig. 11.10** Large venous ulcer overlying the medial malleolus.

**Fig. 11.11** Chronic ulcer failing to respond to treatment. Biopsy, taken from rolled edge, excluded malignant change.

**Table 11.6** Causes of leg ulceration.

*Venous hypertension*
See Table 11.5

*Arterial disease*
Atherosclerosis
Buerger's disease
Giant cell arteritis
Polyarteritis nodosa
Systemic sclerosis

*Small-vessel disease*
Diabetes mellitus
Systemic lupus erythematosus
Rheumatoid arthritis
Systemic sclerosis
Allergic vasculitis

*Abnormalities of blood*
Immune complex disease
Sickle cell anaemia
Cryoglobulinaemia
Pyoderma gangrenosum

*Neuropathy*
Diabetes mellitus
Leprosy
Syphilis
Syringomyelia
Peripheral neuropathy

*Infection*
'Tropical ulcer' (mycobacterium)
Tuberculosis
Deep fungal infections

*Tumour*
Squamous cell carcinoma
Malignant melanoma
Kaposi's sarcoma
Basal cell carcinoma
Lymphoma

*Trauma*
Injury
Factitial
Iatrogenic

**Fig. 11.12** Large, shallow and recalcitrant ulcer complicating rheumatoid arthritis.

the ulcers may be deep and gangrenous. Islands of intact skin are characteristically seen within the ulcer. Claudication may be present and peripheral pulses absent. If the blockage is in the larger arteries.

*Vasculitic* These ulcers start as painful palpable purpuric lesions, turning into small punched-out ulcers. The involvement of larger vessels is heralded by livedo and stellate neurosis that may ulcerate. Sometimes a digit may become gangrenous. The intractable, deep, sharply demarcated ulcers of rheumatoid arthritis are caused by an underlying vasculitis (Fig. 11.12).

*Thrombotic ulcers* Skin infarction (Fig. 11.13), leading to ulceration, may be caused by embolism or by the increased coagulability of polycythaemia or cryoglobulinaemia.

### Differential diagnosis

The main causes of leg ulceration are given in Table 11.6. The most important differences between venous and other leg ulcers are the following.

*Atherosclerotic* These ulcers are more common on the toes, dorsum of foot, heel, calf and shin, and are unrelated to perforating veins. Their edges are often sharply defined, their outline may be polycyclic and

**Fig. 11.13** This ulcer on the foot was not caused by venous insufficiency but cryoglobulins were detected.

*Infective ulcers* Infection is now a rare cause of leg ulcers in the UK but ulcers caused by tuberculosis, leprosy, atypical mycobacteria, diphtheria and deep fungal infections, such as sporotrichosis or chromoblastomycosis, are still seen in the tropics.

*Panniculitic ulcers* These may appear at odd sites, such as the thighs, buttocks or backs of the calves. The most common types of panniculitis that ulcerate are lupus panniculitis, panniculitic T-cell lymphoma, pancreatic panniculitis and erythema induratum (p. 143).

*Malignant ulcers* Those caused by a squamous cell carcinoma (p. 303) are the most common, but both malignant melanomas (p. 306) and basal cell carcinomas (p. 300) can present as flat lesions, which expand, crust and ulcerate. Furthermore, squamous cell carcinoma can arise in any long-standing ulcer, whatever its cause. Ulcers form over CD30 anaplastic large cell lymphomas, panniculitic T-cell lymphomas and tumour stage mycosis fungoides (p . 319).

*Pyoderma gangrenosum* (p. 333) These large and rapidly spreading ulcers may be circular or polycyclic, and have a blue, indurated, undermined or pustular margin. Pyoderma gangrenosum may complicate rheumatoid arthritis, Crohn's disease, ulcerative colitis or blood dyscrasias.

### Investigations

Most chronic leg ulcers are venous, but other causes should be considered if the signs are atypical. In patients with venous ulcers, a search for contributory factors, such as obesity, peripheral artery disease, cardiac failure or arthritis, is always worthwhile. Investigations should include the following.
● Blood glucose.
● Full blood count to detect anaemia, which will delay healing.
● Swabbing for pathogens (p. 154).
● Venography, colour flow duplex scanning and the measurement of ambulatory venous pressure help to detect surgically remediable causes of venous incompetence.

● Doppler ultrasound may help to assess arterial circulation when atherosclerosis is likely. It seldom helps if the dorsalis pedis or posterior tibial pulses can easily be felt. If the maximal systolic ankle pressure divided by the systolic brachial pressure ('ankle brachial pressure index') is greater than 0.8, the ulcer is unlikely to be caused by arterial disease.
● Cardiac evaluation for congestive failure.

### Treatment

Venous ulcers will not heal if the leg remains swollen and the patient chair-bound. Pressure bandages, leg elevation and bed rest take priority over other measures but not for atherosclerotic ulcers with an already precarious arterial supply. A common error is to use local treatment that is too elaborate. As a last resort, admission to hospital for elevation and intensive treatment may be needed, but the results are not encouraging; patients may stay in the ward for many months only to have their apparently well-healed ulcers break down rapidly when they go home.

The list of therapies is extensive. They can be divided into the following categories: physical, local, oral and surgical.

### Physical measures

*Compression bandages and stockings* Compression bandaging, with the compression graduated so that it is greatest at the ankle and least at the top of the bandage, is vital for most venous ulcers; it reduces oedema and aids venous return. The bandages are applied over the ulcer dressing, from the forefoot to just below the knee. Self-adhesive bandages are convenient and have largely replaced elasticated bandages. Bandages can stay on for 2–7 days at a time and are left on at night. Various compression bandaging systems are available, comprising two or three extensible bandages applied over a layer of orthopaedic wool. These require changing only once a week and are very effective. The combined layers give a 40-mmHg compression at the ankle. Once an ulcer has healed, a graduated compression stocking from toes to knee (or preferably thigh) should be prescribed, preferably of class 3, providing pressures of 25–35 mmHg at the ankle. A foam or felt pad may be worn under the stockings to protect vulnerable areas against minor trauma. The stocking should be put on before rising from bed. Care must be taken with all forms of compression to ensure that the arterial supply is satisfactory and not compromised.

*Elevation of the affected limb* Preferably above the hips, this aids venous drainage, decreases oedema and raises oxygen tension in the limb. Patients should rest with their bodies horizontal and their legs up for at least 2 h every afternoon. The foot of the bed should be raised by at least 15 cm; it is not enough just to put a pillow under the feet.

*Walking* Walking, in moderation, is beneficial, but prolonged standing or sitting with dependent legs is not.

*Physiotherapy* Some physiotherapists are good at persuading venous ulcers to heal. Their secret lies in better compliance with therapies such as leg exercises, elevation, gentle massage, intermittent pneumatic compression and graduated compression bandaging. They also teach patients tricks to help them pull on tighter stockings.

*Diet* Many patients are obese and should lose weight.

### Local therapy

Remember that many ulcers will heal with no treatment at all, but if their blood flow is compromised, they will not heal despite meticulous care. In venous ulceration, the blood flow is always compromised.

Local therapy should be chosen to:
- maintain a moist environment;
- absorb excess exudates;
- reduce the pain;
- control the odour;
- protect the surrounding skin;
- remove surface debris;
- promote re-epithelialization; and
- make optimal use of nursing time.

There are many preparations to choose from; those we have found most useful are listed in Formulary 1 (p. 391).

**Fig. 11.14** Clean healing ulcer. Weekly dressing would be suitable.

*Clean ulcers* (Fig. 11.14) Low-adherent dressings are useful in patients with fragile skin. They reduce adherence at the wound bed and allow passage of exudate to an overlying dressing. They are usually made of paraffin tulle, either plain or impregnated with 0.5% chlorhexidine, and need to be changed only once or twice a week. The area should be cleaned gently with arachis oil, 5% hydrogen peroxide or saline before the next dressing is applied. Sometimes, immersing the whole ulcer in a tub of warm water helps to loosen or dissolve adherent crusts. The prolonged use of antiseptics may be harmful.

Semi-permeable films (e.g. Tegaderm, Mefilm) are porous to air and water vapour but not fluids or bacteria, and are suitable for shallow ulcers with low to medium exudate, in which they encourage a moist wound environment and allow healing cytokines in the exudates to do their work. More heavily exudative wounds can be dressed with either alginate or foam dressings. Alginates (e.g. Kaltostat, Sorbsan) produced from the naturally occurring alginic acid found in some seaweeds are highly absorbent, and useful in cavities or undermined wounds but need to be changed daily. Foam dressings are made from polyurethane or silicon and are better in shallow wounds.

Necrotic or sloughy wounds should treated with hydrogel dressings, which promote a moist wound environment, and subsequent débridement of non-viable tissue. Hydrocolloid sheets (e.g. DuoDERM, Granuflex) are almost impermeable to water vapour, and can rehydrate dry eschar while hydrocolloid fibres (e.g. Aquacel) are highly absorbent for exudative wounds.

Medicated bandages (Formulary 1, p. 391) based on zinc paste, with ichthammol, or with calamine and clioquinol, are useful when there is much surrounding eczema, and can be used for all types of ulcers, even infected exuding ones. The bandage is applied in strips from the foot to below the knee. Worsening of eczema under a medicated bandage may signal the development of allergic contact dermatitis to a component of the paste, most often parabens (a preservative) or cetostearyl alcohols.

*Infected ulcers* (Fig. 11.15) The majority of patients will be helped with local treatment alone. Infected

**Fig. 11.15** Infected ulcer with sloughing. Tendon visible at bottom of figure. Hospital admission and frequent dressings needed to save leg.

ulcers have to be cleaned and dressed more often than clean ones, sometimes even twice daily. Useful preparations include 0.5% silver nitrate, 0.25% sodium hypochlorite, 0.25% acetic acid, potassium permanganate (1 in 10,000 dilution) and 5% hydrogen peroxide, all made up in aqueous solution and applied as compresses with or without occlusion. Helpful potions include 1.5% hydrogen peroxide, 20% benzoyl peroxide, 1% silver sulphadiazine and 10% povidone-iodine (Formulary 1, p. 391). The main function of starch polymer beads within cadexomer iodine is to absorb exudate. Although antibiotic tulles are easy to apply and are well tolerated, they should not be used for long periods as they can induce bacterial resistance and sensitize. Resistance is not such a problem with povidone-iodine, and a readily applied non-adherent dressing impregnated with this antiseptic may be useful. Surrounding eczema is helped by weak or moderate strength local steroids, which must never be put on the ulcer itself. Lassar's paste, zinc cream or paste bandages (see above) are suitable alternatives.

### Oral treatment

The following may be helpful.

*Diuretics* Pressure bandaging is more important as the oedema associated with venous ulceration is largely mechanical. Diuretics will combat the oedema of cardiac failure.

*Analgesics* Adequate analgesia is important. Aspirin may not be well tolerated by the elderly. Paracetamol (acetaminophen in the USA) or ibuprofen are often adequate but dihydrocodeine may be required. Analgesia may be needed only when the dressing is changed.

*Antibiotics* Just because bacteria can be isolated from an ulcer does not mean that antibiotics should be prescribed. Ulcers need not be 'sterilized' by local or systemic antibiotics. Short courses of systemic antibiotics should be reserved for spreading infections characterized by an enlarging ulcer, increased redness around the ulcer and lymphangitis. Sometimes they are tried for pain or even odour. Bacteriological guidance is needed and the drugs used include erythromycin and flucloxacillin (streptococcal or staphylococcal cellulitis), metronidazole (*Bacteroides* infection) and ciprofloxacin (*Pseudomonas aeruginosa* infection). Bacterial infection may prejudice the outcome of skin grafting.

*Ferrous sulphate and folic acid* For anaemia.

*Zinc sulphate* May help to promote healing, especially if the plasma zinc level is low.

*Pentoxyfylline* (oxypentifylline) is fibrinolytic, increases the deformability of red and white blood cells, decreases blood viscosity and diminishes platelet adhesiveness. It may speed the healing of venous ulcers if used with compression bandages.

### Surgery

Autologous pinch, split-thickness or mesh grafts have a place. Human skin equivalents comprising a cultured bilayer of epidermal keratinocytes and dermal fibroblasts have been used as grafts with promising results, but this treatment is not widely available. Remember, the cause of the ulcer and slow healing is an inadequate blood supply. Local surgery, like local topical therapy, will not be successful if the skin continues to be deprived of essential nutrients.

Venous surgery on younger patients with varicose veins may prevent recurrences, if the deep veins are competent. Patients with atherosclerotic ulcers should see a vascular surgeon for assessment. Some blockages are surgically remediable.

> **Leaning points**
>
> - An ulcer will never heal, whatever you put on it, if the ankle is oedematous or the blood flow is inadequate
> - Support stockings are better than fancy creams
> - Watch out for contact allergy to local applications
> - Never put topical steroids on ulcers
> - Most ulcers, despite positive bacteriology, are not much helped by systemic antibiotics
> - Avoid compression bandaging if the arterial supply is compromised

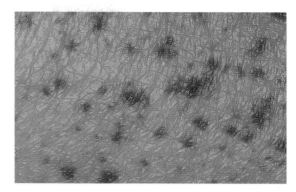

**Fig. 11.16** Typical purpura, which is not abolished by pressure.

## Purpura

Purpura (Fig. 11.16), petechiae and ecchymoses may be caused by a coagulation or platelet disorder, or by an abnormality of the vessel wall or the surrounding dermis. Some common causes are listed in Table 11.7. In general, coagulation defects give rise to ecchymoses and external bleeding. Platelet defects present more often as purpura, although bleeding and ecchymoses can still occur. Vasculitis of small vessels causes purpura, often palpable and painful, but not bleeding; this is discussed in Chapter 8. Purpura from vasodilatation and gravity is seen in many diseases of the legs, especially in the elderly (defective dermis around the blood vessels), and seldom requires extensive investigation.

Cryoglobulinaemia is a rare cause of purpura, which is most prominent on exposed parts. It may also cause cold urticaria (p. 105) and livedo reticularis (p. 148). The condition may be idiopathic, or secondary to myeloma, leukaemia, hepatitis C infection or an autoimmune disease.

### Investigations

The most common cause of purpura is trauma, especially to the thin sun-damaged skin of elderly forearms. When purpura has no obvious cause, investigations should include a platelet count, prothrombin time, APTT, a full blood count and biochemical screen. Electrophoresis is needed to exclude hypergammaglobulinaemia

**Table 11.7** Causes of intracutaneous bleeding.

*Coagulation defects*
Inherited defects (e.g. haemophilia, Christmas disease)
Connective tissue disorders
Disseminated intravascular coagulation
Paraproteinaemias (e.g. macroglobulinaemia)
Acquired defects (e.g. liver disease, anticoagulant
    therapy, vitamin K deficiency, drugs)

*Platelet defects*
Thrombocytopenia
Idiopathic
Connective tissue disorders, especially lupus
    erythematosus
Disseminated intravascular coagulation
Haemolytic anaemia
Hypersplenism
Giant haemangiomas (Kasabach–Merritt syndrome)
Bone marrow damage (cytostatic drugs, leukaemia,
    carcinoma)
Drugs (quinine, aspirin, thiazides and sulphonamides)
Abnormal function
von Willebrand's disease
Drugs (e.g. aspirin)

*Vascular defect*
Raised intravascular pressure (coughing, vomiting,
    venous hypertension, gravitational)
Vasculitis (including Henoch–Schönlein purpura)
Infections (e.g. meningococcal septicaemia, Rocky
    Mountain spotted fever)
Drugs (carbromal, aspirin, sulphonamides, quinine,
    phenylbutazone and gold salts)
Painful bruising syndrome

*Idiopathic*
Progressive pigmented dermatoses (Fig. 11.17)
Lack of support from surrounding dermis
Senile purpura
Topical or systemic corticosteroid therapy
Scurvy (perifollicular purpura)
Lichen sclerosus et atrophicus
Systemic amyloidosis

**Fig. 11.17** This gingery colour is typical of haemosiderin rather than melanin. It is caused by capillary fragility.

and paraproteinaemia. Cryoglobulinaemia should also be excluded. To help detect a consumptive coagulopathy, a coagulation screen, including measurement of fibrinogen and fibrin degradation products, may be necessary. The bleeding time and a Hess tourniquet test for capillary fragility help less often. Skin biopsy will confirm a small vessel vasculitis, if the purpura is palpable.

### Treatment

Treat the underlying condition. Replacement of relevant blood constituents may be needed initially. Systemic steroids are usually effective in vasculitis (Chapter 8).

## Disorders of the lymphatics

### Lymphoedema

The skin overlying chronic lymphoedema is firm and pits poorly. Long-standing lymphoedema may lead to gross, almost furry, hyperkeratosis, as in the so-called 'mossy foot'.

#### Cause

Lymphoedema may be primary or secondary. The primary forms are developmental defects, although signs may only appear in early puberty or even in adulthood. Sometimes lymphoedema involves only one leg. Secondary causes are listed in Table 11.8.

**Table 11.8** Causes of secondary lymphoedema.

*Recurrent lymphangitis*
Erysipelas
Infected pompholyx

*Lymphatic obstruction*
Filariasis
Granuloma inguinale
Tuberculosis
Tumour

*Lymphatic destruction*
Surgery
Radiation therapy
Tumour

*Functional*
Venous stasis
Congestive heart failure
Hypoalbuminemia

*Uncertain aetiology*
Rosacea
Melkersson–Rosenthal syndrome (facial nerve palsy, fissuring of tongue and lymphoedema of lip)
Yellow nail syndrome

### Treatment

Complete decongestive therapy is the best treatment. This consists of multilayer compression bandaging, manual lymphatic drainage by an experienced physiotherapist, lymphoedema pumps, exercise and skin care. Prevention of infection is essential to prevent continued lymphatic damage and antibiotics should be given at the first sign of lymphangitis or erysipelas. If erysipelas recurs, long-term penicillin should be given. Surgery occasionally helps to remove an obstruction or restore drainage.

## Lymphangitis

This streptococcal infection of the lymphatics may occur without any lymphoedema. A tender red line extends proximally. Penicillin, flucloxacillin, cephalexin and erythromycin are usually effective.

## Further reading

Douglas WS & Simpson NB. (1995) Guidelines for the management of chronic venous ulceration: report of a multidisciplinary workshop. *British Journal of Dermatology* **132**, 446–452.

Jones V, Grey JE & Harding KG. (2006) Wound dressings. *British Medical Journal* **332**, 777–780.

Takahashi PY, Kiemele LJ & Jones JP Jr. (2004) Wound care for elderly patients: advances and clinical applications for practicing physicians. *Mayo Clinic Proceedings* **79**, 260–267.

Valencia IC, Falabella A, Kirsner RS & Eaglstein WH. (2001) Chronic venous insufficiency and venous leg ulceration. *Journal of the American Academy of Dermatology* **44**, 401–421.

# 12 Sebaceous and sweat gland disorders

## Sebaceous glands

Most sebaceous glands develop embryologically from hair germs, but a few free glands arise from the epidermis. Those associated with hairs lie in the obtuse angle between the follicle and the epidermis (Fig. 12.1). The glands themselves are multilobed and contain cells full of lipid, which are shed whole (holocrine secretion) during secretion so that sebum contains their remnants in a complex mixture of triglycerides, fatty acids, wax esters, squalene and cholesterol. Sebum is discharged into the upper part of the hair follicle. It lubricates and waterproofs the skin, and protects it from drying; it is also mildly bactericidal and fungistatic. Free sebaceous glands may be found in the eyelid (meibomian glands), mucous membranes (Fordyce spots), nipple, perianal region and genitalia.

Androgenic hormones, especially dihydrotestosterone, stimulate sebaceous gland activity. Human sebaceous glands contain 5α-reductase, 3α- and 17α-hydroxysteroid dehydrogenase, which convert weaker androgens to dihydrotestosterone, which in turn binds to specific receptors in sebaceous glands, increasing sebum secretion. The sebaceous glands react to maternal androgens for a short time after birth, and then lie dormant until puberty when a surge of androgens produces a sudden increase in sebum excretion and sets the stage for acne.

## Acne

Acne is a disorder of the pilosebaceous apparatus characterized by comedones, papules, pustules, cysts and scars.

**Poral occlusion**
Hyperkeratinization
Occlusion (cosmetics,
  oils and tar)
Genetic influence

**Bacterial colonization
of duct**
by *Propionibacterium acnes*
which breaks down sebum

**Dermal inflammation**
due to release of
mediators and contents
of ruptured comedone

↑**Sebum secretion rate**
(androgen-dependent)
Oral contraceptives
  containing progestogens
Genetic influence

**Fig. 12.1** Factors causing acne.

## Prevalence

Nearly all teenagers have some acne (acne vulgaris). It affects the sexes equally, starting usually between the ages of 12 and 14 years, tending to be earlier in females. The peak age for severity in females is 16–17 and in males 17–19 years. Variants of acne are much less common.

## Cause

### Acne vulgaris

Many factors combine to cause acne (Fig. 12.1), characterized by chronic inflammation around pilosebaceous follicles.

- *Sebum* Sebum excretion is increased. However, this alone need not cause acne; patients with acromegaly, or with Parkinson's disease, have high sebum excretion rates but no acne. Furthermore, sebum excretion often remains high long after the acne has gone away.
- *Hormonal* Androgens (from the testes, ovaries, adrenals and sebaceous glands themselves) are the main stimulants of sebum excretion, although other hormones (e.g. thyroid hormones and growth hormone) have minor effects too. Those castrated before puberty, or with androgen insensitivity, never develop acne. In acne, the sebaceous glands respond excessively to what are usually normal levels of these hormones (increased target organ sensitivity). This may be caused by 5α-reductase activity being higher in the target sebaceous glands than in other parts of the body. Fifty per cent of females with acne have slightly raised free testosterone levels – usually because of a low level of sex hormone binding globulin rather than a high total testosterone – but this is still only a fraction of the concentration in males, and its relevance is debatable.
- *Poral occlusion* Both genetic and environmental factors (e.g. some cosmetics) cause the epithelium to overgrow the follicular surface. Follicles then retain sebum that has an increased concentration of bacteria and free fatty acids. Rupture of these follicles is associated with intense inflammation and tissue damage, mediated by oxygen free radicals and enzymes such as elastase, released by white cells.
- *Bacterial Propionibacterium acnes*, a normal skin commensal, plays a pathogenic part. It colonizes the pilosebaceous ducts, breaks down triglycerides releasing free fatty acids, produces substances chemotactic for inflammatory cells and induces the ductal epithelium to secrete pro-inflammatory cytokines via activation of Toll-like receptor 2 (TLR2 see Chapter 2). The inflammatory reaction is kept going by a foreign body reaction to follicular contents of the ruptured follicle and a type IV immune reaction (p. 30) to one or more antigens in the follicular contents.
- *Genetic* The condition is familial in about half of those with acne. There is a high concordance of the sebum excretion rate and acne in monozygotic, but not dizygotic, twins. Further studies are required to determine the precise mode of inheritance.

### Variants of acne

- *Infantile acne* may follow transplacental stimulation of a child's sebaceous glands by maternal androgens.
- *Mechanical*. Excessive scrubbing, picking, or the rubbing of chin straps or a fiddle (Fig. 12.2) can rupture occluded follicles.

**Fig. 12.2** Papulopustular lesions in an odd distribution. The patient played the violin ('fiddler's neck').

• Acne associated with virilization, including clito-romegaly, may be caused by an androgen-secreting tumour of the adrenals, ovaries or testes or, rarely, by congenital adrenal hyperplasia caused by mild 21-hydroxylase deficiency.

• Acne accompanying the polycystic ovarian syndrome is caused by modestly raised circulating androgen levels.

• *Drug-induced* Corticosteroids, androgenic and ana-bolic steroids, gonadotrophins, oral contraceptives, lithium, iodides, bromides, antituberculosis and anti-convulsant therapy can all cause an acneiform rash.

• *Tropical* Heat and humidity are responsible for this variant, which affects white people with a tend-ency to acne.

• Acne due to cosmetics (p. 165).

Cosmetics or other topical preparations may induce comedone formation or precipitate inflammation around vellous hair follicles.

### Presentation

#### Common type

Lesions are confined to the face, shoulders, upper chest and back. Seborrhoea (a greasy skin; Fig. 12.3) is often present. Open comedones (blackheads), because of the plugging by keratin and sebum of the pilosebaceous orifice, or closed comedones (whiteheads), caused by overgrowth of the follicle openings by surrounding epithelium, are always seen. Inflammatory papules, nodules and cysts (Figs 12.4

**Fig. 12.3** The seborrhoea, comedones and scattered inflammatory papules of teenage acne.

**Fig. 12.4** Prominent and inflamed cysts are the main features here.

**Fig. 12.5** Conglobate acne with inflammatory nodules, pustulocystic lesions and depressed scars.

and 12.5) occur, with one or two types of lesion pre-dominating. Depressed or hypertrophic scarring and post-inflammatory hyperpigmentation can follow.

Conglobate (gathered into balls; from the Latin *globus* meaning 'ball') is the name given to a severe form of acne with all of the above features as well as abscesses or cysts with intercommunicating sinuses that contain thick serosanguinous fluid or pus. On resolution, it leaves deeply pitted or hypertrophic scars, sometimes joined by keloidal bridges. Although hyperpigmentation is usually transient, it can per-sist, particularly in those with an already dark skin.

Psychological depression is common in persistent acne, which need not necessarily be severe.

### Variants

• *Infantile* This rare type of acne is present at or appears soon after birth. It is more common in males

**Fig. 12.6** Infantile acne. Pustulocystic lesions on the checks.

**Fig. 12.7** A group of open comedones (blackheads) following the use of a greasy cosmetic.

and may last up to 3 years. Its morphology is like that of common acne (Fig. 12.6) and it may be the forerunner of severe acne in adolescence.

● *Fulminans* Acne fulminans is a rare variant in which conglobate acne is accompanied by fever, joint pains and a high erythrocyte sedimentation rate (ESR).

● *Exogenous* Tars, chlorinated hydrocarbons, oils and oily cosmetics can cause or exacerbate acne. Suspicion should be raised if the distribution is odd or if comedones predominate (Fig. 12.7).

● *Excoriated* This is most common in young girls. Obsessional picking or rubbing leaves discrete denuded areas.

● *Late onset* This too occurs mainly in women and is often limited to the chin (Fig. 12.8). Nodular and cystic lesions predominate. It is stubborn and persistent.

● Acne associated with suppurative hidradenitis and perifolliculitis of scalp (p. 166).

● *Tropical* This occurs mainly on the trunk and may be conglobate. Sweat causes follicular occlusion by causing the perifollicular epidermis to swell.

● *Drug-induced* (Fig. 12.9) Suspicion should be raised when acne, dominated by papulopustules

**Fig. 12.8** Late-onset acne in a woman. Often localized to the chin.

rather than comedones, appears suddenly in a non-teenager and coincides with the prescription of a drug known to cause acneiform lesions (p. 164). Some athletes still use anabolic steroids to enhance their performance.

● *Polycystic ovarian syndrome* Consider this in obese females with oligomenorrhoea or secondary amenorrhoea or infertility. Glucose intolerance, dyslipidaemia and hypertension may be other features.

**Fig. 12.9** Steroid-induced acne in a seriously ill patient.

● *Congenital adrenal hyperplasia* Hyperpigmentation, ambiguous genitalia, history of salt-wasting in childhood and a Jewish background are all clues to this rare diagnosis.

● *Androgen-secreting tumours* These cause the rapid onset of virilization (clitoromegaly, deepening of voice, breast atrophy, male-pattern balding and hirsutism) as well as acne.

## Course

Acne vulgaris clears by the age of 23–25 years in 90% of patients, but some 5% of women and 1% of men still need treatment in their thirties or even forties.

## Investigations

None are usually necessary. Cultures are occasionally needed to exclude a pyogenic infection, an anaerobic infection or Gram-negative folliculitis. Only a few laboratories routinely culture *P. acnes* and test its sensitivity to antibiotics.

Any acne, including infantile acne, that is associated with virilization needs investigation to exclude an androgen-secreting tumour of the adrenals, ovaries or testes, and to rule out congenital adrenal hyperplasia caused by 21-hydroxylase deficiency. Tests should then include the measurement of plasma testosterone, sex hormone-binding globulin, luteinizing hormone (LH), follicle-stimulating hormone (FSH), dehydroepiandrosterone sulphate, androstenedione, 17-hydroxyprogesterone, urinary free cortisol and, depending on the results, ultrasound examination or computed tomography scan of the ovaries and adrenals. Female patients should not be taking the oral contraceptive pill when these hormone levels are measured. Congenital adrenal hyperplasia is associated with high levels of 17-hydroxyprogesterone, and androgen secreting tumours with high androgen levels.

Polycystic ovarian syndrome is characterized by modestly elevated testosterone, androstenedione and dehydroepiandrosterone sulphate levels, a reduced sex hormone-binding level and a LH : FSH ratio of greater than 2.5 : 1. Pelvic ultrasound may reveal multiple small ovarian cysts, although some acne patients have ovarian cysts without biochemical evidence of the polycystic ovarian syndrome.

## Differential diagnosis

Rosacea (p. 170) affects older individuals: comedones are absent; the papules and pustules occur only on the face; and the rash has a centrofacial erythematous background. Pyogenic folliculitis can be excluded by culture. Hidradenitis suppurativa (p. 176) is associated with acne conglobata, but attacks the axillae and groin. Pseudofolliculitis barbae, caused by ingrowing hairs, occurs on the necks of men with curly facial hair and clears up if shaving is stopped. Always suspect cosmetic acne, especially in post-adolescent women with acne limited to the face.

## Treatment

Acne frequently has marked psychological effects. Even those with mild acne need sympathy. An optimistic approach is essential, and regular encouragement worthwhile. Occasionally an underlying cause (p. 163) is found; this should be removed or treated.

**Fig. 12.10** A successful systemic treatment of acne – the picture tells its own story.

At some time most teenagers try anti-acne preparations bought from their pharmacist; local treatment is enough for most patients with comedo-papular acne, although both local and systemic treatment are needed for pustulocystic scarring acne (Fig. 12.10).

*Local treatment* (Formulary 1, p. 389)

**1** Regular gentle cleansing with soap and water should be encouraged, to remove surface sebum.
**2** Benzoyl peroxide. This antibacterial agent is applied only at night initially, but can be used twice daily if this does not cause too much dryness and irritation. It is most effective for inflammatory lesions and is not affected by propionibacterial antibiotic resistance. It is wise to start with a 2.5% or 5% pre-paration, moving up to 10% if necessary. Benzoyl peroxide bleaches coloured materials, particularly towels and flannels.
**3** Retinoids. The vitamin A (retinol) analogues (tretinoin, isotretinoin, adapalene, tazarotene) normalize follicular keratinization, down-regulate TLR2 expression and reduce sebum production. They are especially effective against comedones. Patients should be warned about skin irritation (start with small amounts) and photosensitivity. Concomitant eczema is usually a contraindication to its use. Tretinoin can be prescribed as a lotion, cream or gel. New preparations (in the USA) use microspheres (Retin-A micro) or specially formulated bases (Avita) that minimize irritation. The weakest preparation should be used first, and applied over-night on alternate nights. Sometimes, after a week or two, it will have to be stopped temporarily because of irritation. As with benzoyl peroxide, it may be worth increasing the strength of tretinoin after 6 weeks if it has been well tolerated, especially when closed comedones persist. The combination of benzoyl peroxide in the morning and tretinoin at night has many advocates.

- Isotretinoin 0.05% is made up in a gel base (not available in USA) and applied once or twice daily. It irritates less than the same concentration of tretinoin.
- Adapalene (0.1% or 0.3% gel) is a retinoid-like drug indicated for mild to moderate acne. It appears to work quicker and to be tolerated better than tretinoin.
- Tazarotene (0.5% or 0.1% gel), applied once daily, was found in one study to be more effective than tretinoin (0.1% microsponge).

Topical retinoids should not be prescribed for preg-nant women with acne.
**4** Azelaic acid is bactericidal for *P. acnes*: it is also anti-inflammatory and inhibits the formation of comedones by reducing the proliferation of keratinocytes. It should be applied twice daily, but not used for more than 6 months at a time.
**5** Topical antibiotics: including topical clindamycin, erythromycin and sulfacetamide (Formulary 1, p. 389) but antibacterial resistance of *P. acnes* is a

growing problem, with most erythromycin-resistant strains being cross-resistant to clindamycin. Combining antibiotics with benzoyl peroxide reduces *P. acnes* numbers and the likelihood of resistant strains emerging (Formulary 1, p. 389). The addition of zinc acetate complex to erythromycin enhances the antibiotic's anti-inflammatory effect.

6 Cosmetic camouflage. Cover-ups help some patients, especially females, whose scarring is unsightly. They also obscure post-inflammatory pigmentation. A range of make-ups is available in the UK and USA (Formulary 1, p. 383).

### Systemic treatment (Formulary 2, p. 393)

*Antibiotics* The prevalence of antibiotic-resistant *P. acnes*, particularly to erythromycin, is rising even in patients never previously exposed to it. As well as reducing *P. acnes* numbers, antibiotics also have a direct anti-inflammatory effect so will continue to be beneficial, but wherever possible they should be used in combination with topical benzoyl peroxide or retinoids to limit colonization by antibiotic-resistant bacteria.

• Oxytetracycline and tetracycline. An average starting dosage for an adult is 500 mg twice daily, but up to 1.5 g/day may be needed in resistant cases. The antibiotic should not be used for less than 3 months and may be needed for 1–2 years, or even longer. It should be taken on an empty stomach, 1 h before meals or 4 h after food, as the absorption of these tetracyclines is decreased by milk, antacids and calcium, iron and magnesium salts. The dosage should be tapered in line with clinical improvement, an average maintenance dosage being 250–500 mg/day. Even with long courses, serious side-effects are rare, although candidal vulvovaginitis may force a change to a narrower spectrum antibiotic such as erythromycin.

• Minocycline 50 mg twice daily or 100 mg once or twice daily (in a modified-release preparation) is now preferred by many dermatologists, although it is much more expensive. Absorption is not significantly affected by food or drink. Minocycline is much more lipophilic than oxytetracycline and so probably concentrates better in the sebaceous glands. It can be effective even when oxytetracycline has failed, but can cause abnormalities of liver function and a lupus-like syndrome.

• Doxycycline, 100 mg once or twice daily is a cheaper alternative to minocycline, but more frequently associated with phototoxic skin reactions. A new low-dose preparation (40 mg; Oracea, USA) is given once daily and inhibits acne by stopping inflammation in and around the pilosebaceous follicles without apparently affecting the bacterial flora of the vagina or elsewhere.

Tetracyclines should not be taken in pregnancy or by children under 12 years as they are deposited in growing bone and developing teeth, causing stained teeth and dental hypoplasia. Rarely, the long-term administration of minocycline causes a greyish pigmentation, like a bruise, especially on the faces of those with actinic damage and over the shins.

Erythromycin (dosage as for oxytetracycline) is the next antibiotic of choice but is preferable to tetracyclines in women who might become pregnant. Its major drawbacks are nausea and the widespread development of resistant *Proprionibacteria*, which leads to therapeutic failure.

Trimethoprim is used with or without sulfamethoxazole by some as a third-line antibiotic for acne, when a tetracycline and erythromycin have not helped. White blood cell counts should be monitored. Ampicillin is another alternative.

### Hormonal

Co-cyprindiol, a combined antiandrogen–oestrogen treatment (Dianette: 2 mg cyproterone acetate and 0.035 mg ethinylestradiol), is available in many countries and may help persistent acne in women. Monitoring is as for any patient on an oral contraceptive pill (OCP), and further contraceptive measures are unnecessary. The incidence of venous thromboembolism is higher than for the low-dose OCP, and the course should not go on for more than 3 months after the acne has cleared, at which point the drug should be replaced by a low-oestrogen/low-progestogen oral contraceptive. These drugs are not for males.

A number of combined oral contraceptives have been shown to improve acne. They reduce ovarian androgen synthesis and, by increasing sex hormone-binding globulin, reduce free testosterone levels and sebum production. Ethinyl estradiol 35 µg/norgestimate (Ortho Tri-Cyclen) and ethinyl estradiol 20–35 µg/norethindrone acetate (Estrostep) have been approved for use in acne in the USA.

Spironolactone blocks the androgen receptor, and reduces sebum production. It may be added to the OCP after 3 months if there has been an inadequate response. The usual dosage is 25–100 mg/day with food. In older patients, or those with concomitant medical problems, serum electrolytes should be checked. Pregnancy should be avoided as there is a risk of causing abnormalities of the foetal male genitalia.

Isotretinoin (13-*cis*-retinoic acid; Formulary 2, p. 402) is an oral retinoid, which inhibits sebum excretion, the growth of *P. acnes* and acute inflammatory processes. The drug is usually reserved for severe nodulocystic acne, unresponsive to the measures outlined above. It is routinely given for 4–6 months only, in a dosage of 0.5–1 mg/kg body weight/day; young men with truncal acne usually require the higher dosage. A full blood count, liver function tests and fasting lipid levels should be checked before the start of the course, and then 1 and 4 months after starting the drug. The drug seldom has to be stopped, although abnormalities of liver function rarely limit treatment.

Isotretinoin is highly teratogenic; various national programmes (iPledge in the USA, Pregnancy Prevention Programme in the UK) have been instituted to reduce the risk of women becoming pregnant while taking isotretinoin. Effective contraception must be taken for 1 month before starting isotretinoin, throughout treatment and for 1 month thereafter. Tests for pregnancy are carried out monthly while the drug is being taken, and only a single month's supply of the drug should be prescribed at a time, on receipt of a negative pregnancy test. The recommendations in the USA are especially stringent. Patient, physician and dispensing pharmacy must all be registered with the iPLEDGE programme and, as in the UK, prescriptions are given 1 month at a time on receipt of a negative pregnancy test. Two separate effective forms of birth control must be used at the same time for at least 1 month before starting isotretinoin, while taking it and for 1 month after stopping it. Treatment should start on day 3 of the patient's next menstrual cycle following a negative pregnancy test.

Depression, sometimes leading to suicide, is a rare accompaniment of treatment although causality has yet to be confirmed in a large controlled study.

Nevertheless, patients and their family doctors should be warned about the possible appearance or worsening of depression before starting a course of isotretinoin, and patients should be asked to sign a document that indicates that the issue of adverse psychiatric events has been discussed. The drug should be stopped immediately if there is any concern on this score. The possibility of adverse psychiatric events should be discussed at all visits. This potentially severe accompaniment of isotretinoin treatment has to be balanced against its remarkable efficacy in severe acne. The lives of most patients with conglobate acne have been transformed after successful treatment with isotretinoin.

Other side-effects of isotretinoin include a dry skin, dry and inflamed lips and eyes, nosebleeds, facial erythema, muscle aches, hyperlipidaemia and hair loss; these are reversible and often tolerable, especially if the acne is doing well. Rarer and potentially more serious side-effects include changes in night-time vision and hearing loss. Occasionally, isotretinoin flares acne at first, but this effect is usually short lived and the drug can be continued. It is because of its early side-effects that some dermatologists start isotretinoin in a low dose (e.g. 20 mg/day) and then work up to the target dose if no significant side-effects are reported at review during the first month of treatment. Early review appointments (e.g. at 1 and 2 weeks into treatment) are comforting to both patient and doctor. A useful 'avoidance list' for patients taking isotretinoin is given in Table 12.1.

> **Learning points**
>
> - Never prescribe short courses of many different antibiotics
> - Patients should use a topical retinoid or benzoyl peroxide when they are on antibiotics
> - Avoid tetracyclines in children and pregnant women
> - Make sure that females with acne are not pregnant before you prescribe isotretinoin, and that they do not become pregnant during the course of treatment and for 3 months after it. Only prescribe 1 month of isotretinoin at a time, after confirming a negative pregnancy test. Caution patients not to donate blood or share pills with others
> - Look out for depression in patients taking isotretinoin. If it occurs, stop the drug immediately, seek specialist advice and review your therapeutic options

| Avoid | Reason |
|---|---|
| Pregnancy | Teratogenicity |
| Breast feeding | Unknown effect on baby |
| Giving blood | Teratogenicity in recipient |
| Uncontrolled hyperlipidaemia | Additive side-effects |
| Taking vitamin A and hypervitaminosis A | Additive side-effects |
| Cosmetic procedures | Increased scarring |
| Excessive natural or artificial UVR | Photosensitivity |
| Oral contraceptive with low dose of progesterone – 'minipills' | Ineffective contraception |
| Concomitant antibiotics, unless with permission of prescribing doctor | Intracranial hypertension |

**Table 12.1** Avoidance list for patients taking isotretinoin.

### Physical

Treatment with various lasers, in particular the pulsed dye 585 nm laser, has been tried. While results show some benefit, there are no data on long-term outcomes, or trials comparing lasers with other acne treatments. Peeling procedures and epidermabrasion with gritty soaps peel off more of the stratum corneum than they open comedones, and are not generally recommended,

Cysts can be incised and drained with or without a local anaesthetic.

Intralesional injections of 0.1 mL triamcinolone acetonide (2.5–10 mg/mL) hasten the resolution of stubborn cysts, but can leave atrophy.

### Acne scar treatment

*Dermabrasion* This helps to smooth out facial scars. A high-speed rotating wire brush planes down to a bleeding dermis. Dermabrasion should not be carried out if there are any active lesions and does not help depressed 'ice-pick' scars, which may best be removed with a small punch. Unsightly hyperpigmentation may follow in darker skins. Microdermabrasion is well tolerated but its effects are usually transient.

*Lasers* Skin resurfacing with $CO_2$ and erbium lasers is rapidly replacing dermabrasion and chemical peeling as the best treatment for post-acne scarring. The procedure, which should be delayed until the acne is quiescent, is usually performed under local anaesthesia. Initially, a small test area is treated and then assessed (Fig. 12.11). If the result is satisfactory, the treatment is extended.

*Dermal fillers* Bovine collagen or hyaluronic acid fillers can be injected into depressed scars to improve their appearance. Patients with a history of any autoimmune disorder are excluded from this treatment. Shallow atrophic lesions do better than discrete 'ice-pick' scars. The procedure is expensive and has to be repeated every 6 months as the filler is reabsorbed.

## Rosacea

Rosacea affects the face of adults, usually women. Although its peak incidence is in the thirties and forties, it can also be seen in the young or old. It may coexist with acne but is distinct from it.

**Fig. 12.11** Acne scarring: worth treating a test area with a resurfacing laser.

## Cause and histopathology

The cause is still unknown. Rosacea is often seen in those who flush easily in response to warmth, spicy food, alcohol or embarrassment. Psychological abnormalities, including neuroticism and depression, are more often secondary to the skin condition than their cause. No pharmacological defect has been found that explains these flushing attacks. However, the warmer skin that results may make normal bacteria behave differently, setting off papules, pustules and other inflammation. Sebum excretion rate and skin microbiology are normal. A pathogenic role for the hair follicle mite, *Demodex folliculorum*, or for *Helicobacter pylori* infection of the gastric mucosa has not been proved.

## Clinical course and complications

The cheeks, nose, centre of forehead and chin are most commonly affected; the periorbital and perioral areas are spared (Fig. 12.12). Intermittent flushing is followed by a fixed erythema and telangiectases. Discrete domed inflamed papules, papulopustules

**Fig. 12.13** Marked rhinophyma.

and, rarely, plaques or nodules develop. Rosacea, unlike acne, has no comedones or seborrhoea. It is usually symmetrical. Its course is prolonged, with exacerbations and remissions. Complications include blepharitis, conjunctivitis and, occasionally, keratitis. Rhinophyma, caused by hyperplasia of the sebaceous glands and connective tissue on the nose, is a striking complication (Fig. 12.13) which is more common in males. Lymphoedema, below the eyes and on the forehead, is a tiresome feature in a few cases. Some patients treated with potent topical steroids develop a rebound flare of pustules, worse than the original rosacea, when this treatment is stopped. Many patients have only red skin or flushing and the disease does not necessarily progress. In erythematotelangiectatic rosacea, vascular features predominate, whereas inflammatory lesions are predominant in papulopustular rosacea.

## Differential diagnosis

Acne has already been mentioned. Rosacea differs from it by its background of erythema and telangiectases, and by the absence of comedones. The distribution of the lesions is different too, as rosacea affects the central face but not the trunk. Also rosacea usually appears after adolescence. Sun-damaged

**Fig. 12.12** Typical rosacea with papules and pustules on a background of erythema. Note the patient also has a patch of scaly seborrhoeic eczema on his brow.

**Fig. 12.14** A perioral dermatitis following withdrawal of the potent topical steroid that had been wrongly used to treat seborrhoeic eczema.

**Table 12.2** Overview of first-line treatments for rosacea based on subtype.

*Erythematotelangiectatic type*
Topical metronidazole
Topical azelaic acid
Decrease flushing
Cover-up makeup
Colour-correcting gels (green)
Intense pulsed light

*Papulospustular type*
Combination of topical agent with oral antibiotic
Topical metronidazole
Topical azelaic acid
Topical sulfacetamide/sulphur
Oral tetracyclines

*Phymatous type*
Ablative lasers
Electrosurgery

*Ocular type*
Oral doxycycline
Artifical tears
Lid clensing

skin with or without acne cosmetica causes most diagnostic difficulty. Remember, rosacea affects primarily the central, less mobile parts of the face, whereas sun damage and acne cosmetica are more generalized over the face. Seborrhoeic eczema, perioral dermatitis (Fig. 12.14), systemic lupus erythematosus (p. 137) and photodermatitis should be considered but do not show the papulopustules of rosacea. The flushing of rosacea can be confused with menopausal symptoms and, rarely, with the carcinoid syndrome. Superior vena caval obstruction has occasionally been mistaken for lymphoedematous rosacea.

*Treatment*

Treatment is best directed toward the subtype (Table 12.2). For papulopustular rosacea, tetracyclines, prescribed as for acne (p. 168), are the traditional treatment and are usually effective. Erythromycin is the antibiotic of second choice. Courses should last for at least 10 weeks and, after gaining control with 500–1000 mg/day, the dosage

can be cut to 250 mg/day. The condition recurs in about half of the patients within 2 years, but repeated antibiotic courses, rather than prolonged maintenance ones, are generally recommended. Topical 0.75% metronidazole gel (Formulary 1, p. 390), 15% azelaic acid and sulfacetamide/sulphur lotions (USA only) applied sparingly once or twice daily, are nearly as effective as oral tetracycline and often prolong remission. They can be tried before systemic treatment and are especially useful in treating 'stuttering' recurrent lesions which do not then need repeated systemic courses of antibiotics. Rarely, systemic metronidazole or isotretinoin (p. 394) is needed for stubborn rosacea. Rosacea and topical steroids go badly together (Fig. 12.15). Sunscreens help rhinophyma and even rosacea if sun exposure is an aggravating factor, but changes in diet or drinking habits are seldom of value. Erythematotelangiectatic rosacea responds well to treatment with vascular lasers or intense pulsed light sources. Measures to decrease flushing also help. Various techniques can be used to improve the appearance of disfiguring rhinophymas including surgical excision, cryotherapy, electrocautery and either argon or $CO_2$ laser ablation.

**Fig. 12.15** The result of the prolonged use of potent topical steroids for rosacea. Note the extreme telangiectasia.

---

**Learning point**

Never put strong topical steroids on rosacea. If you do, red faces, skin addiction, rebound flares and a cross dermatologist will all figure in your nightmares

---

## Sweat glands

### Eccrine sweat glands

There are 2–3 million sweat glands distributed all over the body surface but they are most numerous on the palms, soles and axillae. The tightly coiled glands lie deep in the dermis, and the emerging duct passes to the surface by penetrating the epidermis in a corkscrew fashion. Sweat is formed in the coiled gland by active secretion, involving the sodium pump. Some damage occurs to the membrane of the secretory cells during sweating. Initially, sweat is isotonic with plasma but, under normal conditions, it becomes hypotonic by the time it is discharged at the surface, after the tubular resorption of electrolytes and water under the influence of aldosterone and antidiuretic hormone.

In some ways the eccrine sweat duct is like a renal tubule. The pH of sweat is between 4.0 and 6.8; it contains sodium, potassium chloride, lactate, urea and ammonia. The concentration of sodium chloride in sweat is increased in cystic fibrosis, and sweat can be analysed when this is suspected.

Sweat glands have an important role in temperature control, the skin surface being cooled by evaporation. Up to 10 L/day of sweat can be excreted. Three stimuli induce sweating:

**1** Thermal sweating is a reflex response to a raised environmental temperature and occurs all over the body, especially the chest, back, forehead, scalp and axillae.

**2** Emotional sweating is provoked by fear or anxiety and is seen mainly on the palms, soles and axillae.

**3** Gustatory sweating is provoked by hot spicy foods and affects the face.

The eccrine sweat glands are innervated by cholinergic fibres of the sympathetic nervous system. Sweating can therefore be induced by cholinergic and blocked by anticholinergic drugs. Central control of sweating resides in the preoptic hypothalamic sweat centre.

Clinical disorders can follow increased or decreased sweating, or blockage of sweat gland ducts.

### *Generalized hyperhidrosis*

### *Thermal hyperhidrosis*

The 'thermostat' for sweating lies in the preoptic area of the hypothalamus. Sweating follows any rise in body temperature, whether this is caused by exercise, environmental heat or an illness. The sweating in acute infections, and in some chronic illnesses (e.g. Hodgkin's disease), may be a result of a lowering of the 'set' of this thermostat.

### *Other causes of general hyperhidrosis*

● Emotional stimuli, hypoglycaemia, opiate withdrawal and shock cause sweating by a direct or reflex stimulation of the sympathetic system at hypothalamic or higher centres. Sweating accompanied by a general sympathetic discharge occurs on a cold pale skin.

- Lesions of the central nervous system (e.g. a cerebral tumour or cerebrovascular accident) can cause generalized sweating, presumably by interfering directly with the hypothalamic centre.
- Phaeochromocytoma, the carcinoid syndrome, diabetes mellitus, thyrotoxicosis, Cushing's syndrome and the hot flushes of menopausal women have all been associated with general sweating. The mechanisms are not clear.

### Local hyperhidrosis (Fig. 12.16)

Local hyperhidrosis plagues many young adults. The most common areas to be affected are the palms, soles and axillae. Too much sweating there is embarrassing, if not socially crippling. A sodden shirt in contact with a dripping armpit, a wet handshake and stinking feet are hard crosses to bear. Seldom is any cause found, but organic disease, especially thyrotoxicosis, acromegaly, tuberculosis and Hodgkin's disease, should be considered. A blatant anxiety state is occasionally present, but more often an otherwise normal person is understandably concerned about his or her antisocial condition. A vicious circle emerges, in which increased anxiety drives further sweating.

These problems may be no more than one end of the normal physiological range. How many students sitting examinations have to dry their hands before putting pen to paper? It is only when the sweating is gross or continuous that medical advice is sought. Such sweating is often precipitated by emotional stimuli and stops during sleep.

**Fig. 12.16** Severe palmar hyperhidrosis demanding treatment.

### Treatment

#### Topical applications

The most useful preparation for axillary hyperhidrosis is 20% aluminium chloride hexahydrate in an alcohol base (Formulary 1, p. 384). At first it is applied to the dry axillae every night. Soon the interval can be increased, and many need the preparation only once or twice a week. The frequency may have to be cut down if the preparation irritates the skin, which is most likely if it is applied after shaving or when the skin is wet. Aluminium chloride also helps hyperhidrosis of the palms and soles, but it is less effective there.

Potassium permanganate soaks (1 : 10,000 aqueous solution) combat the bacterial superinfection of sweaty feet that is responsible for their foul smell. Patients should soak their feet for 15 min twice a day until the smell has improved and be warned that potassium permanganate stains the skin and everything else brown. Occasionally, glutaraldehyde solutions are used instead, but allergy and yellow-stained skin are potential complications. Topical clindamycin is also effective.

#### Iontophoresis

This is the passage of a low-voltage direct current across the skin. Iontophoresis with tap water or with the anticholinergic drug glycopyronium bromide (glycopyrrolate) may help palmar or plantar hyperhidrosis. Patients attend 2–3 times a week for treatment until the condition improves. Repeated courses or maintenance therapy may be required.

#### Botulinum toxin

This binds to presynaptic nerve membranes and then inhibits the release of acetylcholine. It is now the treatment of choice for severe axillary or plantar hyperhidrosis unresponsive to medical measures. Subdermal aliquots of the toxin are injected into the hyperhidrotic area of the axilla or sole, one region at a single session. Sweating is abolished after a delay of 2–3 days. Repeat injections (about every eighth month) are necessary as the sweating returns when the toxin has gone. Antibodies may form against the toxin and diminish its long-term effectiveness. Botulinum toxin is used less often for palmar hyperhidrosis because of the risk of paralysing the intrinsic muscles of the hand.

### Systemic treatment

Oral anticholinergic agents such as propantheline bromide and glycopyronium bromide (USA) are sometimes tried but their side-effects limit their value.

### Surgery

This is used less nowadays as the above measures are usually effective. However, recalcitrant axillary hyperhidrosis can be treated by removing the vault of the axilla, which bears most of the sweat glands. These can be identified preoperatively by applying starch and iodine, which interact with sweat to colour the sweat gland openings blue. Thoracoscopic sympathetic truncotomy (between the first and second thoracic ganglia) is effective for severe palmar hyperhidrosis alone but is a last resort.

### Hypohidrosis and anhidrosis

#### Anhidrosis caused by abnormality of the sweat glands

*Heat stroke* Caused by sweat gland exhaustion, this is a medical emergency seen most often in elderly people moving to a hot climate. It can also occur in the young, during or after prolonged exercise, especially in hot climates. Patients present with hyperthermia, dry skin, weakness, headache, cramps and confusion, leading to vomiting, hypotension, oliguria, metabolic acidosis, hyperkalaemia, delirium and death. They should be cooled down immediately with cold water, and fluids and electrolytes must be replaced.

*Hypohidrotic ectodermal dysplasia* This rare disorder is inherited as an X-linked recessive trait, in which the sweat glands are either absent or decreased. Affected boys have a characteristic facial appearance, with poor hair and teeth (Figs 13.13 and 13.14), and are intolerant of heat.

*Prematurity* The sweat glands function poorly in premature babies nursed in incubators and hot nurseries.

#### Anhidrosis caused by abnormalities of the nervous system

Anhidrosis may follow abnormalities anywhere in the sympathetic system, from the hypothalamus to the peripheral nerves. It can therefore be a feature of multiple sclerosis, a cerebral tumour, trauma, Horner's syndrome or peripheral neuropathy (e.g. leprosy, alcoholic neuropathy and diabetes). Patients with widespread anhidrosis are heat intolerant, developing nausea, dizziness, tachycardia and hyperthermia in hot surroundings.

#### Anhidrosis or hypohidrosis caused by skin disease

Local hypohidrosis has been reported in many skin diseases, especially those that scar (e.g. lupus erythematosus and morphoea). It may be a feature of Sjögren's syndrome, ichthyosis, psoriasis and miliaria profunda (p. 176).

---

**Learning point**

Aluminium chloride hexahydrate 20% in an alcohol base has now taken over from anticholinergic drugs and surgery for most patients with sweaty armpits and hands. Be sure the skin is dry before it is applied – use a hairdryer if necessary

---

## Interference with sweat delivery

### Miliaria

This is the result of plugging or rupture of sweat ducts. It occurs in hot humid climates, at any age and is common in over-clothed infants in hot nurseries. The physical signs depend on where the ducts are blocked.
- *Miliaria crystallina* This presents as tiny clear non-inflamed vesicles that look like dew. This is the most superficial type.
- *Miliaria rubra* (prickly heat) Tiny erythematous and very itchy papules.

- *Miliaria profunda* These consist of larger erythematous papules or pustules. This is the deepest type.

### Treatment

The best treatment is to move to a cooler climate or into air conditioning. Clothing that prevents the evaporation of sweat (e.g. nylon shirts) should be avoided; cotton is best. Claims have been made for ascorbic acid by mouth, but in our hands it rarely if ever helps. Salicylic acid 2% in isopropyl alcohol applied daily to prone areas has been advocated for prevention. Topical steroids reduce irritation but should only be used briefly. Calamine lotion cools and soothes.

## Apocrine sweat glands

Apocrine glands are limited to the axillae, nipples, periumbilical area, perineum and genitalia. The coiled tubular glands (larger than eccrine glands) lie deep in the dermis, and during sweating the luminal part of their cells is lost (decapitation secretion). Apocrine sweat passes via the duct into the mid-portion of the hair follicle. The action of bacteria on apocrine sweat is responsible for body odour. The glands are innervated by adrenergic fibres of the sympathetic nervous system.

### Hidradenitis suppurativa (apocrine acne)

This is a severe chronic suppurative disorder of the apocrine glands. Many papules, pustules, comedones, cysts, sinuses and scars occur in the axillae, groin and perianal areas. The condition may coexist with conglobate acne. Its cause is unknown, but an underlying follicular abnormality seems likely. Slightly raised androgen levels are found in some affected females. It is probably not an immunodeficiency or a primary infection of the apocrine glands, although *Staphylococcus aureus*, anaerobic streptococci and *Bacteroides* spp. are frequently present. One group of workers has implicated *Streptococcus milleri* as the main pathogen. Treatment is unsatisfactory but should be as for acne vulgaris in the first instance. Systemic antibiotics help early lesions to resolve but are ineffective for chronic draining abscesses and sinuses. Incision and drainage of abscesses, and injections of intralesional triamcinolone (5–10 mg/mL) may reduce the incidence of deforming scars and sinus formation. Topical clindamycin has been shown to prevent new lesions from forming. Infliximab has been used with success; just why it works is uncertain. Systemic antiandrogens help some women and oral retinoids may also help. Severe cases need plastic surgery to remove large areas of affected skin, but patients are often grateful for it, because the disease is painful, messy, unsightly and smelly too.

### Fox–Fordyce disease

This rare disease of the apocrine ducts is comparable to miliaria rubra of the eccrine duct. It occurs in women after puberty. Itchy skin-coloured or light brown papules appear in the axillae and other areas where apocrine glands are found, such as the breasts and vulva. Treatment is not usually necessary but removal of the affected skin, or electrodessication of the most irritable lesions can be considered.

## Further reading

Collin J & Whatling P. (2000) Treating hyperhidrosis. *British Medical Journal* **320**, 1221–1222.

Dahl MV. (2001) Pathogenesis of rosacea. *Advances in Dermatology* **17**, 29–45.

James WD. (2005) Clinical practice. Acne. *New England Journal of Medicine* **352**, 1463–1472.

Kreyden OP, Böni R & Burg G. (2001) *Hyper-hidrosis and Botulinum Toxin in Dermatology*. Karger, Basel.

Mortimer PS & Lunniss PJ. (2000) Hidradenitis suppurativa. *Journal of the Royal Society of Medicine* **93**, 420–422.

Wilkin J, Dahl MV, Detmar M, *et al.* (2002) Standard classification of rosacea: Report of the National Rosacea Society Expert Committee on the Classification and Staging of Rosacea. *Journal of the American Academy of Dermatology* **46**, 584–587.

# 13 Regional dermatology

## The hair

Hair is human plumage: we need just the right amount, in the right places. The twin torments of having too much or too little hair can be understood only when seen against the background of the formation and activity of normal hair follicles.

Hair follicles form before the ninth week of foetal life when the hair germ, a solid cylinder of cells, grows obliquely down into the dermis. Here it is met by a cluster of mesenchymal cells (the placode) bulging into the lower part of the hair germ to form the hair papilla. Eventually, the papilla contains blood vessels bringing nutrients to the hair matrix. The sebaceous gland is an outgrowth at the side of the hair germ, establishing early the two parts of the pilosebaceous unit. The hair matrix, the germinative part of the follicle, is equivalent to the basal cells of the epidermis.

Melanocytes migrate into the matrix and are responsible for the different colours of hair (eumelanin, brown and black; phaeomelanin and trichochromes, red). Grey or white hair is caused by low pigment production and the filling of the cells in the hair medulla with minute air bubbles that reflect light.

The structure of a typical hair follicle is shown in Fig. 13.1.

## Classification

Hairs are classified into three main types.
1 *Lanugo hairs* Fine long hairs covering the foetus, but shed about 1 month before birth.
2 *Vellus hairs* Fine short unmedullated hairs covering much of the body surface. They replace the lanugo hairs just before birth.
3 *Terminal hairs* Long coarse medullated hairs seen, for example, in the scalp or pubic regions. Their growth is often influenced by circulating androgen levels.

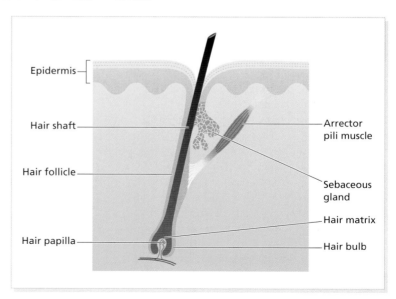

**Fig. 13.1** Anatomy of the hair follicle.

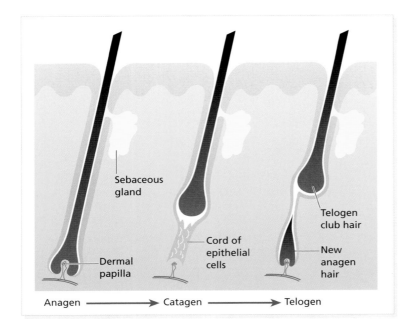

**Fig. 13.2** The hair cycle.

Terminal hairs convert to vellus hairs in male-pattern alopecia, and vellus to terminal hairs in hirsutism. The lips, glans penis, labia minora, palms and soles remain free of hair follicles.

## The hair cycle

Each follicle passes, independently of its neighbours, through regular cycles of growth and shedding. There are three phases of follicular activity (Fig. 13.2).

**1** *Anagen* The active phase of hair production.
**2** *Catagen* A short phase of conversion from active growth to the resting phase. Growth stops, and the end of the hair becomes club-shaped.
**3** *Telogen* A resting phase at the end of which the club hair is shed.

The duration of each of these stages varies from region to region. On the scalp (Fig. 13.3), said to contain an average of 100 000 hairs, anagen lasts for up to 5 years, catagen for about 2 weeks and telogen for about 3 months. As many as 100 hairs may be shed from the normal scalp every day as a normal consequence of cycling. The proportion of hairs in the growing and resting stages can be estimated by looking at plucked hairs (a trichogram). On the scalp, about 85% are normally in anagen and 15% in the telogen phase. The length of hair is determined by the duration of anagen (e.g. the hairs of the eyebrows have shorter cycles than those of the scalp).

Each hair follicle goes through its growth cycles out of phase with its neighbours, so there is no moulting period. However, if many pass into the resting phase (telogen) at the same time, then a

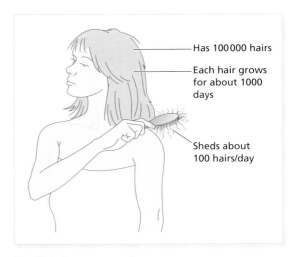

Has 100 000 hairs

Each hair grows for about 1000 days

Sheds about 100 hairs/day

**Fig. 13.3** An average scalp.

**Table 13.1** Some causes of localized alopecia.

| Non-scarring | Scarring |
|---|---|
| Alopecia areata | Burns, radiodermatitis |
| Androgenetic | Aplasia cutis |
| Hair-pulling habit | Kerion, carbuncle |
| Traction alopecia | Cicatricial basal cell carcinoma, lichen planus, lupus erythematosus |
| Scalp ringworm (human) | Necrobiosis, sarcoidosis, pseudopelade |

correspondingly large number will be shed 2–3 months later (p. 184).

There are important racial differences in hair. Asians tend to have straight hair, Negroids woolly hair and Europeans wavy hair. These differences are associated with different cross-sectional shapes (e.g. round, flattened). Mongoloids have less facial and body hair than Mediterranean people who also have more hair than northern Europeans.

## Alopecia

The term means loss of hair and alopecia has many causes and patterns. One convenient division is into localized and diffuse types. It is also important to decide whether or not the hair follicles have been replaced by scar tissue; if they have, regrowth cannot occur. The presence of any disease of the skin itself should also be noted.

## Localized alopecia

Some of the most common types are listed in Table 13.1; only a few can be dealt with in detail.

### Alopecia areata

The lifetime risk of getting alopecia areata is about 2% and, coincidentally, it is the reason for about 2% of consultations in our skin clinics.

### Cause

An immunological basis is suspected because of an association with autoimmune thyroid disease, vitiligo and atopy. Histologically, T lymphocytes cluster like a swarm of bees around affected hair bulbs, having been attracted and made to divide by cytokines

from the dermal papilla. Alopecia areata is probably inherited as a complex genetic trait; sometimes HLA-DQ3, -DR11 or -DR4 act as susceptibility factors, with an increased occurrence in the first-degree relatives of affected subjects and twin concordance. It affects some 10% of patients with Down's syndrome, suggesting the involvement of genes on chromosome 21. Environmental factors may trigger alopecia areata in the genetically predisposed.

### Presentation

A typical patch is uninflamed, with no scaling, but with empty hair follicles (Fig. 13.4). Pathognomonic 'exclamation-mark' hairs may be seen around the edge of enlarging areas. They are broken off about 4 mm from the scalp, and are narrowed and less pigmented proximally (Figs 13.5 and 13.6). Patches

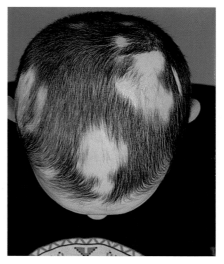

**Fig. 13.4** The characteristic uninflamed patches of alopecia areata.

**Fig. 13.5** Exclamation-mark hairs: pathognomonic of alopecia areata.

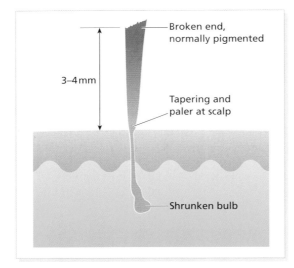

Broken end, normally pigmented

3–4mm

Tapering and paler at scalp

Shrunken bulb

**Fig. 13.6** An exclamation-mark hair.

are most common in the scalp and beard but other areas, especially the eyelashes and eyebrows, can be affected too. An uncommon diffuse pattern is recognized, with exclamation-mark hairs scattered widely over a diffusely thinned scalp. Up to 50% of patients show fine pitting or wrinkling of the nails.

### Course

The outcome is unpredictable. In a first attack, regrowth is usual within a few months. New hairs appear in the centre of patches as fine pale down, and gradually regain their normal thickness and colour, although the new hair may remain white in older patients. Fifty percent of cases resolve spontaneously without treatment within 1 year, and only 10% go on to have severe chronic disease. Subsequent episodes tend to be more extensive and regrowth is slower. Hair loss in some areas may coexist with regrowth in others. A few of those who go on to have chronic disease lose all the hair from their heads (alopecia totalis) or from the whole skin surface (alopecia universalis).

Regrowth is tiresomely erratic but the following suggest a poor prognosis:

1 onset before puberty;
2 association with atopy or Down's syndrome;
3 unusually widespread alopecia; and
4 involvement of the scalp margin (ophiasiform type), especially at the nape of the neck.

### Differential diagnosis

Patches are not scaly, in contrast to ringworm, and are usually uninflamed, in contrast to lupus erythematosus and lichen planus. In the hair-pulling habit of children, and in traction alopecia, broken hairs may be seen but true exclamation-mark hairs are absent. Secondary syphilis can also cause a 'moth-eaten' patchy hair loss. A form of scarring alopecia called 'pseudopelade' (p. 184) can look similar.

### Investigations

None are usually needed. The histology of bald skin shows lymphocytes around and in the hair matrix. Syphilis can be excluded with serological tests if necessary. Organ-specific autoantibody screens provide interesting information but do not affect management.

### Treatment

A patient with a first or minor attack can be reassured about the prospects for regrowth. Topical corticosteroid creams of high potency can be prescribed, but it is difficult to tell whether the regrowth is spontaneous or a result of the creams. The use of systemic steroids should be avoided in most cases, but the intradermal injection of 0.2 ml intralesional

**Fig. 13.7** Regrowth within a patch of alopecia areata after a triamcinolone injection.

triamcinolone acetonide (5–10 mg/ml), raising a small bleb within an affected patch, leads to localized tufts of regrowth (Fig. 13.7). While not affecting the overall outcome, this may be useful to re-establish eyebrows or to stimulate hope. It works so reliably that some patients come regularly for reinjections into eyebrows or small areas of the scalp. The downside of this treatment is dermal atrophy evident as depressed areas at the sites of injections. Mild irritants, such as 0.1–0.25% dithranol, have been used but with limited success. Ultraviolet radiation or even psoralen with ultraviolet A (PUVA) therapy may help extensive cases, but hair fall often returns when treatment stops. Contact sensitizers (e.g. diphencyprone) seemed promising (Figs. 13.8) but the long-term effect of persistent antigen stimulation is worrying; they are still being used only in a few centres under trial conditions. The efficacy of topical immunosuppressive agents (e.g. tacrolimus) has yet to be proved. Wigs are necessary for extensive cases.

## Androgenetic alopecia (male-pattern baldness)

### Cause

Although clearly familial, the exact mode of inheritance has not yet been clarified. The idea of a single autosomal dominant gene, with reduced penetrance in women, now seems less likely than a polygenic type of inheritance. Male-pattern baldness is androgen dependent; in females, androgenetic

**Fig. 13.8** A trial of diphencyprone to one side of the scalp caused some regrowth.

alopecia (female-pattern hair loss), with circulating levels of androgen within normal limits, is seen only in those who are strongly predisposed genetically.

### Presentation

The common pattern in men is the loss of hair first from the temples, and then from the crown (Fig. 13.9). However, in women the hair loss may be much more diffuse, particularly over the crown (Fig. 13.10). In bald areas, terminal hairs are replaced by finer vellus ones.

### Clinical course

Hair loss is relentless, tending to follow the family pattern, with some losing hair quickly and others more slowly. The diffuse pattern seen in women tends to progress slowly.

### Complications

Even minor hair loss may lead to great anxiety and rarely to a monosymptomatic hypochondriasis (p. 343). Bald scalps burn easily in the sun, and may develop multiple actinic keratoses. It has been

**Fig. 13.9** Variations on male-pattern baldness.

**Fig. 13.10** Androgenetic alopecia beginning in the frontal area.

**Table 13.2** Some causes of diffuse hair loss.

Telogen effluvium
Endocrine
    hypopituitarism
    hypo- or hyperthyroidism
    hypoparathyroidism
    high androgenic states
Drug-induced
    antimitotic agents (anagen effluvium)
    retinoids
    anticoagulants
    vitamin A excess
    oral contraceptives
Androgenetic
Iron deficiency
Severe chronic illness
Malnutrition
Diffuse type of alopecia areata

suggested recently that bald men are more likely to have a heart attack and prostate cancer than those with a full head of hair.

### Differential diagnosis

The diagnosis is usually obvious in men, but other causes of diffuse hair loss have to be considered in women (Table 13.2).

### Investigations

None are usually needed. In women, virilization may have to be excluded.

### Treatment

Scalp surgery, hair transplants and wigs are welcomed by some. Topical application of minoxidil lotion may slow early hair loss and even stimulate new growth of hair but the results are not dramatic (Formulary 1, p. 392). Small and recently acquired patches respond best. When minoxidil treatment stops, the new hairs fall out after about 3 months. Antiandrogens help some women with the diffuse type of androgenetic alopecia.

Finasteride (Propecia), an inhibitor of human type II $5\alpha$-reductase, reduces serum and scalp skin levels of dihydrotestosterone in balding men. At the dosage of 1 mg/day, it may increase hair counts and so lead to a noticeable improvement in both frontal and vertex hair thinning. However, the beneficial effects slowly reverse once treatment has stopped. This treatment is not indicated in women or children. Side-effects are rare, but include decreased libido, erectile dysfunction and altered prostate-specific antigen levels.

> **Learning points**
>
> - Be sympathetic even if the hair loss seems trivial to you
> - Reassure your patient that total baldness is not imminent

## Trichotillomania

This is dealt with on p. 346.

## Traction alopecia

### Cause

Hair can be pulled out by several procedures intended to beautify, including hot-combing to straighten kinky hair, tight hairstyles such as a pony tail or 'corn rows', and using hair rollers too often or too tightly.

### Presentation

The changes are usually seen in girls and young women, particularly those whose hair has always tended to be thin anyway. The pattern of hair loss is determined by the cosmetic procedure in use, hair being lost where there is maximal tug. The term 'marginal' alopecia is applied to one common pattern in which hair loss is mainly around the edge of the scalp – at the sides or at the front (Fig. 13.11). The bald areas show short broken hairs, folliculitis and sometimes scarring.

### Clinical course

Patients are often slow to accept that they are responsible for the hair loss, and notoriously slow to alter their cosmetic practices. Even if they do, regrowth is often disappointingly incomplete.

**Fig. 13.11** Traction alopecia. The rollers she thought would help to disguise her thin hair actually made it worse.

### Differential diagnosis

The pattern of hair loss provides the main clue to the diagnosis and if the possibility of traction alopecia is kept in mind there is usually no difficulty. The absence of exclamation-mark hairs distinguishes it from alopecia areata, and of scaling from tinea capitis.

### Treatment

Patients have to stop doing whatever is causing their hair loss. Rollers that tug can be replaced by those that only heat.

## Patchy hair loss caused by skin disease

### Scalp ringworm

Inflammation, often with pustulation, occurs mostly after infection with fungi from animals or soil, and the resultant scarring can be severe. The classic scalp ringworm caught from other human beings causes areas of scaling with broken hairs. The subject is covered in more detail on p. 250.

### Psoriasis

The rough removal of adherent scales can also remove hairs, but regrowth is the rule.

### Scarring alopecia

Hair follicles can be damaged in many ways. If the follicular openings can no longer be seen with a lens, regrowth of hair cannot be expected.

Sometimes the cause is obvious: a severe burn, trauma, a carbuncle or an episode of inflammatory scalp ringworm. Discoid lupus erythematosus (p. 134), lichen planus (p. 72) and morphoea (p. 141) can also lead to scarring alopecia. The term 'pseudopelade' is applied to a slowly progressive, non-inflamed type of scarring which leads to irregular areas of hair loss without any apparent preceding skin disease. If inflammation is present, a biopsy may help to establish the diagnosis.

## Diffuse hair loss

Hair is lost evenly from the whole scalp; this may, or may not, be accompanied by a thinning visible to others (Fig. 13.12). Some of the most common causes are listed in Table 13.2, but often a simple explanation cannot be found.

### Telogen effluvium

#### Cause

Telogen effluvium can be triggered by any severe illness, particularly those with bouts of fever or haemorrhage, by childbirth and by severe dieting. All of these synchronize catagen so that, later on, large numbers of hairs are lost at the same time.

**Fig. 13.12** Diffuse hair loss causing much anxiety.

#### Presentation and course

The diffuse hair fall, 2–3 months after the provoking illness, can be mild or severe. In the latter case Beau's lines (p. 191) may be seen on the nails. Regrowth, not always complete, usually occurs within a few months.

#### Differential diagnosis

This is from other types of diffuse hair loss (Table 13.2). In androgenetic alopecia in females the onset is gradual in mid-adulthood, and hairs remain rather firmly anchored to the scalp. In telogen effluvium the onset is abrupt and follows acute illness, an operation or pregnancy by 1–2 months. Hair fall is prominent and lightly pulling on scalp hairs dislodges many. In diffuse alopecia areata, the hair loss is more patchy, and the onset abrupt with waxing and waning. Shedding may be prominent. 'Exclamation-mark' hairs are often present.

#### Treatment

This condition is unaffected by therapy, but patients can be reassured that their hair fall will be temporary.

### Other causes of diffuse hair loss

The causes mentioned in Table 13.2 should be considered. If no cause is obvious, it is worth checking the haemoglobin, erythrocyte sedimentation rate (ESR), antinuclear antibody, serum iron, thyroxine and thyroid-stimulating hormone (TSH) levels. Also consider checking the serum free testosterone and dihydroepiandrosterone sulphate levels in women with menstrual irregularities or hirsutism. Despite these, often no cause for diffuse alopecia can be found.

## Rare genetic causes of hypotrichosis

More than 300 genetic conditions exist that have hair abnormalities as one component. The *hypohidrotic ectodermal dysplasias* are a group of rare inherited disorders characterized by sparse hair, scanty sweat glands and poor development of the nails and teeth (Figs 13.13 and 13.14). Heat stroke may follow

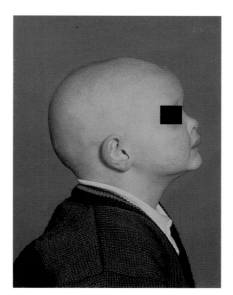

**Fig. 13.13** Hypohidrotic ectodermal dysplasia: minimal scalp hair and characteristic facies.

**Fig. 13.14** The cone-shaped incisors of hypohidrotic ectodermal dysplasia.

inadequate sweat production. One type is inherited as an X-linked recessive. The responsible gene for this type (on chromosome Xq12) has recently been shown to encode for a protein (ectodysplasin) involved in the regulation of ectodermal appendage formation. The genes responsible for the dominant or recessive types encode for the ectodysplasin receptor.

In other inherited disorders the hair may be beaded and brittle (*monilethrix*); flattened and twisted (*pili torti*); kinky (*Menkes' syndrome* caused by mutations in a gene encoding for a copper-transporting membrane protein); like bamboo (*Netherton's syndrome*, caused by a gene on chromosome 5q32 encoding

a serine protease inhibitor); partly broken in many places (*trichorrhexis nodosa*); 'woolly' or 'uncombable'.

## Hirsutism and hypertrichosis

Hirsutism is the growth of terminal hair in a woman (Fig. 13.15), which is distributed in the pattern normally seen in a man. Hypertrichosis is an excessive growth of terminal hair that does not follow an androgen-induced pattern (Fig. 13.16).

**Fig. 13.15** Moderate hirsutism caused by polycystic ovaries.

**Fig. 13.16** Hypertrichosis in a young man of Mediterranean extraction.

## Hirsutism

### Cause

Some degree of hirsutism may be a racial or familial trait, and minor facial hirsutism is common after the menopause. In addition, some patients without a family background of hirsutism become hirsute in the absence of any demonstrable hormonal cause (idiopathic hirsutism). Finally, some patients with hirsutism will have one of the disorders shown in Fig. 13.17, most commonly the polycystic ovarian syndrome.

### Presentation

An excessive growth of hair appears in the beard area, on the chest and shoulder-tips, around the nipples and in the male pattern of pubic hair. Androgenetic alopecia may complete the picture.

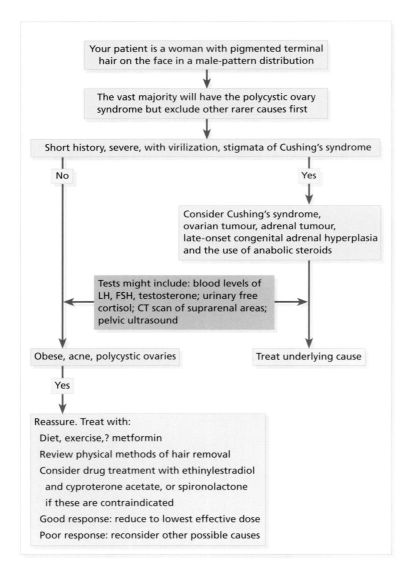

**Fig. 13.17** An approach to hirsutism.
CT, computer tomography;
FSH, follicle-stimulating hormone;
LH, luteinizing hormone.

## Course

Familial, racial or idiopathic hirsutism tends to start at puberty and to worsen with age.

## Complications

Virilization is associated with infertility; psychological disturbances are common.

## Investigations

Significant hormonal abnormalities are not usually found in patients with a normal menstrual cycle.
  Investigations are needed if:
- hirsutism occurs in childhood;
- there are other features of virilization, such as clitoromegaly or voice change;
- the hirsutism is of sudden or recent onset; or
- there is menstrual irregularity or cessation.

  The tests used will include measurement of the serum testosterone, sex hormone-binding globulin, dehydroepiandrosterone sulphate, androstenedione and prolactin. Transvaginal ovarian ultrasound is useful if polycystic ovaries are suspected.

## Treatment (Fig. 13.17)

Any underlying disorder must be treated on its merits. Home remedies for minor hirsutism include commercial depilatory creams (often containing a thioglycollate; p. 188), waxing or shaving, or making the appearance less obvious by bleaching; none removes the hair permanently. Plucking should probably be avoided as it can stimulate hair roots into anagen. The abnormally active follicles, if relatively few, can be destroyed by electrolysis. If the hairs are too numerous for this, the excess can be removed by laser (p. 378). Topical therapy with eflornithine, an inhibitor of ornithine decarboxylase, can slow regrowth. Oral antiandrogens (e.g. cyproterone acetate, Dianette; or spironolactone; Formulary 2, p. 398) may sometimes be helpful, but will be needed long term. Pregnancy must be avoided during such treatment as it carries the risk of feminizing a male fetus.

> **Learning points**
> - Full endocrinological assessment is needed for hirsutism plus virilization
> - Significant hormonal abnormalities are rarely found in patients with a normal menstrual cycle

## Hypertrichosis

The localized type is most commonly seen over melanocytic naevi including Becker's naevi (Fig. 13.18). It can also affect the sacral area – as a 'satyr's tuft' – in some patients with spina bifida. Excessive amounts of hair may grow near chronically inflamed joints or under plaster casts. Repeated shaving does not bring on hypertrichosis although occupational pressure may do so (e.g. from carrying weights on the shoulder).
  Generalized hypertrichosis is much less common. Some causes are listed in Table 13.3.

### Hair cosmetics

Hair can be made more attractive by dyeing, bleaching and waving, but there is often a price to be paid for beauty. Some hair dyes based on

**Fig. 13.18** A typical Becker's naevus with marked localized hypertrichosis within a patch of hyperpigmentation.

**Table 13.3** Some causes of generalized hypertrichosis.

Anorexia nervosa, starvation
Drug-induced (minoxidil, diazoxide, ciclosporin)
Cutaneous porphyrias (p. 328)
Foetal alcohol and foetal phenytoin syndromes
Hypertrichosis lanuginosa (both congenital type and
    acquired types are very rare – the latter signals an
    internal malignancy)
Some rare syndromes (e.g. Cornelia de Lange syndrome –
    hypertrichosis, microcephaly and mental deficiency –
    and Hurler's syndrome)

paraphenylenediamine are allergens (p. 87). Bleaches can weaken the hair shafts.

Permanent waving solutions reduce disulphide bonds within hair keratin and so allow the hair to be deformed before being reset in a new position. The thioglycollates in use to dissolve disulphide bonds are also popular as chemical hair removers. If used incorrectly, either too strong or for too long, or on hair already damaged by excessive bleaching or waving, thioglycollate waving lotions can cause hairs to break off flush with the scalp. This hair loss, which can be severe although temporary, may be accompanied by an irritant dermatitis of the scalp.

## The nails

The structure of the nail and nail bed is shown in Fig. 13.19. The hard keratin of the nail plate is formed in the nail matrix, which lies in an invagination of the epidermis (the nail fold) on the back of the terminal phalanx of each digit. The matrix runs from the proximal end of the floor of the nail fold to the distal margin of the lunule. From this area the nail plate grows forward over the nail bed, ending in a free margin at the tip of the digit. Longitudinal ridges and grooves on the undersurface of the nail plate dovetail with similar ones on the upper surface of the nail bed. The nail bed is capable of producing small amounts of keratin which contribute to the nail and which are responsible for the 'false nail' formed when the nail matrix is obliterated by surgery or injury. The cuticle acts as a seal to protect the potential space of the nail fold from chemicals and from infection. The nails provide strength and protection for the terminal phalanx. Their presence helps with fine touch and with the handling of small objects.

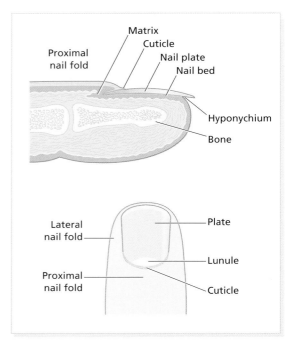

**Fig. 13.19** The nail and nail bed.

The rate at which nails grow varies from person to person: fingernails average between 0.5 and 1.2 mm per week, while toenails grow more slowly. Nails grow faster in the summer, if they are bitten, and in youth. They change with ageing from the thin, occasionally spooned nails of early childhood to the duller, paler and more opaque nails of the very old. Longitudinal ridging and beading are particularly common in the elderly.

### Effects of trauma

Permanent ridges or splits in the nail plate can follow damage to the nail matrix. Splinter haemorrhages (Fig. 13.20), the linear nature of which is determined by longitudinal ridges and grooves in the nail bed, are most commonly seen under the nails of manual workers and are caused by minor trauma. They may also be a feature of psoriasis of the nail and of subacute bacterial endocarditis. Larger subungual haematomas (Fig. 13.21) are usually easy to identify but the trauma that caused them may have escaped notice and dark areas of altered blood can raise worries about the presence of a subungual melanoma.

**Fig. 13.20** Gross splinter haemorrhages caused by trauma.

Jan. 9    Apr 9    July 7

**Fig. 13.21** A subungual haematoma of the big toe. Although there was no history of trauma we were happy to watch this grow out over 6 months as the appearance was sudden, the colour was right and the nail folds showed no pigment.

Chronic trauma from sport and from ill-fitting shoes contributes to haemorrhage under the nails of the big toes, to the gross thickening of toenails known as *onychogryphosis* (Fig. 13.22) and to in-growing nails. *Onycholysis*, a separation of the nail plate from the nail bed (Fig. 13.23), may be a result of minor trauma although it is also seen in nail psoriasis (see Fig. 5.8), phototoxic reactions, repeated

**Fig. 13.22** Onychogryphosis.

immersion in water, after the use of nail hardeners and possibly in thyroid disease. Usually, no cause for it is found. The space created may be colonized by yeasts, or by bacteria such as *Pseudomonas aeruginosa*, which turns it an ugly green colour.

Some nervous habits damage the nails. Bitten nails are short and irregular; some people also bite their cuticles and the skin around the nails. Viral warts can be seeded rapidly in this way. In the common habit tic nail dystrophy, the cuticle of the thumbnail is the target for picking or rubbing. This repetitive trauma causes a ladder pattern of transverse ridges and grooves to run up the centre of the nail plate (Fig. 13.23).

Lamellar splitting of the distal part of the fingernails, so commonly seen in housewives, has been attributed to repeated wetting and drying (Fig. 13.23).

Attempts to beautify nails can lead to contact allergy. Culprits include the acrylate adhesive used with artificial nails and formaldehyde in nail hardeners. In contrast, contact dermatitis caused by allergens in nail polish itself seldom affects the fingers but presents as small itchy eczematous areas where the nail plates rest against the skin during sleep. The eyelids, face and neck are favourite sites.

## The nail in systemic disease

The nails can provide useful clues for general physicians.
● *Clubbing* (Fig. 13.24) A bulbous enlargement of the terminal phalanx with an increase in the angle between the nail plate and the proximal fold to

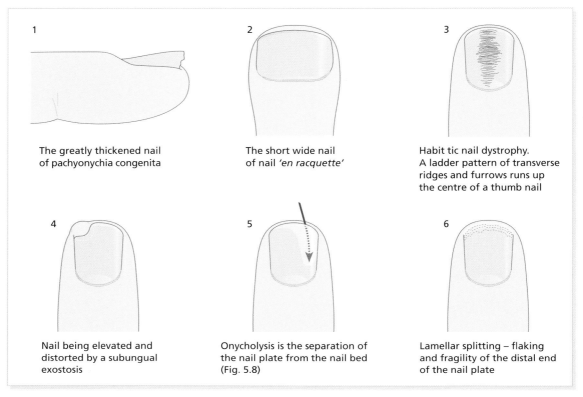

1 The greatly thickened nail of pachyonychia congenita

2 The short wide nail of nail *'en racquette'*

3 Habit tic nail dystrophy. A ladder pattern of transverse ridges and furrows runs up the centre of a thumb nail

4 Nail being elevated and distorted by a subungual exostosis

5 Onycholysis is the separation of the nail plate from the nail bed (Fig. 5.8)

6 Lamellar splitting – flaking and fragility of the distal end of the nail plate

**Fig. 13.23** Some nail plate abnormalities.

over 180° (Fig. 13.25). Its association with chronic lung disease and with cyanotic heart disease is well known. Rarely, clubbing may be familial with no underlying cause. The mechanisms involved in its formation are still not known.

**Fig. 13.24** In this case, severe clubbing was accompanied by hypertrophic pulmonary osteoarthropathy.

In clubbing the finger tip is bulbous

The normal angle between the proximal part of the nail and the skin of the finger below is eliminated

**Fig. 13.25** Clubbing.

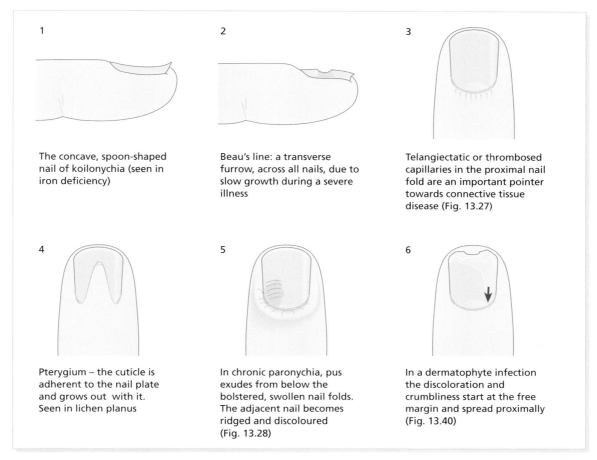

1

The concave, spoon-shaped nail of koilonychia (seen in iron deficiency)

2

Beau's line: a transverse furrow, across all nails, due to slow growth during a severe illness

3

Telangiectatic or thrombosed capillaries in the proximal nail fold are an important pointer towards connective tissue disease (Fig. 13.27)

4

Pterygium – the cuticle is adherent to the nail plate and grows out with it. Seen in lichen planus

5

In chronic paronychia, pus exudes from below the bolstered, swollen nail folds. The adjacent nail becomes ridged and discoloured (Fig. 13.28)

6

In a dermatophyte infection the discoloration and crumbliness start at the free margin and spread proximally (Fig. 13.40)

**Fig. 13.26** Some other nail changes.

- *Koilonychia* A spooning and thinning of the nail plate, indicating iron deficiency (Fig. 13.26).
- *Colour changes* The 'half-and-half' nail, with a white proximal and red or brown distal half, is seen in a minority of patients with chronic renal failure. Whitening of the nail plates may be related to hypoalbuminaemia, as in cirrhosis of the liver. Some drugs, notably antimalarials, antibiotics and phenothiazines, can discolour the nails.
- *Beau's lines* Transverse grooves that appear synchronously on all nails a few weeks after an acute illness, and which grow steadily out to the free margin (Fig. 13.26).
- *Connective tissue disorders* Nail fold telangiectasia or erythema is a useful physical sign in dermatomyositis, systemic sclerosis and systemic lupus erythematosus (Fig. 13.27). In dermatomyositis, the

cuticles become shaggy, and in systemic sclerosis loss of finger pulp leads to overcurvature of the nail plates. Thin nails, with longitudinal ridging and sometimes partial onycholysis, are seen when the peripheral circulation is impaired, as in Raynaud's phenomenon.

## Nail changes in the common dermatoses

### Psoriasis

Most patients with psoriasis have nail changes at some stage; severe nail involvement is more likely in the presence of arthritis. The best-known nail change is pitting of the surface of the nail plate (see Fig. 5.7). Almost as common is psoriasis under the nail plate, showing up as red or brown

**Fig. 13.27** Large tortuous capillary loops of the proximal nail fold signal the presence of a connective tissue disorder.

areas resembling oil spots, often with onycholysis bordered by obvious discoloration (see Fig. 5.8). There is no effective topical treatment for psoriasis of the nails.

> **Learning point**
>
> Do not waste time and money treating asymptomatic nail psoriasis or onycholysis with antifungals

### Eczema

Some patients with itchy chronic eczema bring their nails to a high state of polish by scratching. In addition, eczema of the nail folds may lead to a coarse irregularity with transverse ridging of the adjacent nail plates.

### Lichen planus

Some 10% of patients with lichen planus have nail changes. Most often this is a reversible thinning of the nail plate with irregular longitudinal grooves and ridges. More severe involvement may lead to pterygium in which the cuticle grows forward over the base of the nail and attaches itself to the nail plate (Fig. 13.26). The threat of severe and permanent nail changes can sometimes justify treatment with systemic steroids.

### Alopecia areata

The more severe the hair loss, the more likely there is to be nail involvement. A roughness or fine pitting is seen on the surface of the nail plates and the lunulae may appear mottled.

## Infections

### Acute paronychia

The portal of entry for the organisms concerned, usually staphylococci, is a break in the skin or cuticle as a result of minor trauma. The subsequent acute inflammation, often with the formation of pus in the nail fold or under the nail, requires systemic treatment with flucloxacillin, cephalexin or erythromycin (Formulary 2, p. 394) and appropriate surgical drainage.

### Chronic paronychia

#### Cause

A combination of circumstances can allow a mixture of opportunistic pathogens (yeasts, Gram-positive cocci and Gram-negative rods) to colonize the space between the nail fold and nail plate, producing a chronic dermatitis. Predisposing factors include a poor peripheral circulation, wet work, working with flour, diabetes, vaginal candidosis and overvigorous cutting back of the cuticles.

#### Presentation and course

The nail folds become tender and swollen (Figs 13.26 and 13.28) and small amounts of pus are discharged at intervals. The cuticular seal is damaged and the adjacent nail plate becomes ridged and discoloured. The condition may last for years.

#### Differential diagnosis

In atypical cases, consider the outside chance of an amelanotic melanoma. Paronychia should not be confused with a dermatophyte infection in which the nail folds are not primarily affected.

**Fig. 13.28** Paronychia with secondary nail ridging.

## Investigations

Test the urine for sugar, check for vaginal and oral candidosis. Pus should be cultured.

## Treatment

Manicuring of the cuticle should cease. Treatment is aimed at both the infective and dermatitic elements of the condition. The hands should be kept as warm and as dry as possible, and the damaged nail folds packed several times a day with an imidazole cream (Formulary 1, p. 388). Highly potent topical corticosteroid creams applied for 3 weeks also help. If there is no response, and swabs confirm that *Candida* is present, a 2-week course of itraconazole should be considered (Formulary 2, p. 396).

## *Dermatophyte infections* (Figs 13.26 and 16.40)

### Cause

The common dermatophytes that cause tinea pedis can also invade the nails (p. 248).

### Presentation

Toe nail infection is common and associated with tinea pedis. The early changes often occur at the free edge of the nail and spread proximally. The nail plate becomes yellow, crumbly and thickened. Usually, only a few nails are infected but occasionally all are. The finger nails are involved less often

and the changes, in contrast to those of psoriasis, are usually confined to one hand. Nail infection in patients with HIV infections often involve the proximal subungual skin without distal involvement.

### Clinical course

The condition seldom clears spontaneously.

### Differential diagnosis

Psoriasis has been mentioned. Yeast and mould infections of the nail plate, much more rare than dermatophyte infections, can look similar. Coexisting tinea pedis favours dermatophyte infection of the nail.

### Investigations

The diagnosis is confirmed by microscopic examination of potassium hydroxide-treated nail clippings (p. 40). Cultures should be carried out in a mycology laboratory.

### Treatment

This is given on p. 251. Remember that most symptom-free fungal infections of the toe nails need no treatment at all.

## Tumours

• *Periungual warts* are common and stubborn. Cryotherapy must be used carefully to avoid damage to the nail matrix, but is painful.

• *Periungual fibromas* (see Fig. 24.5) arise from the nail folds, usually in late childhood, in patients with tuberous sclerosis.

• *Glomus tumours* can occur beneath the nail plate. The small red or bluish lesions are exquisitely painful if touched and when the temperature changes. Treatment is surgical.

• *Subungual exostoses* (Fig. 13.22) protrude painfully under the nail plate. Usually secondary to trauma to the terminal phalanx, the bony abnormality can be seen on X-ray and treatment is surgical.

• *Myxoid cysts* (Fig. 13.29) occur on the proximal nail folds, usually of the fingers. The smooth

**Fig. 13.29** Myxoid cyst creating a groove in the nail.

**Fig. 13.30** The curved slow-growing greenish-yellow nails of the yellow nail syndrome.

domed swelling contains a clear jelly-like material that transilluminates well. A groove may form on the adjacent nail plate. Cryotherapy, injections of triamcinolone and surgical excision all have their advocates.

Malignant melanoma should be suspected in any subungual pigmented lesion, particularly if the pigment spreads to the surrounding skin (Hutchinson's sign Fig. 14.13). Subungual haematomas may cause confusion but 'grow out' with the nail (Fig. 13.21). The risk of misdiagnosis is highest with an amelanotic melanoma, which may mimic chronic paronychia or a pyogenic granuloma.

### Some other nail abnormalities

A few people are born with one or more nails missing. In addition, there are many conditions, either inherited or associated with chromosomal abnormalities and usually rare, in which nail changes form a minor part of the clinical picture. Most cannot be dealt with here.

In the rare *nail–patella syndrome*, the thumb nails, and to a lesser extent those of the fingers, are smaller than normal. Rudimentary patellae, renal disease and iliac spines complete the syndrome, which is inherited as an autosomal dominant trait linked with the locus controlling ABO blood groups.

*Pachyonychia congenita* is also rare and inherited as an autosomal dominant trait. The nails are grossly thickened, especially peripherally, and have a curious triangular profile (Fig. 13.23). Hyperkeratosis may occur on areas of friction on the legs and feet.

Permanent loss of the nails may be seen with the dystrophic types of *epidermolysis bullosa* (p. 129).

In the *yellow nail syndrome* (Fig. 13.30) the nail changes begin in adult life, against a background of hypoplasia of the lymphatic system. Peripheral oedema is usually present and pleural effusions may occur. The nails grow very slowly and become thickened and greenish-yellow; their surface is smooth but they are overcurved from side to side.

*The nail 'en racquette'* is a short broad nail (Fig. 13.23), usually a thumbnail, which is seen in some 1–2% of the population and inherited as an autosomal dominant trait. The basic abnormality is shortness of the underlying terminal phalanx.

## The mouth and genitals

Mucous membranes are covered with a modified stratified squamous epithelium that lacks a stratum corneum. This makes them moist and susceptible to infection, and to conditions not seen elsewhere. In contrast, the skin around them is like that on other body sites, and develops the standard range of skin disorders. It follows that the diagnosis of puzzling mouth or genital changes is often made easier by looking for skin disease elsewhere.

**Table 13.4** Some common tongue problems.

| Condition | Cause | Treatment |
|---|---|---|
| Furred tongue | Hypertrophy of the filiform papillae | Brush the tongue |
| Black hairy tongue (Fig. 13.31) | Pigmentation and hypertrophy of filiform papillae caused by bacterial overgrowth | Brush the tongue |
| Smooth tongue | Nutritional deficiency, sprue, malabsorption | Vitamins, nutrition |
| Fissured tongue | Congenital, Down's syndrome, ageing changes | No treatment needed |
| Median rhomboid glossitis | Developmental defect and candidosis Smoking and dentures worsen | No treatment needed |
| Geographic tongue (Fig. 13.32) | Familial, atopic, psoriasis | Topical steroids |
| Varices | Blue compressible blebs of veins | No treatment needed |
| Hairy leucoplakia (see Fig. 16.36) | Epstein–Barr virus infection in patients with HIV/AIDS | Highly active retroviral therapies (HAART) |
| Herpetic glossitis | Painful fissures without vesicles | Aciclovir group (p. 397) |
| Macroglossia | Developmental, tumours, infections, amyloidosis, thyroid | Treat the cause |
| Glossodynia | Trauma, *Candida*, menopause, diabetes, nutritional, dry mouth | Treat the cause, use tricyclic antidepressants |

**Fig. 13.31** Black hairy tongue.

**Fig. 13.32** Geographic tongue.

## The mouth

The mouth can harbour an enormous range of diseases, affecting each of its component structures. Inflammatory and infectious disorders of the mouth are usually either red or white – leading to the terms erythroplakia and leucoplakia, respectively. These are descriptive terms but not diagnoses. A biopsy will help sort out the non-dysplastic causes, such as lichen planus and *Candida* infections, from the dysplastic ones that are the precursors of carcinoma.

Some skin diseases cause ulceration in the mouth. These ulcers are accompanied by skin diseases elsewhere on the body; making a diagnosis there is easier than in the mouth. In other patients with mouth ulcers, the course of the ulcers or erosions, and their size and location in the mouth, provide diagnostic clues. Table 13.4 lists some common tongue troubles.

### *Lichen planus*

#### *Cause*

The cause of oral lichen planus is unknown (see Chapter 6). However, some 40% of patients with symptomatic lichen planus of the mouth have relevant allergies, diagnosable by patch testing.

These are usually to metals (especially gold and mercury) and flavourings such as cinnamon, peppermint and spearmint. Lichen planus also results from drug reactions, liver disease and bone marrow transplantation.

### Presentation

When a lichen planus-like cutaneous eruption is present, finding lichen planus in the mouth confirms the diagnosis, and vice versa. In the mouth, typically, there is a lace-like whitening of the buccal mucosae (see Fig. 6.4), but sometimes this laciness is not present. Oral lichen planus can also be red, and can ulcerate. A 'desquamative gingivitis' may occur, in which the mucosa shears off with friction, such as that from brushing the teeth or eating an apple. Desquamative gingivitis can also result from pemphigus or pemphigoid (p. 197). Often, oral lichen planus is asymptomatic and more of a curiosity than a problem for the patient.

### Course

Oral lichen planus can last for years – even for a lifetime. Asymptomatic lichen planus does not usually progress to the symptomatic form.

### Differential diagnosis

In its classic lace-like state, the appearance of oral lichen planus is diagnostic. Dysplastic leucoplakias are more likely to be focal, appearing on only a portion of the mucosae, gingivae or lips. They are also more likely to be red and symptomatic, and shown by those who have smoked cigarettes or chewed tobacco. *Candida albicans* infections may occasionally be considered, but their white patches scrape off.

### Investigations

A potassium hydroxide (KOH) examination and a culture will rule out candidasis. Biopsy will determine if a white patch is dysplastic or not. The histology of lichen planus, as seen in the skin, may be less typical in the mouth, and may even suggest a dermatitis. Patch testing may be useful as allergic causes can be cured by allergen elimination. Liver function tests, and tests for hepatitis B, hepatitis C and antimitochondrial antibodies are often recommended.

### Treatment

If asymptomatic, no treatment is necessary. High-potency topical steroids, in gel or ointment bases, are worth a try if the lesions are painful or ulcerated. Failing that, a few patients require oral prednisone; they should be referred to a dermatologist or specialist in oral medicine. Topical tacrolimus ointment may help, but treatment with this new agent is experimental.

### Complications

Watch out for carcinoma, even if previous biopsies have shown no dysplasia. The risk is highest in the ulcerative forms, and the overall risk for development of squamous cell carcinoma in oral lichen planus is probably 1–5%. It should be suspected if an area becomes thickened, nodular or ulcerates.

## Candidiasis

### Cause and presentation

Infections with *Candida albicans* appear suddenly, on the tongue, lips or other mucosae, in the 'pseudomembranous form' (also called thrush; see Fig. 16.47). Small lesions are more common than large ones. About 15% of infants develop thrush on the tongue, lips or buccal mucosa. Sometimes candidiasis appears as red sore patches under dentures, or as angular chelitis (perlèche).

### Course

If the candidiasis is a complication of systemic antibiotic therapy, treatment will be curative. Immunosuppressed and denture-wearing patients often have recurrent disease.

### Differential diagnosis

Many tongues are coated with desquamated epithelial cells that create a yellow wet powder on

**Table 13.5** Some possible causes underlying oral candidiasis in adults.

Antibiotic treatment
HIV infection
Myelodysplastic syndromes
  leukaemia
  lymphoma
  thymoma
Chemotherapy
Inhalation of corticosteroids for asthma
Widespread metastatic malignancy
Vitamin deficiency
Inflammatory bowel disease
Xerostomia
Previous radiation therapy to mouth
Diabetes
Addison's disease
Myasthenia gravis
Dentures
Chronic mucocutaneous candidiasis (on skin and nails
  too; p. 252)

their surface. This srapes off easily, and shows no inflammation underneath. Lichen planus, oral hairy leucoplakia and dysplastic leucoplakia may cause confusion.

*Investigations*

Thrush does not normally occur in healthy adults, in whom the appearance of candidiasis needs more investigation than just a simple diagnosis by appearance, KOH examination or culture. Table 13.5 lists some possible underlying causes.

*Treatment*

Topical and systemic imidazoles are the treatments of choice. Creams and solutions can be used, but sucking on a clotrimazole troche (Formulary 1, p. 388) three times daily is better. Some patients are best treated with fluconazole, 150 mg once daily for 1–3 days. If an underlying condition is present, this should be identified and treated. Patients with 'denture sore mouth' should scrub their dentures each night with toothpaste and a toothbrush, sleep without dentures, and swish a teaspoonful of nystatin solution around the dentureless mouth three times a day.

*Contact stomatitis*

This underdiagnosed problem usually causes a transient soreness, associated with a diffuse redness of the lips and buccal gingivae. Mouthwashes, hard sweets (candies) and hot pizzas are common causes of the irritant type, whereas cinnamon, vanilla, peppermint, spearmint and dentifrices are the most common causes of allergic contact stomatitis. When local stomatitis or ulcers occur near a gold tooth filling, gold allergy should be suspected, but patch testing is needed before recommending that the filling be removed.

*Ulcers*

One problem with oral ulcers (as with ulcers elsewhere) is the usual lack of a primary lesion, such as a bulla, papule or plaque. Ulcers are often secondary reactions which rob the clinician of the chance to make a morphological diagnosis. The history, the location of the ulcers within the mouth, their duration and the presence of coexisting non-oral signs or symptoms, especially of the skin, are then all-important clues to the underlying diagnosis.

*Bullous diseases*

Pemphigus and pemphigoid are most likely (see Chapter 9). Pemphigus causes large painful long-lasting erosions (see Fig. 9.3). The whole mouth can be involved, but more often it affects just the lips, buccal mucosa or tonsillar pillars. Desquamative gingivitis can occur. The ulcers are large, appear without warning and last months. A biopsy may show separation of keratinocytes (acantholysis) and should not be taken from an ulcer, but from normal-appearing mucosa next to an active area. Direct immunofluorescence (biopsy normal mucosa) shows antibody rimming each keratinocyte.

Cicatricial (scarring) pemphigoid affects the mucous membranes predominantly, but occasionally affects the skin too. The eyelid conjunctiva and other mucosae can also be affected; scarring often results (see Fig. 9.8). Cicatricial pemphigoid is also a cause of desquamative gingivitis. Biopsy shows a subepidermal bulla, and direct immunofluorescence

**Fig. 13.33** Aphthous ulcer of the labial mucosa.

a linear band of IgG and C3 at the dermal–mucosal junction.

### Aphthae

#### Presentation

These common small oval painful mouth ulcers arise, usually without an obvious cause, most often in 'movable mucosae' such as the gutters of the mouth, tongue or cheek (Fig. 13.33). An area of tenderness changes into a small red papule that quickly turns into a grey 2–5 mm painful ulcer with a red areola. Herpetiform aphthae occur in groups of 2–5 tiny painful ulcers. Major aphthae (periadenitis mucosa necrotica) are usually larger than 1 cm across and tend to appear in the back of the mouth.

#### Course

Small ulcers heal in a week or two; the pain stops within days. Major aphthae may persist for months.

#### Differential diagnosis

Recurrent herpes simplex infections mimic herpetiform apthae but, in the latter, cultures are negative and blisters are not seen. Behçet's disease causes confusion in patients with major aphthae. In fact, a diagnosis of Behçet's is often wrongly made in patients with recurrent aphthae of all sorts, when the patient has some other skin disease or joint pain. Patients with true Behçet's disease should have

at least two of these other findings: genital ulcers, pustular vasculitis of skin, synovitis, uveitis or meningoencephalitis.

#### Investigations

Usually none are needed. Occasional associations include Crohn's disease, ulcerative colitis, gluten-sensitive enteropathy, cyclical neutropenia, other neutropenias, HIV infection and deficiencies of iron, vitamin $B_{12}$ or folate.

#### Treatment

Prevention is best. Trauma, such as aggressive tooth brushing, hard or aggravating foods, and stress should be avoided if relevant. The application of a topical corticosteroid gel, such as fluocinonide, to new lesions may shorten their course. In severe or complex cases, consider referral.

### Some other oral lumps, bumps and colour changes

- Mucocoeles are collections of mucin following the rupture of a minor salivary gland duct. They are blue-tinted soft translucent nodules, usually of the lips, and arise suddenly without pain.
- Fordyce spots are ectopic sebaceous glands, appearing as pinhead-sized whitish-yellow papules on the labial mucosa (Fig. 13.34).
- Yellow patches in the mouth may suggest pseudo-xanthoma elasticum.

**Fig. 13.34** Fordyce spots are ectopic sebaceous glands.

**Fig. 13.35** Venous lake.

● Brown macules on the lips should trigger thoughts about the dominantly inherited Peutz–Jeghers syndrome (see Fig. 19.12) and its bowel polyps and tumours.

● Neurofibromas may occur, especially in patients with widespread cutaneous neurofibromatosis.

● Telangiectases may suggest hereditary haemorrhagic telangiectasia. These patients may also have telangiectases in their intestinal tract leading to gastrointestinal bleeding, and arteriovenous fistulae – especially in the lungs – that may lead to cerebral embolism.

● Venous lakes are blue or black papules on the lips (Fig. 13.35). These melanoma-like lesions worry patients and doctors alike, but pressure with a diascope or glass slide causes them to blanch.

● Multiple, somewhat translucent, papules may suggest Cowden's syndrome. These are fibromas. Patients with Cowden's syndrome have facial papules and nodules (tricholemmomas and fibromas), fibrocystic disease of the breasts and a great propensity to develop malignant tumours of the breast, thyroid and other organs.

● Patients with the multiple mucosal neuroma syndrome have neuromas in their mouths, and 75% of those with this autosomal dominantly inherited disorder also have medulary carcinoma of the thyroid. Many also develop phaeochromocytomas. Many small bumps appear along the lips, tongue and buccal mucosae.

● Pyogenic granulomas of the gingiva appear as quick-growing red bleeding papules. They are reactive proliferations of blood vessels, and often develop in pregnancy ('pregnancy tumours').

● Fibromas may result from dentures, or from resolving or indolent pyogenic granulomas, but can also appear without reason, usually on the gingiva of adults. Tooth bites may cause fibromas to appear on the tongue and on the buccal mucosae. Cowden's disease should be considered if multiple lesions are present.

● Warts in the mouth are not uncommon.

● The differential diagnosis of oral papules and nodules also includes lipomas, keloids, giant cell granulomas, granular cell tumours, myxomas, xanthomas, haemangiomas, myomas, neural tumours and a host of uncommon benign growths.

### *Squamous cell carcinoma*
(Fig. 13.36; see also p. 303)

#### *Cause*

Predisposing factors include smoking or chewing tobacco products, and the 'straight-shot' drinking of alcohol. Cancer can also occur in the plaques and ulcers of lichen planus. Lip cancers may be sun-induced.

#### *Presentation*

A thickening or nodule develops, usually on the lower lip, and often in a field of actinic chelitis (rough scaling mucosa from sun damage). Inside the mouth, the tongue is the most common site to be affected, often on its undersurface. The cancer itself appears either as an indurated ulcer with steep

**Fig. 13.36** Squamous cell carcinoma in a heavy smoker.

edges, or as a diffuse hardness or nodule. Red or white thickened plaques are common precursors, and the cancer may be surrounded by these changes.

### Course

Unfortunately, cancer of the mouth often goes undetected. Its symptoms are excused by the patient as aphthous ulcers or denture sores, and its signs are not seen by the physicians who scan the skin. Cancers grow, and squamous cell carcinomas of the mouth are no exception. Plaques and hard areas may ulcerate.

### Differential diagnosis

Confusion occurs with ulcerative lichen planus and other causes of white and red patches. Biopsy will differentiate a squamous cell carcinoma from these other conditions.

### Treatment

Dermatologists often treat lip cancers by a wedge excision through all layers of the lip, with primary repair. Oral surgeons or otolaryngologists usually remove intra-oral cancers. Metastatic disease may require radiotherapy or chemotherapy.

### Complications

Squamous cell carcinomas of the lip caused by sun exposure carry a much better prognosis than the others. Left untreated, squamous cell carcinomas are prone to metastasize to regional lymph nodes and elsewhere. The overall 5-year survival for intra-oral squamous cell carcinoma is about 40–50%.

---

**Learning points**

- Mouths talk, but don't expect one to tell you its diagnosis
- Leucoplakia is not a diagnosis. Find the cause of your patient's white spots
- Aphthae are small and heal quickly. Consider pemphigus or another bullous disease if your patient has many, persisting or large erosions in the mouth
- A mouth ulcer may be cancerous

---

## The genitals

The genital area is richly supplied with cutaneous nerves. This means that skin disease there makes life more miserable than might be expected from its extent or apparent severity. In addition, patients often feel a special shame when their genitals harbour skin diseases. Skin diseases seen elsewhere may afflict this area, but the patient will often hide them from the examining physician. Many never seek treatment.

### Benign conditions

An array of problems can plague the genitals; Table 13.6 lists some of them.

**Table 13.6** Some benign genital problems.

| | |
|---|---|
| Pearly penile papules | Pinhead-sized angiofibromas of the glans penis |
| Fordyce spots | Ectopic sebaceous glands of the glans penis |
| Angiokeratomas | Black papules of scrotum |
| Balanitis | Many types, but poor hygiene is common |
| Warts (condyloma accuminata) | Cauliflower-like growths of moist genital skin (see Chapter 16) |
| Fixed drug eruptions | Red plaques or ulcers can be localized to the penis (see Chapter 25) |
| Lichen planus (Fig. 13.37) | Look for lesions in the mouth or on the skin to confirm the diagnosis |
| Psoriasis | Often favours the glans penis |
| Paget's disease | Intra-epithelial adenocarcinoma appearing as a marginated red plaque |
| Infections | Syphilis, herpes simplex, chancroid, lymphogranuloma venereum |

**Fig. 13.37** White lace-like appearance of vulval lichen planus.

## Vulvovaginitis

Inflammatory diseases of the vagina often also affect the vulva, but the vagina alone can be affected. Vaginitis causes discharge, odour, painful intercourse and itching or burning sensations. The differential diagnosis includes candidiasis, trichomoniasis, bacterial vaginosis, cytolytic vaginosis and atrophic vaginitis. The diagnosis can be made by the appearance of the discharge, both grossly and under the microscope. Most patients with vaginitis obtain their care from gynaecologists. Swabs for microbiological examination are essential.

## Lichen sclerosus (see Chapter 10)

### Cause

This is unknown but local conditions have a role; not only does skin develop the disease after being transplanted into affected areas, but the disease also goes away when the grafted skin is returned to a distant site.

### Presentation

The affected areas on the vulva, penis (Fig. 13.38), perineum and/or perianal skin show well-marginated white thin fragile patches with a crinkled surface. Itching can be severe, especially in women. The fragility of the atrophic areas may lead to purpura and erosions. Scratching can cause lichenification, and diagnostic confusion.

**Fig. 13.38** Lichen sclerosus of the foreskin, carrying the risk of causing phimosis.

Women are more commonly afflicted than men, but pre-adolescent girls and boys also can develop this problem. In girls, the white patches circling the vulva and anus take on an hourglass shape around the orifices (Fig. 13.39).

### Course

As time goes on, scarring occurs. In adult women, the clitoral prepuce may scar over the clitoris, and the vaginal introitus may narrow, preventing enjoyable sexual intercourse. Scarring is rare in girls and boys; treatment may prevent it occurring in adults.

### Differential diagnosis

The sharply marginated white patches of vitiligo can afflict the vulva and penis but lack atrophy, and typical vitiligo may be found elsewhere on the body. Neurodermatitis may be superimposed upon lichen sclerosus after incessant scratching.

### Investigations

Biopsy is often unnecessary but the appearances

**Fig. 13.39** Lichen sclerosus of the perineum in a prepubescent girl.

are distinctive. The epidermis is thin, the basal layer shows damage, and the papillary dermis contains a homogeneous pink-staining material and lymphocytes.

### Treatment

At first sight it might seem unwise to rub potent topical steroids onto atrophic thin occluded skin. Yet treatment with potent topical steroids not only reduces itch, pain and misery, but also reverses hypopigmentation and atrophy by shutting down its cause. However, atrophy, striae and other complications can develop on untreated adjacent skin if the medication spreads there. Ointments are preferable to creams. Only small amounts (15 g) should be dispensed. After a course of 8–12 weeks, weaker topical steroids can be used to maintain a remission.

### Complications

Scarring can destroy anatomical structures and narrow the vaginal opening. Squamous cell carcinomas may develop in men as well as women. Any focal thickening needs a biopsy.

## Vulval and scrotal pruritus

### Cause

Itching of the genital skin is usually caused by skin disease, or by rubbing, sweating, irritation or occlusion. Once started, genital itching seems able to continue on its own.

### Presentation

The vulva and scrotum contain nerves that normally transmit pleasurable sensations. However, itching itself is not pleasurable, although scratching is. A torturing itch may be present all day, but more frequently appears or worsens at night. Once scratching has started, it perpetuates itself. The history is of an incessant and embarrassed scratching. Examination may show normal skin, or the tell-tale signs of excoriations and lichenification.

### Differential diagnosis

Itch is part of many inflammatory skin diseases. In the groin its most common causes are tinea, *Candida*, erythrasma, atopic dermatitis, psoriasis, pubic lice, intertrigo and irritant or allergic contact dermatitis. However, patients with 'essential' pruritus show no skin changes other than those elicited by scratching. Sometimes the cause is psychogenic, but one should be reluctant to assume that this is the cause. Biopsy rarely helps. Look for clues by hunting for skin disease at other body sites.

### Treatment

Low-potency topical corticosteroids sometimes help by suppressing secondary inflammation; however, atrophy sometimes quickly occurs, and then the itch is replaced by a burning sensation. A better approach is to eliminate the trigger factors for itch – such as hot baths, tight clothing, rough fabrics, sweating, cool air, the chronic wetness of vaginal secretions, menstrual pads and soaps. Antipruritic creams, such as doxepin cream, pramoxine cream or menthol in a light emollient base, help to abort the itch–scratch–itch cycles. Many patients benefit from systemic antihistamines or tricyclic drugs such as amitriptyline or doxepin.

**Table 13.7** Nine common groin dermatoses.

| Condition | Clinical comments |
| --- | --- |
| Tinea cruris | Involves the groin but seldom the scrotum |
| Candidiasis | Beefy red with satellite papules and pustules |
| Erythrasma | Brown patches of the upper thighs |
| Irritant contact dermatitis | Burning sensations may predominate |
| Allergic contact dermatitis | The scrotum may be oedematous |
| Inverse psoriasis | Beefy red marginated plaques extend up the gluteal fold |
| Seborrhoeic dermatitis | Look at the scalp for disease there, to confirm the diagnosis |
| Neurodermatitis | It feels wonderful to scratch an itchy groin |
| Intertrigo | Skin breaks down from maceration |

## Complications

Atrophy is common but hard to see. Lichenification creates leathery thickenings, marked with grooves resembling fissures.

## Dermatoses

The skin of the groins and genitalia is susceptible to many inflammatory skin diseases. They are listed here (Table 13.7), but discussed in other chapters.

> **Learning point**
>
> 'Jock itch' (tinea) affects the thighs and inguinal folds. Consider other diagnoses for rashes of the groin by examing other sites

## Malignant conditions

### Squamous cell carcinoma

#### Cause

Human papilloma viruses, especially HPV types 6, 11, 16 and 18, often play a part. These are sexually transmitted, so the risk of carcinoma of the vulva or penis is greatest in those who have had many sexual partners. Squamous cell carcinoma of the glans penis is especially common in the uncircumcised. Smegma can incite inflammation leading to both phimosis and carcinoma. Exposure to tar also predisposes to scrotal carcinoma. Other predisposing factors are immunosuppression, lichen sclerosus and, possibly, lichen planus. Cancer can also develop from bowenoid papulosis – growths on the penis that resemble dark seborrhoeic keratoses clinically, and Bowen's disease histologically. The female equivalent is vulvar intra-epithelial neoplasia.

#### Presentation

In men, a glistening irregular red moist patch (Fig. 13.40; Bowen's disease or erythroplasia of Queyrat) develops on an uncircumcised penis, either on the glans or on the inner prepuce. Maceration may make it look white until evaporation reveals its true colour. It enlarges slowly, and invasion and tumour formation may not occur for years in immunocompetent men. In women, the precursor lesion is often Bowen's disease presenting as a sharply marginated, very slowly growing, mildly hyperkeratotic or slightly scaling, irregularly shaped red patch or plaque that is usually a single lesion on one labia or in the perineum. This may become huge (up to 10 cm diameter). Sometimes, cancer of the

**Fig. 13.40** Erythroplasia of Queyrat.

penis or labia resembles a large wart destroying the underlying tissue. Biopsy confirms the diagnosis.

*Course*

Eventually the precursor lesions become frankly invasive and capable of metastasizing. Invasive carcinomas present either as bleeding ulcerated indurated plaques, or as tumorous nodules.

*Treatment*

Mohs' micrographic excision (p. 373) is probably the best treatment for small and minimally invasive carcinomas, but partial penectomy is indicated if the tumour is large. Precursor lesions such as warts, bowenoid papulosis, vulvar intra-epithelial neoplasia and Bowen's disease can be destroyed with laser surgery (p. 378) or cryotherapy (p. 374). In some patients with minimally invasive carcinomas, topical applications of the cytokine inducer imiquimod cream or the chemotherapeutic 5-fluorouracil cream can be curative. It is hoped that immunization with the new HPV vaccine will prevent infections with the oncogenic wart viruses and relegate genital squamous cell carcinomas to the history books.

## Further reading

Baran R, Dawber RPR, de Berker DAR, Haneke E & Tosti A. (2001) *Baran and Dawber's Diseases of the Nails and their Management*, 3rd edn. Blackwell Science, Oxford.

Bruce AJ & Rogers RS. (2004) Oral manifestations of sexually transmitted diseases. Review. *Clinical Dermatology* **22**, 520–527.

Edwards L. (2004) *Genital Dermatology Atlas*. Lippincott Williams & Wilkins, Philadelphia.

Hordinsky MK, Sawaya ME & Scher RK. (2000) *Atlas of the Hair and Nails*. Churchill Livingstone, Philadelphia.

Lynch PJ & Edwards L. (1994) *Genital Dermatology*. Churchill Livingstone, Edinburgh.

MacDonald Hull SP, Wood ML, Hutchinson PE, Sladden M & Messenger AG. (2003) Guidelines for the management of alopecia areata. *British Journal of Dermatology* **149**, 692–699.

Margesson JJ. (2006) Vulvar disease pearls. Review. *Dermatologic Clinics* **24**, 145–155.

Ridley CM, Oriel JD & Robinson A. (2000) *Vulval Disease*. Arnold, London.

Scully C. (2006) Clinical practice. Aphthous ulceration. Review. *New England Journal of Medicine* **355**, 165–172.

# 14 Racially pigmented skin

In the 40,000 years since our common ancestors left Africa, human skin colour has diverged widely. A dark skin protect against skin cancer and photolysis of folate (necessary for foetal development), while pale skin allows for Vitamin D synthesis and the prevention of rickets. These two competing evolutionary pressures should favour a range of skin colours dependent on different ultraviolet (UV) exposure. This has been confirmed by comparing data taken from satellite measurements of UV irradiance of the earth, with reflectance spectrophotometry measurements from the skin of different races (Table 14.1). Around three quarters of the variation in human pigmentation is accounted for by UV irradiation. Ultraviolet irradiation is generally highest at the equator and decreases with increasing latitude, although high altitude and dry air increase irradiance for given latitutdes.

No colour defines normal skin. No race or skin colour has a monopoly on skin disease. The same skin diseases occur in all races. Because of both genetic and environmental differences, skin diseases in those with pigmented skin often differ from those with non-pigmented skin in their incidence, prevalence, appearance and behaviour. They also differ in the types of cosmetic impairment they produce. For example, an acne papule in a white person can cause a transient mild tan or pink colour after the inflammation subsides, but the same papule may produce a long-lasting black macule in an African-American with darker skin.

## Skin types

For the most part, melanin determines the colour of the skin. Other determinants that modify colour are capillary blood flow, carotene, lycopene, dermal collagen and the amounts of absorbed or reflected colours of light. As discussed in detail in Chapter 2, each melanocyte supplies melanin to about 30 nearby keratinocytes regardless of race, so it is the type, amount, and distribution of melanin in keratinocytes that determine the colour of the skin. Tyrosinase in melanosomes converts tyrosine to dopa and then dopa to dopaquinone. This generates eumelanin, which is a dark brown–black colour. Eumelanin is plentiful in the dark skin of Africans and East Indians. Pheomelanin is yellow–red and forms when dopaquinone combines with cysteine or glutathione (p. 272). It is more plentiful in freckles in the light skin of Celtic populations of northern Europe.

Because people of the same race may have a darker or lighter skin, dermatologists use skin typing numbers to grade baseline pigmentation. These skin types range from the pale, white, sunburning skin of type I individuals to the dark brown or black, never sun-burning skin of type VI individuals. Skin types are assigned by the criteria listed in Table 18.1.

**Table 14.1** Skin colour (measured by reflectance at 685nm) and latitude. Lower numbers represent darker skin. Adapted from Jablonski and Chaplin, *Journal of Human Evolution* (2000).

|  | Skin colour | Approximate Latitude |
| --- | --- | --- |
| Kenya | 32 | 0° (Equator) |
| Papua New Guinea (Goroka) | 33 | 6°S |
| Ethiopian Highlands | 34 | 8°N |
| South Africa (San) | 44 | 22°S |
| Libya (Fezzan) | 44 | 24°N |
| South Africa | 51 | 32°S |
| Northern England | 67 | 54°N |
| Greenland (dietary Vitamin D) | 56 | 60°N |

## Racial differences in structure and function

Despite obvious differences in colour, the skin of the various races is remarkably similar in structure and function. However, the epidermis is often thicker in dark skin, perhaps because it is less photodamaged. The stratum corneum of Negroid skin may be more compact and contain higher concentrations of lipids. Functional differences in sweating may be ascribed to acclimatization and climate. The production of sebum may be higher in Negroid skin, but these differences, if any, are small.

Fibroblasts are larger and more numerous in black than in white skin and the collagen bundles are finer and stacked more closely together. The fibroblasts may also be more active. This, combined with the decreased collagenase activity of black skin, predisposes it to form keloids.

Negroid hair is more likely to be spiral (coil with a decreasing diameter outwards), rather than straight, wavy or helical (coil with a constant diameter). Negroid hair shafts tend to be more elliptical, and hair follicles more curved. Mongoloid hair has the largest cross-sectional area, while Caucasoid hair of western Europeans has the smallest. Native Americans and Mayan Indians have hair with large round cross-sections.

Darker skin seems more resistant to irritation, but this has been hard to prove by scientific study. Erythema is difficult to see in dark skin, so visual measures of irritation falsely underestimate the degree of inflammation. Chemicals penetrate black skin at about the same rate as they penetrate white skin, and skin irritants produce comparable irritation if this is measured with surrogate markers such as the rate of transepidermal water loss across irritated skin.

## Hyperpigmentation

Inflammation often leaves either dark or light spots; in other words, either it increases melanocyte activity, or it increases epidermal turnover so that melanocytes inject less pigment into the surrounding keratinocytes. Although these areas are not scars, patients often refer to them as such and, like scars, they can be unsightly and persistent (Fig. 14.1).

**Fig. 14.1** Postinflammatory hyperpigmentation. Inflammation often stimulates pigment cells to produce excessive melanin, so that previously inflamed areas are marked long afterwards with dark patches.

For example, acne causes hyperpigmented macules when papules and pustules resolve. Like the acne itself, these marks are hard to hide, and the facial appearance worsens progressively as they accumulate. For this reason, acne in coloured skin calls for more aggressive treatment but, unfortunately, irritation from acne treatments can also induce hyperpigmentation. Less irritating retinoids such as adapalene are often preferred, and systemic antibiotics tend to be prescribed more quickly and generously. Azelaic acid preparations lighten the skin while opening comedones and reducing papule counts, so agents containing it are useful for mild cases.

Any inflammation can leave dark spots, but in all races these are especially prominent and persistent in diseases that damage basal melanocytes and lead to pigmentary incontinence, such as lichen planus (p. 72), erythema dyschromicum perstans (p. 215) and erythema multiforme (p. 110).

Treatment for hyperpigmentation is twofold. First, the primary disease should be suppressed or cured. Secondly, the darker spots can be treated with a 'bleaching agent' such as 4% hydroquinone cream. Proprietary creams containing hydroquinone plus a retinoid, a glucocorticosteroid, or all three are available. Again, care has to be taken not to irritate the skin with treatments designed to lighten it. Hydroquinone in concentrations greater than 4% can be compounded but carries a risk of inducing irreversible exogenous pigmentation, ochronosis. This darkens the skin and prompts applications of even more hydroquinone.

# Hypopigmentation

Areas of skin with inflammation or an increased epidermal turnover can leave light spots. These are not completely depigmented, and so can be distinguished from vitiligo by their appearance as well as by their history.

## Pityriasis alba

### *Presentation*

Pityriasis alba appears as poorly marginated, light patches on pigmented skin (Chapter 19, p. 283). Although it occurs in skin types I and II, it is far more easily seen in darker skin types as the contrast is greater (Fig. 14.2 and 19.6). Sometimes there is fine superficial scaling – hence the term pityriasis. Many patients are children with atopic dermatitis elsewhere. Examination under Wood's light highlights the pigmentary abnormality. Other provokers of pityriasis alba are bites, sunburn (even among the dark-skinned), mechanical irritation from scrubbing, or other forms of eczematous dermatitis.

**Fig. 14.2** Pityriasis alba. Sometimes the epidermis proliferates at slightly different rates, so less pigment gets injected into some keratinocytes than others. The cheeks of an atopic child are particularly prone.

**Fig. 14.3** Vitiligo. Note the complete loss of pigment and the mirror-like symmetry.

### *Course*

The higher the skin type number, the more resistant this disorder is to treatment. Most children with the disease improve at puberty.

### *Differential diagnosis*

In vitiligo (p. 281) the spots are much whiter, much more sharply marginated and always without scaling (Fig. 14.3). Pityriasis versicolor (p. 254) is also more sharply marginated and is usually scaly. A potassium hydroxide (KOH) examination of scraping from these scales should be carried out if there is doubt. Sarcoidosis and leprosy should also be kept in mind.

### *Treatment*

If mild eczema is the provoking factor, treatment with a weak corticosteroid such as hydrocortisone 0.5% or 1%, or a cream containing a calcineurin inhibitor such as pimecrolimus, is often prescribed. However, the pigmentary abnormality will take months to improve. Syndets (synthetic balanced detergents) can

**Fig. 14.4** Vitiligo. If just on the hands, it may have been set off by depigmenting chemicals.

be used to wash the face as they are often less irritating than alkaline soaps. Moisturizers can be applied twice daily, and after face washing. Tanning does not help: too often it accentuates the contrast.

### Leprosy (Hansen's disease)

This is discussed in Chapter 16. Patients with tuberculoid and borderline tuberculoid leprosy often present with lighter patches, sometimes with a subtle erythema at their edges (Fig. 16.10). Palpate for nerve enlargement, test the skin for pinprick anaesthesia, or stain skin biopsy sections for mycobacteria (may be hard to find organisms in tuberculoid forms). Asians seem especially prone to leprosy.

### Vitiligo

This disorder is discussed in Chapter 19. It can occur in any skin type, but is especially disfiguring in those with a dark skin (Figs 14.4 and 14.5). Furthermore, many cultures assume that patients with depigmented areas of skin carry leprosy, and therefore those with vitiligo may be thrown out of society, for example into an 'untouchable' class. Vitiliginous skin is prone to sunburn.

## Conditions more common in coloured skin

About two-thirds of Negroids have a 'demarcation line', also called 'Forcher's line', running down the

**Fig. 14.5** Vitiligo. The pigmented macules in the porcelain-white patches are areas where pigment cells have migrated to the skin surface from hair follicles. Phototherapy regimens work by encouraging this.

ventral sides of their arms and forearms, and often also on their thighs. These lines are normal: they signify no disease, and need no treatment. Most Negroids also have a line of a different shade about 1 cm in width running from the umbilicus to the pubis. If dark, this line is called a 'linea nigra': if light, it is a 'linea alba'.

### Dermatosis papulosa nigra (p. 292)

Negroids are prone to develop small black seborrhoeic keratoses on their faces (Fig. 14.6 and 20.7). Although these are harmless, patients dislike them. Unfortunately, attempts to remove them with cryosurgery, electrosurgery, acids or even lasers can leave white or brown macules that are even more unsightly.

**Fig. 14.6** Dermatosis papulosa nigra.  These small facial seborrheic keratoses which so commonly occur on the faces of Negroids.  Removing them may leave unsatisfactory white scars.

## Pseudofolliculitis barbae ('hair bumps')

This is common in African-Americans and other Negroids, and is related to the curliness of their hair. The hair either exits the follicle below the skin surface, or curls around and 'ingrows' into the dermis, where it elicits a foreign body reaction.

### Presentation

The patient is usually a black male, but black women and persons of other colours are also affected. Often the person is unaffected, or only minimally affected, until he or she shaves. Shortly thereafter, papules and pustules develop at the shave site, most typically in the beard area (Fig. 14.7). Comedones are not seen. Sometimes inflammatory nodules develop; often a hair can be found curled up within them. Hairs sometimes grow sideways.

### Course

Long hair simply does not ingrow. If shaving stops, the number of inflammatory lesions lessens.

**Fig. 14.7** Pseudofolliculitis barbae (shaving bumps). These are due to ingrown hairs.

If shaving is resumed, the process recurs. Individual lesions resolve, often leaving scars or hyperpigmented macules. Long-standing cases may have scars and scar-distorted follicles that are even more prone to inflammation.

### Differential diagnosis

Acne vulgaris can mimic this disorder, as both occur on the face and neck. Acne is associated with comedones, and with papules and pustules on non-hair-bearing areas such as the forehead and temples. Darker skinned individuals tend to use oily cosmetics to produce a desirable sheen on their faces, and sometimes these can produce acne cosmetica (p. 164).

### Treatment

It is easy to advise patients to stop shaving, but they may not want a beard. A compromise lets the hair grow slightly longer than the length provided by a close shave. Special electric razors are widely available. They cut the hair above the skin surface to prevent ingrowth from below, and depend on daily shaving to prevent the ingrowth from above. Some find that daily aggressive rubs with a washcloth dislodge early ingrown hairs. Others prefer to dissolve hair with chemical depilatories. These leave a blunt edge on the hair end, rather than the spear-like point left by razors. Laser treatments target the pigment in hair follicles. Unfortunately in dark skin they may destroy surface pigment along with the hair bulb, leaving white marks. Some doctors prescribe topical retinoids and systemic antibiotics, but the rationale and efficacy of this is questionable. Hot compresses and topical steroids may reduce inflammation.

## Infections

People with pigmented skin acquire the same infections as other people, yet their cutaneous manifestations and prognosis may be different. Post-inflammatory pigment changes are common after many infections, including impetigo, herpes simplex, tineas and pityriasis versicolor.

### Tinea capitis (p. 250)

#### Cause

For some reason, the scalps and hairs of black children are especially prone to infection with *Trichophyton tonsurans*. This fungus invades the hair shaft as well as the stratum corneum. It is transferred from person to person by direct contact, or via contaminated fomites such as brushes, combs, barber's instruments and pillows.

#### Presentation and course

Presentations vary, depending upon the amount of cell-mediated immunity. Inflammation is usually mild, and the disorder mimics seborrhoeic dermatitis (Fig. 14.8). Fine scaling covers some or all of the hair-bearing areas of scalp. In some patients, the fungus weakens the hair shaft, so that it breaks off at the surface of the scalp – the remaining proximal hair appearing as 1–3 mm long black dots ('black dot ringworm'). A patchy alopecia develops in these patients. If host resistance is greater, discernible inflammation may create pink plaques or follicular pustules. Cervical lymph nodes may then enlarge. Kerions from *T. tonsurans* (see Fig. 16.42) are rare. Adults seem resistant to infection, perhaps because of the antifungal effects of sebum. Untreated infections persist, and organisms can be spread to others.

#### Differential diagnosis

The disorder is so common that 'seborrhoeic dermatitis' of the scalp in a black child aged 4–7 years

**Fig. 14.8** Tinea capitis. This is the seborrhoeic form where inflammation is slight and hair loss and scaling prevail. Culture scale and short hairs for fungus.

is likely to be tinea capitis until proved otherwise. Although arthroconidia or hyphae can be seen inside the hair on KOH mounts, the presence of many other pigment granules, bubble-like abnormalities, superimposed scales and hair accretions often fools the non-cognoscenti. The organism does not fluoresce, so examination with a Wood's light is not helpful except to rule out infecting fluorescent fungi such as *Microsporum canis*. The diagnosis is best made by culture of the hair and scales on Sabouraud's agar containing the antibiotic cycloheximide to prevent overgrowth of bacteria. Some paediatricians scrub the scalp with a new toothbrush or wet cotton applicator, and then brush the acquired scale and hair into the culture dish (plucked hairs should not be cultured because they often break off at the point of infection, leaving uninfected hairs on the culture medium).

Other hair breakage syndromes can mimic tinea capitis with patchy alopecia. This is especially true of hair that has been straightened, as the chemicals used to do this weaken the hair bonds. Traction alopecia (p. 183), trichotillomania and other alopecias may also be considered, but these seldom have associated scalp scaling. When the infection is accompanied by inflammation, traction alo-pecia, bacterial folliculitis, chemical folliculitis and 'pomade acne' from oils may be considered. If kerions develop, they are often misdiagnosed as bacterial abscesses. Think, too, of discoid lupus erythematosus and lichen planopilaris in atypical patients with scarring.

Because the disease occasionally occurs in neonates, infants and adults, the disorder may then suggest other causes of scaling scalps such as cradle cap, psoriasis and dandruff. 'Dry scalp' in adults may be tinea, but in black adults 'dry scalp' more com-monly results from alcohol in hair care products.

### Treatment

Most clinicians practising in endemic areas start treatment without waiting for culture results. This reduces time lost from school, scarring and the poten-tial to infect others. Oral treatment is essential as the infecting organism invades the hair follicles where they are not reached by topical agents. Microsize griseofulvin is the oral antifungal of choice. It is given at a daily dose of 20–25 mg/kg until cultures are negative, which is often 6–8 weeks. Gastrointestinal upset, vomiting and headaches are the most common side-effects. Itraconazole, fluconazole and terbinafine work too.

As part of the treatment, children should use a shampoo that inhibits the growth of fungal spores. These include shampoos containing selenium sul-phide, zinc pyrithione and ketoconazole. Otherwise, spores in the distal part of hairs may reinfect the child or infect other children. Some experts suggest that family members should use these shampoos too.

## Dissecting folliculitis

Bacteria can also cause boggy, inflamed scalps in African-Americans. The scalp is tender, hair loss is common and pressure on the boggy scalp causes pus to exude from sinus tract openings nearby and far away. Many patients also have acne conglobata (p. 164), hidradenitis suppurativa (p. 176), or both. Culture and antibiotics help, but some patients also need temporary systemic steroid treatment and isotretinoin. Scarring and keloid formation often follow.

## Alopecia (hair loss)

The hair of most Negroids is curly which makes it difficult to brush, comb, wash and set because it tends to form knots. As a consequence, most African-Americans do not shampoo their hair daily or even weekly. This leads to seborrhoeic dermatitis and an itchy scalp. Therapeutic shampoos often cannot be used frequently enough. Instead, patients apply topical antifungal agents and corticosteroid solutions, lotions and foams.

Black-skinned individuals with curly hair often try to straighten it by using 'hair relaxers', or to create permanent waves through chemical treatments. These work by dissolving disulphide bonds and then reforming them after the hair is styled. Not all bonds reform, so chemically treated hair is 'weaker'. Broken hairs and patchy hair loss are therefore common. 'Texturizers' use these chemicals too, in weaker concentrations, to 'loosen' a curl and make it more manageable and straighter.

Traction on hair can cause alopecia (traction alopecia; Chapter 13). In Negroids this often follows vigorous combing, brushing, using fork-like 'Afro picks', and styling into tight ponytails, tight braids, microbraids, twists or 'corn rows' that pull on hair (Fig. 14.9). Hair curlers and hairpiece wigs or extenders woven into the natural hair can also produce traction leading to hair loss with patchy alopecia, a receding frontal hairline and decreased hair density.

**Fig. 14.9** Traction alopecia. The tight braids have caused hair loss.

Thermal hairstyling depends upon high temperatures delivered to styled hair by curling irons, flat irons and hot combs. These can damage hair. Hair loss can also follow the use of oils to make hair more manageable. On the scalp, they can produce a follicular inflammation and pustules leading to hair loss and scarring (pomade acne).

## Keloids

Keloids are thick scars. Some cultures intentionally provoke keloids as a decoration similar to a tattoo. Men and women develop them equally easily, although earlobe piercing gives the current edge to women (Fig. 14.10). Black patients develop keloids much more often than people with type I skin. Chinese patients are also slightly more prone to keloids.

**Fig. 14.10** Keloids. These arose after ears were pierced for jewelry.

**Fig. 14.11** Postsurgical keloid. Small keloids even developed where the skin was pierced by sutures used to close the excision site.

### Cause

Keloids usually follow trauma. A typical patient is 10–30 years old and develops a thickening of skin at the site of a previous wound or surgery (Fig. 14.11). The injury may be major or trivial. Some keloids seem to appear spontaneously. Keloids occur after burns, bites, piercings, surgery, acne pustules, vaccinations and even tattooing. Acne keloidalis nuchae occurs almost exclusively in blacks as small, skin-coloured, hard, discrete and agminated papules at the nape of the neck associated with hair loss there. The provoking factor is assumed to be the inflammation of pseudofolliculitis (p. 209).

Fibroblasts in keloids produce more collagen and tend to proliferate more than normal fibroblasts, perhaps because of the stimulating effect of transforming growth factor β.

### Presentation

Itching or pain is common. Keloids commonly erupt on the shoulders, upper chest, upper back, upper arms and earlobes. As opposed to hypertrophic scars, keloids often do not develop until weeks, months or years after the injury. They extend beyond the confines of the original wound and seem to invade the surrounding skin rather than expand locally.

### Course

Keloids may enlarge, and over decades may regress.

Some are self-perpetuating, especially on the chest where they can become larger, harder, trabeculated, itching and deforming thick scars.

## Treatment

Treatments are complicated by the tendency of keloids to regrow after their removal. Intralesional injection of corticosteroids, such as triamcinolone acetonide at a concentration of at least 10–20 mg, soften the keloid after one or more treatments and also decrease the intensity of pain and itch. Injection of interferon-α2b has been advocated too. Excision is frequently followed by regrowth unless the surgical wound is injected with corticosteroids or X-irradiated monthly for several months. Silicone gel dressings applied continuously to the wound site may also prevent recurrence. Although cryotherapy with liquid nitrogen flattens a small number of keloids, it is often contraindicated in deeply pigmented individuals because it destroys pigment cells, leaving whiter skin at the sites treated.

## Melanomas and other tumours

As might be predicted, individuals with a dark skin are less likely to develop non-melanoma skin cancers. Melanin in the skin confers natural protection against ultraviolet radiation. Basal cell carcinomas are rare, but sometimes occur on sun-exposed areas. Other risk factors are albinism, ulcers, sebaceous naevus (p. 298), prior radiation exposure, traumas, immunosuppression and scars. Squamous cell carcinomas are more common, and usually arise in areas of chronic inflammation such as scars, ulcers, discoid lupus erythematosus or draining sinus tracts. In Negroids and Asians, basal cell carcinomas tend to be pigmented ('black pearly' appearance).

In Hispanic, Asian and black persons, melanomas (p. 306) tend to develop on non-sun-exposed skin, such as that on the soles, palms, mouth, nail bed or nail matrix. About 90% of black persons have at least one pigmented naevus, and usually these are on the extremities. The incidence of melanomas on the soles of black-skinned patients approaches the incidence of melanomas on the soles of others, but melanomas of the sole make up more than 50% of all

**Fig. 14.12** Acral melanoma. Be especially wary of odd pigmentation of the hands and feet in patients with dark skins.

melanomas of blacks, compared with 5% in whites. Most melanomas in blacks are of the acral lentiginous type (Fig. 14.12). They are sharply marginated, irregular brown macules or patches. Melanomas in black patients tend to be thicker tumours at the time of diagnosis, and thus melanomas in black patients have an overall poorer prognosis and higher mortality than melanomas in white patients. The same is true to a lesser extent for Hawaiians, Hispanics and Asians.

Black people often have longitudinal pigmented streaks in their nails, so the finding of these does not cause the concern for melanoma that arises when these are seen in white people. Yet, melanomas around the nails are not uncommon in persons with skin types V and VI (Fig. 14.13). When they occur, they are often misdiagnosed as paronychia, or as subungual haematomas, or ignored until they are advanced. Hutchinson's sign is an increased pigmentation of skin of the proximal nail fold in association with a subungual melanoma. Unfortunately, this sign is not always present in whites or in blacks with nearby melanomas. Other clues suggesting melanoma as the origin of longitudinal melanonychia are width greater than 3 mm, variable pigmentation, rapid

**Fig. 14.13** Subungual melanoma. The tumour is in the proximal nail fold and has caused a longitudinal band of pigment and a groove in the nail plate. Note the pigmentation of the proximal nail fold (positive Hutchinson's sign).

increase in size and the presence of just a single streak. Nail bed or nail matrix biopsy should be performed if there is diagnostic doubt.

## Other considerations

Erythema is difficult to see in black skin, the overlying pigmentation masking the erythema to give a purplish hue. Furthermore, many types of eczema have a tendency to surround and involve hair follicles, leading to evenly spaced, skin-coloured papules resembling goose flesh. If accompanied by itching, this appearance should suggest eczema in black skin rather than other forms of folliculitis.

Pityriasis rosea (p. 71) tends to be itchier in black people, and to leave long-standing black macules of post-inflammatory hyperpigmentation. For that reason, systemic steroids are sometimes given (do not forget to rule out syphilis!).

Cutaneous T-cell lymphoma occurs about twice as often in Negroids than in Caucasoids. Persisting pruritic hypopigmented patches may prompt biopsies.

Sarcoidosis (p. 325) is up to 18 times more common in black than in white people. Its skin man-

ifestations include erythema nodosum, widespread non-scaling papules, flesh-coloured or blue–red nodules on the trunk, bulbous purple nodules and plaques on the face or ears (lupus pernio), inflammation in scars (scar sarcoid), soft swellings on the cheeks with overlying telangiectases (angiolupoid sarcoid) and lesions resembling psoriasis or ichthyosis. Sarcoidosis imitates many skin diseases, but biopsy will show its typical granulomas.

Melasma (p. 286) can be severe in pigmented skin. At least half of Hispanic women develop melasma during pregnancy. Patients can apply creams containing up to 4% hydroquinone. Sun protection is essential. Because they are so seldom sunburned, many black patients do not apply sunscreens regularly or practise sun avoidance and may need special instructions.

Atopic dermatitis may be severe, especially in Asians. Their eyelid dermatitis is particularly common and resists the usual treatments. In Negroid patients, eczemas tend to show follicular papules. Subtle cases may even be diagnosed as folliculitis rather than recognized as an eczema.

Warts occur in pigmented people too. Treatments such as cryotherapy can cause complications. Melanocytes are particularly sensitive to destruction by cold, so the treatment of warts in pigmented patients is more likely to leave an obvious leucoderma. Surgeons must consider the increased risk of keloid formation, especially in keloid-prone areas of skin such as the upper chest, upper back and shoulders.

Black-skinned infants may develop infantile acropustulosis. Pinhead pink macules on the hands and feet become vesicles or pustules, and the itching leads to fretful days and nights. Topical steroids can help, and the disorder typically resolves by the age of 2 years.

Mongolian spots (p. 217) arise from dermal melanocytic naevi. These slate-grey to slightly blue patches are found among the majority of black infants and in many Mongoloids and other pigmented races, often on the lower back.

Lichen nitidus occurs most commonly in black skin. Pinhead-sized uniformly distributed shiny flat-topped skin-coloured papules occur on the genitals, abdomen, or flexor surfaces of the extremities. The lesions do not itch, and skin biopsy establishes the diagnosis. No treatment is necessary; the disease is asymptomatic and goes away after 2–3 months.

## Erythema dyschromicum perstans

This is a chronic progressive disorder of unknown cause. Some call it the 'ashy dermatosis' because of its distinctive slate-grey colour. Most patients are Hispanic or Asian, but the disorder can occur in other people with darker skins. Some believe the condition to be a macular variant of lichen planus.

### Presentation and course

Many slate-grey, usually asymptomatic patches develop on the trunk and extremities. They may cover large areas of the body. The scalp, palms, soles and mucous membranes are spared. Biopsy shows pigmentary incontinence, with melanin packed into dermal histiocytes. Pigmentation is chronic, as the word 'perstans' suggests.

### Differential diagnosis

Post-inflammatory hyperpigmentation is hard to disregard. In fact, sometimes slightly raised, subtle pink smooth plaques arise before pigment changes become evident at the sites. Fixed drug reactions (p. 360) are slate-grey between their active phases, but arise from obvious urticaria-like wheals and are associated with taking a drug. Photodermatoses (p. 270), some reactions to tick bites and urticaria pigmentosa (p. 317) may also show grey or brown patches.

### Treatment

There is no effective treatment other than cosmetic cover-up. Sun tanning may mask lesions by darkening the skin around and over them.

## Cultural marks

Different societies decorate their skins in different ways. Some practise rituals that scar or mark the skin. These may surprise physicians from other cultures. Asians, for example, may practise coining, cupping or moxibustion. Coining produces linear petechiae and ecchymoses after a coin or other instrument is rubbed hard against oil-coated skin. Cupping produces petechiae in perfect circles after suction has been created inside a bell-like device attached to skin. Asians and African societies sometimes burn the skin (moxibustion) to treat various maladies including eczemas. One must keep these 'cultural treatments' in mind before accusing a parent of child abuse.

## Further reading

Gloster HM & Neal K. (2006) Skin cancer in skin of color. *Journal of the American Academy of Dermatology* **55**, 741–760.

Jablonski NG. (2006) *Skin, a Natural History.* University of California Press, Berkeley, 76–96.

Nordlund JJ, Ortonne JP, Cesstari T, Grimes P & Chan H. (2006) Confusions about color: formatting a more precise lexicon for pigmentation, pigmentary disorders, and abnormalities of 'chromatics'. *Journal of the American Academy of Dermatology* **54**, S291–297.

Rendon M, Berneburg M, Arellano I & Picardo M. (2006) Treatment of melasma. *Journal of the American Academy of Dermatology* **12**, S272–280.

Shaffer JJ, Taylor SC & Cook-Bolden F. (2002) Keloidal scars: a review with critical look at therapeutic options. *Journal of the American Academy of Dermatology* **46**, 63S–97S.

Taylor SC. (2002) Skin of color: biology, structure, function, and implications for dermatologic disease. *Journal of the American Academy of Dermatology* **46**, 41S–62S.

Taylor SC, Burgess CM, Callendar VD, *et al.* (2006) Postinflammatory hyperpigmentation: evolving combination strategies. *Cutis* **78**, 6–19.

# 15 Dermatology of different age groups

Shakespeare knew how the skin changes with age: from the shining morning face of youth to the dry hand, yellow cheek and white beard of old age. In this chapter, we bring together the skin conditions encountered in different age groups, and add two more to Shakespeare's seven ages – those of the foetus and the pregnant woman.

## Foetal skin

*In utero*, the skin remains one cell thick until weeks 4–6, when two layers can be seen; by weeks 8–11, there are three layers. Hair follicles start to appear at about 9 weeks, as do nails. Sebaceous glands arrive by 14 weeks, and pigmentation by 4–6 months. Free nerve endings begin to develop in the skin at about 7 weeks but the central connections required for a foetus to appreciate pain are not complete until 23–25 weeks.

Some families are at high risk of having a child with an intolerable genetic skin disorder. Prenatal diagnosis coupled with genetic counselling is then required, as early as possible so that selective termination is easy and safe. In the past, a foetal skin biopsy was sometimes taken under ultrasound guidance to help such families. However, this technique cannot be undertaken before 15 weeks' gestation and has gradually been superseded by DNA-based diagnostic screening of amniotic fluid cells (at 12–15 weeks) or chorionic villi samples (at 10–12 weeks). This type of testing has been used for conditions such as epidermolysis bullosa (p. 128), severe ichthyoses including harlequin foetus (p. 49) and oculocutaneous albinism (p. 280). Preimplantation diagnosis is for the future.

## Infancy (first year of life)

At birth, the skin is covered, wholly or partly, with a whitish slimy layer: the vernix caseosa. This comes off over the first few days, although some think that 'cradle cap' (scaling of the scalp during the first weeks of life) is caused by its localized persistence.

An infant's skin is often mottled at birth (cutis marmorata) and peripheral cyanosis is common, as is a generalized erythema lasting for a day or two. The term 'harlequin skin change' refers to an appearance seen in a few babies when they lie on their side; the uppermost part of their body becomes pale and is sharply demarcated from a redder lower half.

Preterm infants may be covered with fine lanugo hairs. In full-term babies there is usually some loss of scalp hair over the first few weeks. Multiple milia (tiny white epidermal cysts) are seen in about half of all babies. The tiny yellowish papules on the face of many babies are sebaceous glands that have hypertrophied under the influence of maternal androgens that have passed via the placenta. Neonatal acne (p. 164) may have the same trigger.

Rarely, maternal autoantibodies pass through the placenta. The child of a mother with subacute lupus erythematosus (p. 134) and anti Ro (SS-A) antibodies, for example, may develop an elevated, often annular erythema (neonatal lupus erythematosus). This clears over the first few months, but may be associated with congenital heart block.

Other important changes seen at birth include those resulting from underlying genetic disorders. A 'collodion baby' (p. 49) for example, whose shiny smooth skin looks almost as though it has been painted with collodion, may have an underlying non-bullous ichthyosiform erythroderma or lamellar ichthyosis (p. 49). Incontinentia pigmenti (p. 353) is in its linear vesicular stage at birth. In the severe junctional type of epidermolysis bullosa (p. 128), the newborn child has a mixture of large raw areas and flaccid blisters. In contrast, in tuberous

**Fig. 15.1** Mongolian spot.

sclerosis (p. 351), tiny white patches may be the only manifestation at birth.

Common birthmarks include congenital melanocytic naevi (p. 294), Mongolian spots (Fig. 15.1) and haemangiomas (port-wine stains, salmon patches, p. 314). Capillary cavernous haemangiomas (strawberry naevi) appear within a few weeks of birth and then tend to regress slowly over the next few years (p. 315).

The stratum corneum is fully formed at birth, and so barrier function is normal except in premature babies. Nevertheless, newborn skin tolerates irritants poorly. Primary irritant reactions are common after prolonged contact with faeces and urine in the napkin and perianal areas, although severe napkin (diaper) dermatitis has become much less common since the introduction of disposable napkins (p. 85). True allergic contact eczema is rare in infancy. Atopic eczema (p. 91) commonly starts before the age of 6 months, often appearing on the face with a patchy non-specific distribution elsewhere.

There is large surface area : body weight ratio in babies and the risk of side-effects from absorption of topically applied medications (e.g. topical corticosteroids and scabicides) is increased.

Sadly, practitioners may see signs suggestive of physical abuse. Contusions, abrasions, lacerations, burns and scalds associated with broken bones or other evidence of trauma are classic features of the battered baby, but the signs may be more subtle. In any event, disorders responsible for the blisters and raw areas, such as epidermolysis bullosa (p. 128), or for bruising (Table 11.7), such as a coagulation or platelet defect, must be excluded.

## Childhood

Parents soon learn that nurseries and schools are mixed blessings for health. Snuffles, coughs and colds are usually considered an inevitable part of the growing-up process and essential for the development of an effective immune system. However, exposure and close contact at school also bring a host of skin infections and infestations (e.g. impetigo, p. 222; warts, p. 235; molluscum contagiosum, p. 243; head lice, p. 258; and scabies, p. 262). Such unwelcome guests are seldom accepted passively by mothers who require full explanations to lessen blame.

Atopic dermatitis (p. 91) is common in children. A recent survey in a semi-rural community in Scotland revealed a 1-year period prevalence of 8% in children aged 2–11 years. Even before the advent of corticosteroid treatment, retarded growth in children with atopic dermatitis was well recognized. It is thought to be caused by a decreased frequency and size of growth hormone pulses during sleep which is presumably interrupted by scratching. Nevertheless, the amount of corticosteroids prescribed in this age group should be carefully monitored (p. 369), just as with children with asthma, as these drugs retard growth.

Both boys and girls may be seen by family doctors with symptoms and signs that might indicate sexual abuse. Vulval and perianal soreness and inflammation for which no other cause, especially threadworms, can be found should be considered suspicious. Anogenital warts (p. 236) should also ring alarm bells although some are innocently acquired. The situation is usually more clear-cut if a sexually transmitted disease such as gonorrhoea, herpes simplex or even HIV infection is found. Suspicion is increased if there is delay in seeking medical help, if the accompanying person's explanation for the appearance is not compatible with the signs and if the child discloses the cause. However, it is again important to note, as with battered babies, that skin conditions such as psoriasis (p. 54), lichen

**Fig. 15.2** Lichen sclerosus.

sclerosus (p. 201 and Fig. 15.2) and Crohn's disease in childhood can be mistaken for evidence of sexual abuse. Of course, this is a highly charged area and the diagnosis of sexual abuse, just as with non-accidental injury, should be a multidisciplinary exercise involving paediatricians, family doctors, dermatologists and social workers.

Trichotillomania or hair-pulling habit in children is described on p. 346.

## Adolescence

A sudden increase in androgen and oestrogen levels leads to sexual maturation. The skin changes of adolescence include the appearance of pubic, facial and axillary hair, and increasing activity of the sebaceous glands. The adolescent growth spurt can be vigorous enough to cause stretch marks (Fig. 15.3 and 26.2) or retarded by the presence of severe atopic eczema (p. 91).

**Fig. 15.3** Adolescent striae.

The skin disorders of adolescents often operate against a background of social and examination stress. Personal appearance has become important, so that minor skin conditions can have a disproportionate effect on quality of life. Even a mild greasiness of the skin and hair can cause much embarrassment, worsened by the presence of acne (p. 162) – which itself may be subjected to regular picking – and/or seborrhoeic dermatitis (p. 97). Smelly armpits and heavy eccrine sweating of the palms (p. 174) can have the same effect. Neurotic excoriations (p. 345) and other forms of dermatitis artefacta (p. 344) are also triggered by stress.

Sexual awakening leads to close contact with others and so to a high incidence of infections and infestations, such as scabies (p. 262). Cosmetics and jewellery become popular, and can lead to contact allergy to materials such as nickel (p. 87), especially if skin piercing is involved.

## Young adults

The quest for independence and work usually precedes the hunt for a social partner. Whichever comes first, personal appearance assumes even more importance with early male-pattern baldness (p. 181) and hirsutism (p. 185) becoming reasons for consultation. Stubborn acne causes increasing depression, and management is both tricky and time-consuming.

Many women notice changes in their skin and hair during the menstrual cycle. These range from the development of a few acne spots in the premenstrual phase to textural (greasy/dry) changes. Premenstrual exacerbations of psoriasis, rosacea, atopic dermatitis, recurrent oral aphthous ulcers and herpes simplex are also well recognized. 'Auto-immune progesterone dermatitis' is the name given to various reaction patterns in the skin that occur regularly in the premenstrual period: eczema, urticaria, erythema multiforme and dermatitis herpetiformis. Exogenous challenge with progesterone reproduces the picture.

Finally, there is the problem of selecting the right job. Young adults with atopic eczema, for example, or psoriasis on their hands will react badly to contact with irritants (p. 9), and so should avoid jobs in catering, engineering and hairdressing.

# Pregnancy

Some of the many skin changes that can occur during pregnancy are listed below.

**1** *Pigmentation* The skin tends to darken generally. This is most obvious on the nipples, genitalia and in the midline of the lower abdomen (the linea nigra). Melosma of pregnancy (p. 286) – an irregular pigmentation of the face – is common.

**2** *Skin tags* ( p. 293).

**3** *Vascular changes* include oestrogen-induced spider naevi and palmar erythema. Varicose veins may become troublesome.

**4** *Stretch marks* (Fig. 15.4) Common on the abdomen. After childbirth they change from red lines to permanent silvery ones.

**5** *Decreased cell-mediated immunity* may lead to candidal and other infections. Genital and perianal warts may be luxuriant but should not be treated with podophyllin.

**6** *Itching* with no obvious skin cause is common in the third trimester and may be caused by cholestasis.

**7** *Pre-existing skin diseases* react unpredictably to pregnancy. Usually, atopic eczema, psoriasis and acne tend to improve.

**8** *Skin disorders specific to pregnancy* include the following.

- *Polymorphic eruption of pregnancy* (Fig. 15.4) Itchy red urticarial papules and plaques or vesicles appear, usually in the third trimester, mainly on the abdomen and tending to follow the lines of stretch marks. They clear when, or soon after, the baby is born. The rash carries no risk of damaging the baby.
- *Prurigo of pregnancy* Many itchy and scratched papules come up, often at about 25 weeks. They too tend to clear, although more slowly, after childbirth, but may come back in subsequent pregnancies. Again, the baby is unharmed.
- *Pemphigoid gestationis* (p. 124) A rare disorder, related to pemphigoid (p. 123), with autoantibodies directed against the same targets. Erythematous urticarial papules, plaques and bullae appear, especially around the umbilicus. It may occur at any time in the pregnancy (including the postpartum period) and recur in subsequent pregnancies. The baby may be born prematurely and be of low birth weight. The diagnosis is confirmed by finding a linear band of complement (3 in skin biopsies).

## Middle age

As far as the skin goes, the most consistent and distressing middle age crisis is menopausal flushing or 'hot flushes' (p. 149). A sudden feeling of intense heat, discomfort and sweating, accompanied by blotchy erythema on the face, neck, upper chest and breasts, lasts for 3–5 min. Some women also develop palpitations, headaches and nausea. Hormone replacement therapy with oestrogens is the most effective treatment.

Keratoderma climactericum (p. 52), most commonly seen in middle-aged women around the menopause, may also occur in men and women of other ages, many of whom are obese.

Male-pattern baldness (androgenetic alopecia; p. 181) is becoming more prevalent and occurring at an earlier age than 50 years ago. The burgeoning number of hair clinics are testimony to the fact that many men do not suffer this indignity lightly. Androgenetic alopecia in women, much more common than generally thought, usually causes a more diffuse hair loss, especially over the crown.

**Fig. 15.4** Polymorphic eruption of pregnancy with stretch marks. Widespread urticated papules.

Whereas the prevalence of atopic eczema declines sharply in middle age, the discoid and asteatotic types (p. 101) appear.

## Old age

Shakespeare's 'last scene of all' does not single out the skin, because it perhaps puts up with the ravages of time better than the eyes and the teeth. However, the skin is certainly not exempt from problems in old age and the list below is not exhaustive. The first section lists those changes that are essentially 'cosmetic'; many are discussed in detail in Chapter 22. The second section includes disorders that are most common in old age; they are described in detail elsewhere in this book.

### Cosmetic changes of old age (Chapter 22)

- Atrophy, sagging and wrinkling.
- Coarse wrinkling of facial skin because of long-term cigarette smoking.
- Dryness.
- Photodamage (exposed skin only) including elastosis, cutis rhomboidalis nuchae and irregular pigmentation.
- Senile/solar lentigines ('liver spots', p. 284).
- Hair loss and greying of hair (because of loss of pigment in the hair shaft, secondary to depletion of melanocytes in the hair bulb and outer root sheath).
- Slowed nail growth.

## Skin conditions common in old age

- Xerosis/asteatotic eczema (p. 101)/senile pruritus (p. 332).
- Seborrhoeic keratoses (p. 291).
- Precancerous lesions (e.g. actinic keratoses, p. 299).
- Skin cancers (Chapter 20).
- Hirsutism (p. 185).
- Pemphigoid (p. 123).
- Shingles with post-herpetic neuralgia (p. 240).
- Actinic reticuloid (p. 272).
- Slow healing of leg ulcers (p. 152) and pressure sores (p. 151).
- Scabies in homes for the elderly (p. 262).

## Further reading

Black MM, McKay M, Braude PR, Vaughn Jones SA & Margesson LJ. (2001) *Obstetric and Gynecologic Dermatology*, 2nd edn. Elsevier Mosby, London.

Eichenfield LF, Frieden IJ & Esterly NB. (2001) *Textbook of Neonatal Dermatology*. Elsevier Saunders, Philadelphia.

Harper J, Oranje A & Prose N. (2005) *Textbook of Pediatric Dermatology*, 2nd edn. Blackwell Publishing, Oxford.

Norman RA, ed. (2001) *Geriatric Dermatology*. Parthenon, New York.

# **16** Infections

## Bacterial infections

### Resident flora of the skin

The surface of the skin teems with micro-organisms, which are most numerous in moist hairy areas, rich in sebaceous glands. Organisms are found, in clusters, in irregularities in the stratum corneum and within the hair follicles. The resident flora is a mixture of harmless and poorly classified staphylococci, micrococci and diphtheroids. *Staphylococcus epidermidis* and aerobic diphtheroids predominate on the surface, and anaerobic diphtheroids (*Propionibacteria* sp.) deep in the hair follicles. Several species of lipophilic yeasts also exist on the skin. The proportion of the different organisms varies from person to person but, once established, an individual's skin flora tends to remain stable and helps to defend the skin against outside pathogens by bacterial interference or antibiotic production. Nevertheless, overgrowth of skin diphtheroids can itself lead to clinical problems. The role of *Propionibacteria* in the pathogenesis of acne is discussed on p. 63. Overgrowth of aerobic diphtheroids causes trichomycosis axillaris, pitted keratolysis and erythrasma.

### *Trichomycosis axillaris*

The axillary hairs become beaded with concretions, usually yellow, made up of colonies of commensal diphtheroids. Clothing becomes stained in the armpits. Topical antibiotic ointments, or shaving, will clear the condition, and frequent washing with antibacterial soaps will keep it clear.

### *Pitted keratolysis*

The combination of unusually sweaty feet and occlusive shoes encourages the growth of diphtheroid organisms that can digest keratin. The result is a cribriform pattern of fine punched-out depressions on the plantar surface (Fig. 16.1), coupled with an unpleasant smell (of methane-thiol). Fusidic acid or mupirocin ointment is usually effective, and antiperspirants (Formulary 1, p. 382) can also help. Occlusive footwear should be replaced by sandals and cotton socks if possible.

### *Erythrasma*

Some diphtheroid members of the skin flora produce porphyrins when grown in a suitable medium. Overgrowth of these strains is sometimes the cause of symptom-free macular wrinkled slightly scaly pink, brown or macerated white areas, most often found in the armpits or groins, or between the toes. In diabetics, larger areas of the trunk may be involved. Diagnosis is helped by the fact that the porphyrins produced by these diptheroids fluoresce coral pink with Wood's light. Topical fusidic acid or miconazole will clear the condition.

**Fig. 16.1** Pitted keratolysis of the heel.

## Staphylococcal infections

*Staphylococcus aureus* is not part of the resident flora of the skin other than in a minority who carry it in their nostrils, perineum or armpits. Carriage rates vary with age. Nasal carriage is almost invariable in babies born in hospital, becomes less frequent during infancy and rises again during the school years to the adult level of roughly 30%. Rather fewer carry the organism in the armpits or groin. Staphylococci can also multiply on areas of diseased skin such as eczema, often without causing obvious sepsis. A minor breach in the skin's defences is probably necessary for a frank staphylococcal infection to establish itself; some strains are particularly likely to cause skin sepsis. Of concern is the rise in incidence of methicillin-resistant *Staphylococcus aureus* (MRSA) in the community and in hospitalized patients. This can result in abscesses and furunculosis as well as other infections. Prevention of emerging resistant strains is with a combination of scrupulous hygiene, patient isolation, antiseptic agents and restriction of the 'blind' use of antibiotics.

**Fig. 16.2** Widespread impetigo due to *Staph. aureus* with erosions and cruising.

## Impetigo

### Cause

Impetigo may be caused by staphylococci, streptococci, or by both together. As a useful rule of thumb, the bullous type is usually caused by *Staphylococcus aureus*, whereas the crusted ulcerated type is caused by β-haemolytic strains of streptococci. Both are highly contagious. Exfoliative toxins produced by *S. aureus* cleave the cell adhesion molecule desmoglein 1 (pp. 12, 120). If the toxin is localized this produces the blisters of bullous impetigo, but if generalized leads to more widespread blistering as in the staphylococcal scalded skin syndrome.

### Presentation

A thin-walled flaccid clear blister forms, and may become pustular before rupturing to leave an extending area of exudation and yellowish varnish-like crusting (Fig. 16.2). Lesions are often multiple, particularly around the face. The lesions may be more obviously bullous in infants. A follicular type of impetigo (superficial folliculitis) is also common.

### Course

The condition can spread rapidly through a family or class. It tends to clear even without treatment.

### Complications

Streptococcal impetigo can trigger an acute glomerulonephritis.

### Differential diagnosis

Herpes simplex may become impetiginized, as may eczema. Always think of a possible underlying cause such as this. Recurrent impetigo of the head and neck, for example, should prompt a search for scalp lice.

### Investigation and treatment

The diagnosis is usually made on clinical grounds. Gram stains can be performed or swabs taken and sent to the laboratory for culture, but treatment must not be held up until the results are available.

Systemic antibiotics (such as flucloxacillin, erythromycin or cefalexin) are needed for severe cases or if a nephritogenic strain of streptococcus is suspected (penicillin V). For minor cases the removal of crusts by compressing them and application of a topical antibiotic such as neomycin, fusidic acid (not available in the USA), mupirocin or bacitracin will suffice (Formulary 1, p. 388).

> **Learning points**
>
> ● Look for head lice in the patient with recurrent impetigo of the head and neck
> ● The skin changes of the scalded skin syndrome, and of the toxic shock syndrome, are caused by staphylococcal exotoxins. Look for the primary infection elsewhere

### Ecthyma

This term describes ulcers forming under a crusted surface infection. The site may have been that of an insect bite or of neglected minor trauma. The bacterial pathogens and their treatment are similar to those of impetigo. Whereas in impetigo the erosion is at the stratum corneum, in ecthyma the ulcer is full thickness, and thus heals with scarring.

### Furunculosis (boils)

#### Cause

A furuncle is an acute pustular infection of a hair follicle, usually with *Staphylococcus aureus*. Adolescent boys are especially susceptible to them.

#### Presentation and course

A tender red nodule enlarges, and later may discharge pus and its central 'core' before healing to leave a scar (Fig. 16.3). Fever and enlarged draining nodes are rare. Most patients have one or two boils only, and then clear. The sudden appearance of many furuncles suggests a virulent staphylococcus including strains of community-aquired MRSA. A few unfortunate persons experience a tiresome sequence of boils (chronic furunculosis), often because of susceptibility of follicles or colonization of nares or groins to pathogenic bacteria. Immunodeficiency is rarely the problem.

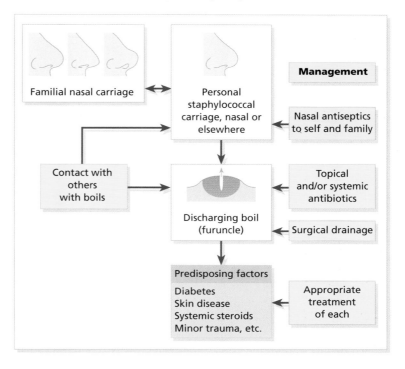

**Fig. 16.3** Chronic furunculosis.

*Complications*

Cavernous sinus thrombosis is an unusual complication of boils on the central face. Septicaemia may occur but is rare.

*Differential diagnosis*

The diagnosis is straightforward but hidradenitis suppurativa (p. 176) should be considered if only the groin and axillae are involved.

*Investigations in chronic furunculosis*

● General examination: look for underlying skin disease (e.g. scabies, pediculosis, eczema).
● Test the urine for sugar. Full blood count.
● Culture swabs from lesions and carrier sites (nostrils, perineum) of the patient and immediate family. Test both to identify the organism and to evaluate sensitivity to various antibiotics.
● Immunological evaluation only if the patient has recurrent or unusual internal infections too.

*Treatment*

● Acute episodes will respond to simple incision and drainage. An appropriate systemic antibiotic is needed when many furuncles are erupting, when fever is present or when the patient is immuno-suppressed.
● In chronic furunculosis, treat carrier sites such as the nose and groin twice daily for 6 weeks with an appropriate topical antiseptic or antibiotic (e.g. chlorhexidine solution, mupirocin cream or clindamycin solution). Treat family carriers in the same way.
● In stubborn cases, add 6 weeks of a systemic antibiotic chosen to cover organism's proven sensitivities.
● Daily bath using an antiseptic soap.
● Improve hygiene and nutritional state, if faulty.

*Carbuncle*

A group of adjacent hair follicles becomes deeply infected with *Staphylococcus aureus*, leading to a swollen painful suppurating area discharging pus from several points. The pain and systemic upset are greater than those of a boil. Diabetes must be excluded. Treatment needs both topical and systemic antibiotics. Incision and drainage have been shown to speed up healing, although it is not always easy when there are multiple deep pus-filled pockets. Consider the possibility of a fungal kerion (p. 250) in unresponsive carbuncles.

### Scalded skin syndrome

In this condition the skin changes resemble a scald. Erythema and tenderness are followed by the loosening of large areas of overlying epidermis (Fig. 16.4). In children, the condition is usually caused by a toxin produced by staphylococcal infection elsewhere (e.g. impetigo or conjunctivitis). Organisms in what may be only a minor local infection release exfoliative toxins that cleave the superficial skin adhesion molecule desmoglein 1 (p. 12, 120) to disrupt adhesion high in the epidermis, causing the stratum corneum to slough off. With systemic antibiotics the outlook is good. The disorder affects children and patients with renal failure; most adults have antibodies to the

**Fig. 16.4** Staphylococcal scalded skin syndrome in a child. The overlying epidermis is loosening in the red areas.

toxin, and therefore are protected. In adults with widespread exfoliation, consider toxic epidermal necrolysis, which is usually drug induced. The damage to the epidermis in toxic epidermal necrolysis is full thickness, and a skin biopsy will distinguish it from the scalded skin syndrome (p. 224).

### Toxic shock syndrome

A staphylococcal toxin is also responsible for this condition, in which fever, a rash – usually a widespread erythema – and sometimes circulatory collapse are followed a week or two later by characteristic desquamation, most marked on the fingers and hands. Many cases have followed staphylococcal overgrowth in the vagina of women using tampons. Systemic antibiotics and irrigation of the underlying infected site are needed.

## Streptococcal infections

### Erysipelas

The first warning of an attack is often malaise, shivering and a fever. After a few hours the affected area of skin becomes red, and the eruption spreads with a well-defined advancing edge. Blisters may develop on the red plaques (Fig. 16.5). Untreated, the condition can even be fatal, but it responds rapidly to systemic penicillin, sometimes given intravenously. The causative streptococci usually gain their entry through a split in the skin (e.g. between the toes or under an ear lobe).

**Fig. 16.5** Erysipelas – note sharp spreading edge, here demarcated with a ballpoint pen.

Episodes can affect the same area repeatedly and so lead to persistent lymphoedema. Low dosage long-term oral penicillin V will usually cut down the frequency of recurrences. The cause of the original skin split, perhaps a minor tinea pedis, should be treated too.

> **Learning points**
>
> - Unlike lightning, erysipelas often strikes in the same place twice
> - Shivering and malaise precede the rash – and that is when the penicillin should be given
> - Recurrent bouts may need long-term prophylactic penicillin

### Cellulitis

This inflammation of the skin occurs at a deeper level than erysipelas. The subcutaneous tissues are involved and the area is more raised and swollen, and the erythema less marginated than in erysipelas. Cellulitis often follows an injury and favours areas of hypostatic oedema. Streptococci, staphylococci or other organisms may be the cause. Treatment is elevation, rest – sometimes in hospital – and systemic antibiotics, sometimes given intravenously.

### Necrotizing fasciitis

A mixture of pathogens, usually including streptococci and anaerobes, is responsible for this rare condition, which is a surgical emergency. Diabetics and post-surgical patients are predisposed. At first the infection resembles a dusky, often painful, cellulitis, but it quickly turns into an extending necrosis of the skin and subcutaneous tissues. Classically, the central area of skin involvement becomes anaesthetic because of cutaneous nerve damage. A deep 'stab' incision biopsy through the skin into the fascia may be necessary to establish the diagnosis and to obtain material for bacteriological culture. A magnetic resonance imaging (MRI) scan may help to establish how far the infection has spread. The prognosis is often poor despite early wide surgical débridement and prompt intravenous antibiotic administration, even when given before the bacteriological results are available.

## Erysipeloid

It is convenient to mention this here, but the causative organism is *Erysipelothrix insidiosa* and not a streptococcus. It infects a wide range of animals, birds and fish. In humans, infections are most common in butchers, fishmongers and cooks, the organisms penetrating the skin after a prick from an infected bone. Such infections are usually mild, and localized to the area around the inoculation site. The swollen purple area spreads slowly with a clear-cut advancing edge. With penicillin, the condition clears quickly; without it, resolution takes several weeks.

## Cat-scratch disease

The infective agent is the bacillus *Rochalimaea henselae*. A few days after a cat bite or scratch, a reddish granulomatous papule appears at the site of inoculation. Tender regional lymphadenopathy follows some weeks later and lasts for several weeks, often being accompanied by a mild fever. The glands may discharge before settling spontaneously. There is no specific treatment.

## Meningococcal infection

*Neisseria meningitides* is a Gram-negative coccus that commonly colonizes the upper respiratory tract. Usually it is only responsible for local infections such as conjunctivitis, but for unknown reasons it may rarely become invasive and cause a severe and life-threatening disease. Meningitis and septicaemia are not always easy to recognize in their early stages when their symptoms can be very similar to common illnesses such as influenza. The signs and symptoms do not appear in any order and some may not appear at all. Acute meningococcal septicaemia can present as a fulminating disease with septic shock and meningitis or more non-specifically with rigors, leg pain, headache, stiff neck, vomiting and pallor. A haemorrhagic rash with petechiae and then purpura (with no blanching or change on diascopy), found mainly on the trunk and limbs, is characteristic. An unwell, feverish child with these skin signs should be considered highly likely to have meningococcal disease. Diagnosis is confirmed by the isolation of *N. meningitidis* from blood or cerebrospinal fluid, but treatment with high-dose intravenous benzylpenicillin should be started as soon as the diagnosis is suspected. Rifampicin prophylaxis can be used for close contacts.

> **Learning point**
>
> Trust your instincts; if you suspect meningitis or septicaemia seek hospital help *immediately*

## Spirochaetal infections

### Syphilis

*Cause*

Infection with the causative organism, *Treponema pallidum*, may be congenital, acquired through transfusion with contaminated blood, or by accidental inoculation. The most important route, however, is through sexual contact with an infected partner, and the incidence is currently rising sharply, with concurrent HIV infection.

*Presentation*

*Congenital syphilis* If there is a high standard of antenatal care and testing, syphilis in the mother will be detected and treated during pregnancy, so congenital syphilis will be rare. Otherwise, stillbirth is a common outcome, although some children with congenital syphilis may develop the stigmata of the disease only in late childhood.

*Acquired syphilis* The features of the different stages are given in Fig. 16.6. After an incubation period (9–90 days), a primary chancre develops at the site of inoculation. Often this is genital, but oral and anal chancres are not uncommon. A typical chancre is a painless, button-like ulcer of up to 1 cm in diameter accompanied by local lymphadenopathy. Untreated it lasts about 6 weeks and then clears leaving an inconspicuous scar.

The secondary stage may be reached while the chancre is still subsiding. Systemic symptoms and a generalized lymphadenopathy usher in eruptions that at first are macules and inconspicuous, and later papules and more obvious. Lesions are distributed

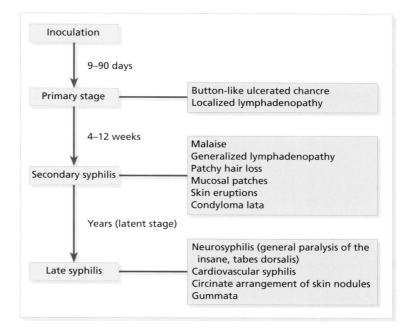

**Fig. 16.6** The stages of syphilis.

symmetrically and are of a coppery ham colour. Sometimes they resemble pityriasis rosea or guttate psoriasis. Classically, there are obvious lesions on the palms and soles. Annular lesions are not uncommon. Condylomata lata are moist papules in the genital and anal areas. Other signs include a 'moth-eaten' alopecia and mucous patches in the mouth.

The skin lesions of late syphilis may be nodules that spread peripherally and clear centrally, leaving a serpiginous outline. Gummas are granulomatous areas; in the skin they quickly break down to leave punched-out ulcers that heal poorly, leaving papery white scars.

*Clinical course*

Even if left untreated, most of those who contract syphilis have no further problems after the secondary stage has passed. Others develop the cutaneous or systemic manifestations of late syphilis such as gummas and dementia.

*Differential diagnosis*

The skin changes of syphilis can mimic many other skin diseases. Always consider the following.

1 *Chancre* Chancroid (multiple and painful), herpes simplex, anal fissure, cervical erosions.
2 *Secondary syphilis*
  ● Eruption – measles, rubella, drug eruptions, pityriasis rosea, lichen planus, psoriasis
  ● Condylomas – genital warts, haemorrhoids
  ● Oral lesions – aphthous ulcers, candidiasis
  ● Alopecia – tinea, trichotillomania, traction alopecia
3 *Late syphilis* Bromide and iodide reactions, other granulomas, erythema induratum.

*Investigations*

The diagnosis of syphilis in its infectious (primary and secondary) stages has traditionally been confirmed using dark-field microscopy to show up spirochaetes in smears from chancres, oral lesions or moist areas in a secondary eruption.

Serological tests for syphilis become positive only some 5–6 weeks after infection (usually a week or two after the appearance of the chancre). The non-treponemal (rapid plasma reagin [RPR] and Venereal Disease Research Laboratory [VDRL]) tests are 78–86% sensitive in primary and 100% sensitive in secondary syphilis, but may produce false positive results. Positive results are thus confirmed with more specific treponemal tests such as the fluorescent treponemal antibody/absorption (FTA/ABS) and *T. pallidum* particle agglutination (TPPA) tests, although HIV infection may cause false negative results. Serological tests may not become negative after treatment if an infection has been present for more than a few months and thus cannot be relied on to differentiate between active and successfully treated infections.

Patients with syphilis should be screened for concurrent sexually transmitted infections, including gonorrhoea and HIV.

### Treatment

This should follow the current national recommendations (see www.guidelines.gov). Penicillin is still the treatment of choice, given parenterally for 10 days in early syphilis and 17 days in late-stage disease or in early syphilis with neurological involvement. Doxycycline for 14 days or azithromycin for 10 days are alternatives for those with penicillin allergy. Patients with concomitant HIV infection need longer treatment and higher doses. Lumbar puncture is indicated in later stages as a guide to treatment. The use of long-acting penicillin injections overcomes the ever-present danger of poor compliance with oral treatment. Every effort must be made to trace and treat infected contacts.

---

**Learning points**

- Syphilis is still around. Remember that today's general was yesterday's lieutenant
- It is still worth checking for syphilis in perplexing rashes

---

### Yaws

Yaws is distributed widely across the poorer parts of the tropics. The spirochaete, *Treponema pallidum* ssp. *pertenue*, gains its entry through skin abrasions. After an incubation period of up to 6 months, the primary lesion, a crusting and ulcerated papule known as the 'mother yaw', develops at the site of inoculation; later it may enlarge to an exuberant raspberry-like swelling which lasts for several months before healing to leave an atrophic pale scar. In the secondary stage, other lesions may develop in any area but do so especially around the orifices. They are not unlike the primary lesion but are smaller and more numerous ('daughter yaws'). Hyperkeratotic plaques may appear on the palms and soles. The tertiary stage is characterized by ulcerated gummatous skin lesions, hyperkeratosis of the palms and soles, and a painful periostitis that distorts the long bones. Serological tests for syphilis are positive. Treatment is with penicillin.

### Lyme disease

The spirochaete *Borrelia burgdorferi* is responsible for this condition, named after the town in the USA where it was first recognized. It is transmitted to humans by ticks of the genus *Ixodes*, commonly harboured by deer. The site of the tick bite becomes the centre of a slowly expanding erythematous plaque or ring ('erythema migrans'; Fig. 16.7). Later, many annular non-scaly plaques may develop. In the USA, a few of those affected develop arthritis and heart disease, both of which are less common in European cases. Other internal complications include meningitis and cranial nerve palsies. Treated early, the condition clears well with a 21-day course of oral

**Fig. 16.7** A tick bite was followed by erythema migrans.

amoxicillin or doxycycline. Patients affected systemically need longer courses of parenteral antibiotics. Infection can be confirmed by serology, although this is usually negative in the first few weeks after innoculation. Individuals living in endemic areas may have positive serological tests, probably as a result of minor infection that resolved spontaneously. Serial testing may be necessary to sort this out in patients with atypical rashes.

## Other infections

### Cutaneous anthrax

This condition is usually acquired through contact with infected livestock or animal products such as wool or bristles. Previously rare in industrialized countries, its importance increased after the infectious agent was used in the USA for a bioterrorism attack.

Anthrax has two main clinical variants: the often fatal inhalational anthrax, which is outside the scope of this book, and cutaneous anthrax. The incubation period of the latter is usually 2–5 days. A skin lesion then appears on an exposed part, often in association with a variable degree of cutaneous oedema, which can sometimes be massive, especially on the face. Within a day or two, the original small painless papule shows vesicles that quickly coalesce into a larger single blister. This ruptures to form an ulcer with a central dark eschar, which falls off after 1–2 weeks, leaving a scar. The skin lesions are often accompanied by fever, headache, myalgia and regional lymphadenopathy. The mortality rate for untreated cutaneous anthrax is up to 20%; with appropriate antibiotic treatment, this falls to less than 1%.

Cultures of material taken from the vesicle may be positive in 12–48 h; a Gram stain will show Gram-positive bacilli, occurring singly or in short chains. Quicker results may be obtained by a direct fluorescent antibody test, or by an enzyme-linked immunosorbent assay (ELISA) – both of which are currently available only at reference laboratories. Before the results are available it is wise to assume that the organism is penicillin and tetracycline resistant, and to start treatment with ciprofloxacin at 400 mg intravenously every 12 h or, for milder cases, ciprofloxacin 500 mg orally every 12 h. The latter regimen is suitable for prophylactic use in those who are known to have been exposed to spores. A switch to an alternative regimen can be made once the antibiotic sensitivity of the organism has been established. At present, anthrax vaccine is in short supply; it requires six injections over 18 months, with subsequent boosters, to prevent anthrax. The spores of *Bacillus anthracis*, the causative organism, are highly resistant to physical and chemical agents.

### Gonococcal septicaemia

Skin lesions are important clues to the diagnosis of this condition, in which the symptoms and signs of classic gonorrhoea are usually absent. The patient, usually a menstruating woman with recurring fever and joint pains, develops sparse crops of skin lesions, usually around the hands and feet. The grey, often haemorrhagic, vesicopustules are characteristic. Rather similar lesions are seen in chronic meningococcal septicaemia.

## Mycobacterial infections

### Tuberculosis

Most infections in the UK are caused by *Mycobacterium tuberculosis*. *Mycobacterium bovis* infection, endemic in cattle, can be spread to humans by milk, but human infection with this organism is now rare in countries where cattle have been vaccinated against tuberculosis and the milk is pasteurized. The steady decline of tuberculosis in developed countries has been reversed in some areas where AIDS is especially prevalent. Dormant tuberculosis of the skin can also be reactivated by systemic corticosteroids, immunosuppressants and new anti-TNF biological agents.

### Inoculation tuberculosis

Inoculation into skin causes a wart-like lesion at the site. Systemic spread to the skin (lupus vulgaris; Fig. 16.8) can follow from an underlying infected lymph node, or from a pulmonary lesion. Lesions occur most often around the head and neck. A reddish-brown scaly plaque slowly enlarges, and can damage deeper tissues such as cartilage, leading to ugly mutilation. Scarring and contractures may follow.

**Fig. 16.8** A plaque with the brownish tinge characteristic of lupus vulgaris. Diascopy was positive.

Diascopy (p. 39) shows up the characteristic brownish 'apple jelly' nodules. The clinical diagnosis should be confirmed by biopsy.

### Scrofuloderma

The skin overlying a tuberculous lymph node or joint may become involved in the process. The subsequent mixture of lesions (irregular puckered scars, fistulae and abscesses) is most commonly seen in the neck.

### Tuberculides

A number of granulomatous skin eruptions have, in the past, been attributed to a reaction to internal foci of tuberculosis. Of these, the best authenticated – by finding mycobacterial DNA by polymerase chain reaction (PCR) – are the 'papulonecrotic tuberculides' – recurring crops of firm dusky papules, which may ulcerate, favouring the points of the knees and elbows. Most tuberculosis-like granulomas of the face are forms of granulomatous rosacea.

### Erythema induratum (Bazin's disease)

In erythema induratum, deep purplish ulcerating nodules occur on the backs of the lower legs, usually in women with a poor 'chilblain' type of circulation. Sometimes this is associated with a tuberculous focus elsewhere. Erythema nodosum (p. 112) may also be the result of tuberculosis elsewhere.

### Investigations

Biopsy for:
- microscopy (tuberculoid granulomas);
- bacteriological culture;
- detection of mycobacterial DNA by PCR;

Mantoux test
Chest X-ray.

### Treatment

The treatment of all types of cutaneous tuberculosis should be with a full course of a standard multidrug antituberculosis regimen. There is no longer any excuse for the use of one drug alone.

### Prevention

Outbreaks of pulmonary tuberculosis are reminders that this disease has not yet been conquered and that vigilance is important. Bacillus Calmette–Guérin (BCG) vaccination of schoolchildren, immunization of cattle and pasteurization of milk remain the most effective protective measures.

## Leprosy

### Cause

*Mycobacterium leprae* was discovered by Hansen in 1874, but has still not been cultured *in vitro*, although it can be made to grow in some animals (e.g. armadillos, mouse foot-pads). In humans the main route of infection is through nasal droplets from cases of lepromatous leprosy although, interestingly, some cases have occurred from eating infected armadillos.

### Epidemiology

Some 15 million people worldwide have leprosy. Most live in the tropics and subtropics, but the ease of modern travel means that some cases are seen in northern Europe and the USA.

### Presentation

The range of clinical manifestations and complications

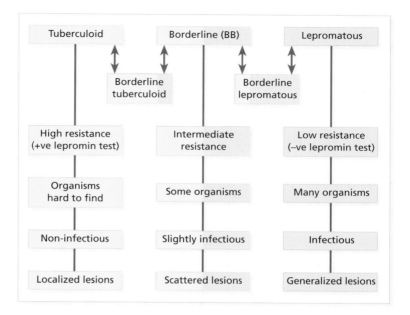

Fig. 16.9 The spectrum of leprosy: tuberculoid to lepromatous.

| Tuberculoid | Borderline (BB) | Lepromatous |
|---|---|---|
| ↕ Borderline tuberculoid | ↕ Borderline lepromatous | |
| High resistance (+ve lepromin test) | Intermediate resistance | Low resistance (−ve lepromin test) |
| Organisms hard to find | Some organisms | Many organisms |
| Non-infectious | Slightly infectious | Infectious |
| Localized lesions | Scattered lesions | Generalized lesions |

depends upon the immune response of the patient (Fig. 16.9). Those with a high resistance develop a paucibacillary tuberculoid type (Fig. 16.10) and those with low resistance a multibacillary lepromatous type. Nerve thickening is earlier and more marked in the tuberculoid than lepromatous type (Fig. 16.11). Between the extremes lies a spectrum of reactions classified as 'borderline'. Those most

Fig. 16.10 Tuberculoid leprosy: subtle depigmentation with a palpable erythematous rim at the upper edge.

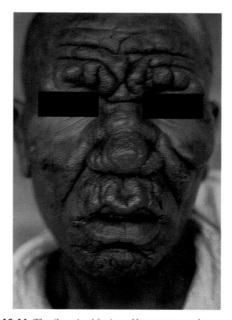

Fig. 16.11 The 'leonine' facies of lepromatous leprosy.

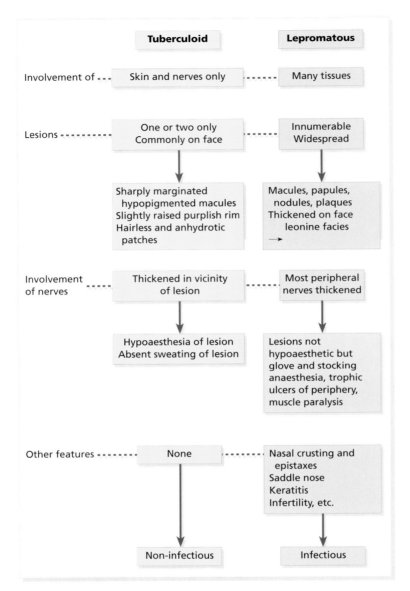

**Fig. 16.12** Tuberculoid vs. lepromatous leprosy.

like the tuberculoid type are known as borderline tuberculoid (BT) and those nearest to the lepromatous type as borderline lepromatous (BL). The clinical differences between the two polar types are given in Fig. 16.12.

*Differential diagnosis*

*Tuberculoid leprosy* Consider the following – in none of which is there any loss of sensation:

- vitiligo (p. 281) – loss of pigment is usually complete;
- pityriasis versicolor (p. 254) – scrapings show mycelia and spores;
- pityriasis alba (p. 207) – a common cause of scaly hypopigmented areas on the cheeks of children;
- post-inflammatory depigmentation of any cause; and

*Borderline leprosy* Consider sarcoidosis, granuloma annulare, necrobiosis lipoidica.

*Lepromatous leprosy* Widespread leishmaniasis can closely simulate lepromatous leprosy. The nodules seen in neurofibromatosis and mycosis fungoides, and multiple sebaceous cysts, can cause confusion, as can the acral deformities seen in yaws and systemic sclerosis. Leprosy is a great imitator.

### Investigations

● Biopsy of skin or sensory nerve.
● Skin or nasal smears, with Ziehl–Neelsen or Fité stains, will show up the large number of organisms seen in the lepromatous type.
● Lepromin test. This is of no use in the diagnosis of leprosy but, once the diagnosis has been made, it will help to decide which type of disease is present (positive in tuberculoid type).

### Treatment

The emergence of resistant strains of *M. leprae* means that it is no longer wise to treat leprosy with dapsone alone. It should now be used in combination (multi-drug therapy-MDT), usually with rifampicin, and also with clofazimine for lepromatous leprosy. Rifampin is rapidly bactericidal, making patients non-infectious and able to return to the community. However, their management should remain in the hands of physicians with a special interest in the disease. Tuberculoid forms are usually treated for 6 months; multibacillary leprosy needs treatment for at least 1 year.

Special care is needed with the two types of lepra reaction that can occur during treatment.
● Type 1 (reversal) reactions are seen mainly in BT disease (Fig. 16.13). Lesions become red and angry, and pain and paralysis follow neural inflammation. Treatment is with salicylates, chloroquine, non-steroidal and steroidal anti-inflammatory drugs. Nerve palsies need prompt treatment with corticosteroids to preserve function.
● Type 2 reactions are common in lepromatous leprosy and include erythema nodosum, nerve palsies, lymphadenopathy, arthritis, iridocyclitis, epididymo-orchitis and proteinuria. They are treated with the drugs used for type 1 reactions, and also with thalidomide.

The household contacts of lepromatous patients

**Fig. 16.13** Type 1 reversal reaction. The posterior auricular nerve is grossly swollen.

are at risk of developing leprosy and should be followed up. Child contacts may benefit from prophylactic therapy and BCG inoculation.

### Other mycobacterial infections

Mycobacteria are widespread in nature, living as environmental saprophytes. Some can infect humans.

### Mycobacterium marinum

*Mycobacterium marinum* lives in water. Human infections have occurred in epidemics centred on infected swimming pools and brackish water. Another route of infection is through minor skin breaches in those who clean out tropical fish tanks (Fig. 16.14). After a 3-week incubation period, an indolent abscess or ulcerated nodule forms at the site of inoculation; later nodules may develop along the draining lymphatics (sporotrichoid spread; Fig. 16.15 and p. 254). The lesions heal spontaneously, but slowly. Resolution may be speeded by an 8-week course of co-trimoxazole or minocycline. Should these fail, rifampicin in combination with ethambutol is worth a trial.

**Fig. 16.14** Dead tropical fish picked out of the tank by the patient shown in Fig. 16.15.

**Fig. 16.16** Leishmaniasis acquired in the Middle East.

**Fig. 16.15** The sporotrichoid spread of an atypical mycobacterial infection.

### *Mycobacterium ulcerans*

Infections are confined to certain humid tropical areas where the organism lives on the vegetation, and are most common in Uganda (Buruli ulcers). The necrotic spreading ulcers, with their undermined edges, are usually found on the legs. Drug therapy is often disappointing and the treatment of choice is probably the surgical removal of infected tissue.

## *Leishmaniasis*

Leishmania organisms are protozoa whose life cycle includes stages in phlebotomus flies, from which they are transmitted to humans. Different species, in different geographical areas, cause different clinical pictures.
- *Leishmania tropica* is found around the Mediterranean coast and in southern Asia; it causes chronically discharging skin nodules (oriental sores; Fig. 16.16).
- *Leishmania donovani* causes kala-azar, a disease characterized by fever, hepatosplenomegaly and anaemia. The skin may show an irregular darkening, particularly on the face and hands.
- *Leishmania mexicana* and *L. braziliensis* are found in Central and South America. They also cause deep sores, but up to 40% of those infected with *L. braziliensis* develop 'episodic' destructive metastatic lesions in the mucosa of the nose or mouth (éspundia).

### *Diagnosis*

This is confirmed by:
- histology – amastigote parasites, granulomatous reaction;
- touch smear – amastigote parasites;
- culture; and
- PCR tests.

### *Treatment*

The aims of treatment are to accelerate healing, and thus avoid disfiguring scars, and in New World leishmaniasis to prevent metastatic spread to the oropharynx which would result in mucocutaneous disease. Single nodules often resolve spontaneously and may not need treatment. Destructive measures, including cryotherapy, are sometimes used for localized skin lesions. The topical application of paromomycin (15%) plus methylbenzethonium chloride (12%) is beneficial.

Intralesional or intravenous antimony compounds are still the treatment of choice for most types of leishmaniasis (e.g. sodium stibogluconate

20 mg/kg/day for 20 days) with regular blood tests and electrocardiographic monitoring.

## Viral infections

The viral infections dealt with here are those that are commonly seen in dermatology clinics. A textbook of infectious diseases should be consulted for details of systemic viral infections, many of which – like measles and German measles – have their own specific rashes.

### Viral warts

Most people will have a wart at some time in their lives. Their prevalence is highest in childhood, and they affect an estimated 4–5% of schoolchildren in the UK.

### *Cause*

Warts are caused by the human papilloma virus (HPV), which has still not been cultured *in vitro*. Nevertheless, around 'types' of the virus are now recognized by DNA sequencing; each has its own range of clinical manifestations. HPV-1, 2 and 4, for example, are found in common warts, whereas HPV-3 is found in plane warts, and HPV-6, 11, 16 and 18 are most common in genital warts. Infections occur when wart virus in skin scales comes into contact with breaches in the skin or mucous membranes or when immunity is suppressed and dormant viruses escape from their resting place in the outer root sheaths of hairs.

### *Presentation*

Warts adopt a variety of patterns (Fig. 16.17), some of which are described below.

*Common warts* (Figs 16.18 and 16.19) The first sign is a smooth skin-coloured papule, often more easily felt than seen. As the lesion enlarges, its irregular hyperkeratotic surface and vertical shoulders give it the classic 'warty' appearance. Common warts usually occur on the hands but are also often on the face and genitals. They are more often multiple than single. Pain is rare.

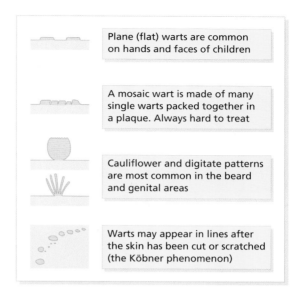

| | |
|---|---|
| | Plane (flat) warts are common on hands and faces of children |
| | A mosaic wart is made of many single warts packed together in a plaque. Always hard to treat |
| | Cauliflower and digitate patterns are most common in the beard and genital areas |
| | Warts may appear in lines after the skin has been cut or scratched (the Köbner phenomenon) |

**Fig. 16.17** Viral warts – variations on the theme.

**Fig. 16.18** Typical common warts on the fingers.

**Fig. 16.19** Multiple hand warts in a fishmonger showing the Köbner phenomenon.

**Fig. 16.20** Solitary plantar wart on the heel. (Courtesy of Dr E.C. Benton, The Royal Infirmary of Edinburgh, Edinburgh, UK.)

**Fig. 16.21** Group of warts under the forefoot pared to show mosaic pattern.

*Plantar warts* These have a rough surface, which protrudes only slightly from the skin and is sur-rounded by a horny collar (Fig. 16.20). On paring, the presence of bleeding capillary loops allows plantar warts to be distinguished from corns. Often multiple, plantar warts can be painful.

*Mosaic warts* (Fig. 16.21) These rough marginated plaques are made up of many small, tightly packed but discrete individual warts. They are most com-mon on the soles but are also seen on palms and around finger nails. Usually they are not painful.

*Plane warts* (Fig. 16.22) These smooth flat-topped papules are most common on the face and brow, on the backs of the hands and on the shaven legs of

**Fig. 16.22** Plane warts resolving with inflammation.

women. Usually skin-coloured or light brown, they become inflamed as a result of an immunological reaction, just before they resolve spontaneously. Lesions are multiple, painless and, like common warts, are sometimes arranged along a scratch line.

*Facial warts* These are most common in the beard area of adult males and are spread by shaving. A digitate appearance is common. Lesions are often ugly but are painless.

*Anogenital warts (condyloma acuminata)* (Fig. 16.23) Papillomatous cauliflower-like lesions, with a moist macerated vascular surface, can appear anywhere in this area. They may coalesce to form huge fungat-ing plagues causing discomfort and irritation. The vaginal and anorectal mucosae may be affected. The presence of anogenital warts in children raises the spectre of sexual abuse, but is usually caused by autoinoculation from common warts elsewhere.

## Course

Warts resolve spontaneously in the healthy as the immune response overcomes the infection. This happens within 6 months in some 30% of patients,

**Fig. 16.23** Multiple penile warts in an immunosuppressed patient.

**Fig. 16.24** Spontaneous resolution of a group of plantar warts. The blackness is caused by capillary thrombosis.

and within 2 years in 65%. Such spontaneous resolution, sometimes heralded by a punctate blackening caused by capillary thrombosis (Fig. 16.24), leaves no trace. Mosaic warts are notoriously slow to resolve and often resist all treatments. Warts persist and spread in immunocompromised patients (e.g. those on immunosuppressive therapy or with lymphoreticular disease). Seventy per cent of renal allograft recipients will have warts 5 years after transplantation.

## Complications

1 Some plantar warts are very painful.
2 Epidermodysplasia verruciformis is a rare inherited disorder in which there is a universal wart infection, usually with HPV of unusual types. An impairment of cell-mediated immunity (p. 30) is commonly found and ensuing carcinomatous change frequently occurs.
3 Malignant change is otherwise rare, although infection with HPV types 16 and 18 predisposes to cervical carcinoma. HPV infections in immunocompromised patients (e.g. renal allograft recipients) have also been linked with skin cancer, especially on light-exposed areas.

## Differential diagnosis

Most warts are easily recognized. The following must be ruled out.
● *Molluscum contagiosum* (p. 243) are smooth, dome-shaped and pearly, with central umbilication.
● *Plantar corns* are found on pressure areas; there is no capillary bleeding on paring. They have a central keratotic core and are painful.
● *Granuloma annulare* lesions (p. 325) have a smooth surface, as the lesions are dermal, and their outline is often annular.
● *Condyloma lata* are seen in syphilis. They are rare but should not be confused with condyloma acuminata (warts). The lesions are flatter, greyer and less well defined. If in doubt, look for other signs of secondary syphilis (p. 227) and carry out serological tests.
● *Amelanotic melanomas, squamous cell carcinomas and other epithelial malignancies* can present as verrucose nodules – those in patients over the age of 40 years should be examined with special care. Mistakes have been made in the past.

## Treatment

Many warts give no trouble, need no treatment and go away by themselves. Otherwise treatment will depend on the type of wart. In general terms, destruction by cryotherapy is less likely to cause scars than excision or electrosurgery.

### Palmoplantar warts

Regression of warts and prevention of their recurrence depends on establishment of cell-mediated immunity. Both induction of immunity and elicitation of cytotoxic responses are hindered by the insulation of wart virus in relatively inaccessible upper epidermis. Irritating the warts or 'blowing them up' with cryotherapy helps induce immunity by bringing wart virus and immune cells together.

For now, home treatment is best, with one of the many wart paints or plasters now available (Formulary 1, p. 388). Most contain salicylic acid (12–20%). The success rate is good if the patient is prepared to persist with regular treatment. Paints should be applied once daily, after moistening the warts in hot water for at least 5 min. After drying, dead tissue and old paint are removed with an emery board or pumice stone. Enough paint to cover the surface of the wart, but not the surrounding skin, is applied and allowed to dry. Warts on the plantar surface should be covered with plasters although this is not necessary elsewhere. Side-effects are rare if these instructions are followed. Wart paints should not be applied to facial or anogenital skin, or to patients with adjacent eczema.

If no progress is being made after the regular and correct use of a salicylic acid wart paint for 12 weeks, then a paint containing formaldehyde or glutaraldehyde is worth trying. A useful way of dealing with multiple small plantar warts is for the area to be soaked for 10 min each night in a 4% formalin solution, although a few patients become allergic to this.

Cryotherapy with liquid nitrogen (at −196°C) is more effective than the less cold dry ice or dimethyl ether or propane techniques; however, it is painful. The wart is sprayed with liquid nitrogen until a small frozen halo appears in the surrounding normal skin (Fig. 16.25). The use of two freeze–thaw cycles increases the clearance rate of plantar warts but not of hand warts. If further treatments are necessary, the optimal interval is 3 weeks. The cure rate is higher if plantar warts are pared before they are frozen, but this makes no difference to warts elsewhere. If there has been no improvement after four or five treatments there is little to be gained from further freezings.

A few minutes tuition from a dermatologist will help practitioners wishing to start cryotherapy. Blisters should not be provoked intentionally, but occur from time to time, and will not alarm patients who have been forewarned.

**Fig. 16.25** A wart treated with cryotherapy: area includes a small frozen halo of normal surrounding skin.

### Anogenital warts

Women with anogenital warts, or who are the partners of men with anogenital warts, should have their cervical cytology checked regularly as the wart virus can cause cervical cancer.

The focus has shifted towards self-treatment using podophyllotoxin (0.5% solution or 0.15% cream) or imiquimod (5% cream). Both are irritants and should be used carefully according to the manufacturer's instructions. Imiquimod is an immune response modifier that induces keratinocytes to produce cytokines, leading to wart regression, and may help to build cell-mediated immunity for long-lasting protection. It is applied as a thin layer three times weekly and washed off with a mild soap 6–10 h after application. Podophyllin paint (15%) is used much less often now. It should be applied carefully to the warts and allowed to dry before powdering with talcum. On the first occasion it should be washed off with soap and water after 2 h but, if there has been little discomfort, this can be increased stepwise to 6 h. Treatment is best carried out weekly by a doctor or nurse, but not by the patient. Podophyllin must not be used in pregnancy. Cryotherapy, electrosurgery and laser treatment are all effective treatments in the clinic.

Prevention of anogenital warts may soon be possible with the recent development of a successful vaccine against the relevant HPV subtypes. This appears to be highly effective at preventing HPV infection, and subsequent cervical dysplasia and cancer.

*Facial common warts*

These are best treated with electrocautery or a hyfrecator, but also surrender to careful cryotherapy. Scarring is an unwanted complication. Shaving, if essential, should be with a brushless foam and a disposable razor.

*Plane warts*

On the face these are best left untreated and the patient or parent can be reasonably assured that spontaneous resolution will occur. When treatment is demanded, the use of a wart paint, tretinoin gel or imiquimod cream is reasonable. Gentle cryotherapy of just a few warts may help to induce immunity.

*Solitary, stubborn or painful warts*

These can be removed under local anaesthetic with a curette, although cure is not assured with this or any other method, and a scar often follows. Surgical excision is never justifiable (Fig. 16.26). Bleomycin can also be injected into such warts with success but this treatment should only be undertaken by a specialist.

**Fig. 16.26** Multiple scars following the injudicious surgical treatment of warts.

> **Learning points**
>
> - Do not hurt children by using cryotherapy without a good trial of a wart paint first
> - Treat most common warts with a wart paint for 12 weeks before referring
> - Do not leave scars; nature does not
> - Avoid podophyllin during pregnancy
> - Do not miss an amelanotic malignant melanoma

## Varicella (chickenpox)

*Cause*

The herpes virus varicella-zoster is spread by the respiratory route; its incubation period is about 14 days.

*Presentation and course*

Slight malaise is followed by the development of papules, which turn rapidly into clear vesicles on a pink base (dewdrops on a rose petal). Vesicles soon become pustules and then umbilicate. Over the next few days the lesions crust and then clear, sometimes leaving white depressed scars. Lesions appear in crops, are often itchy, and are most profuse on the trunk and least profuse on the periphery of the limbs (centripetal). Second attacks are rare. Varicella can be fatal in those who are immunologically compromised.

*Complications*

- Pneumonitis, with pulmonary opacities on X-ray.
- Secondary infection of skin lesions.
- Haemorrhagic or lethal chickenpox in leukaemics and other immunocompromised children and adults.
- Scarring.

*Differential diagnosis*

Smallpox, mainly centrifugal anyway, has been universally eradicated, and the diagnosis of chickenpox is seldom in doubt.

*Investigations*

None are usually needed. The Tzanck smear (p. 41) is positive.

*Treatment*

Aciclovir, famciclovir and valaciclovir (Formulary 2, p. 397) should be reserved for severe attacks and

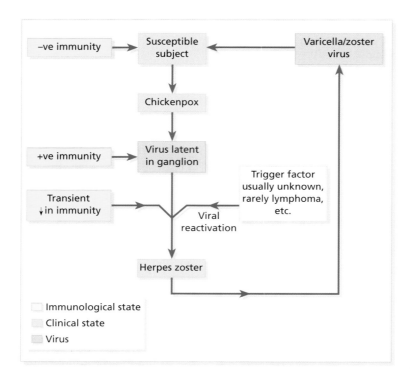

**Fig. 16.27** Zoster–varicella relationships.

for immunocompromised patients; for the latter, prophylactic aciclovir can also be used to prevent disease if given within a day or two of exposure. In mild attacks, calamine lotion topically is all that is required. A live attenuated vaccine is now available, and is being more widely used. It is not universally effective and should not be given to patients with immunodeficiencies, therapeutic immunosuppression or blood dyscrasias who might not be able to resist even the attenuated organism.

## Herpes zoster

### Cause

Shingles is caused by the herpes virus varicella-zoster. An attack is a result of the reactivation, usually for no obvious reason, of virus that has remained dormant in a sensory root ganglion since an earlier episode of chickenpox (varicella). The incidence of shingles is highest in old age, and in conditions such as Hodgkin's disease, AIDS and leukaemia, which weaken normal defence mechanisms. Shingles does not occur in epidemics; its clinical manifestations are caused by virus acquired in the past. However, patients with zoster can transmit the virus to others in whom it will cause chickenpox (Fig. 16.27).

### Presentation and course

Attacks usually start with a burning pain, soon followed by erythema and grouped, sometimes blood-filled, vesicles scattered over a dermatome. The clear vesicles quickly become purulent, and over the space of a few days burst and crust. Scabs usually separate in 2–3 weeks, sometimes leaving depressed depigmented scars.

Zoster is characteristically unilateral (Fig. 16.28). It may affect more than one adjacent dermatome. The thoracic segments and the ophthalmic division of the trigeminal nerve are involved disproportionately often.

It is not uncommon for a few pock-like lesions to be found outside the main segment of involvement, but a generalized chickenpox-like eruption accompanying segmental zoster should raise suspicions

**Fig. 16.28** Herpes zoster of the left ophthalmic division of the trigeminal nerve. No nasociliary involvement (see text); this is reassuring.

of an underlying immunocompromised state or malignancy, particularly if the lesions are unusually haemorrhagic or necrotic.

## Complications

- Secondary bacterial infection is common.
- Motor nerve involvement is uncommon, but has led to paralysis of ocular muscles, the facial muscles, the diaphragm and the bladder.
- Zoster of the ophthalmic division of the trigeminal nerve can lead to corneal ulcers and scarring. A good clinical clue here is involvement of the nasociliary branch (vesicles grouped on the side of the nose).
- Persistent neuralgic pain, after the acute episode is over, is most common in the elderly.

## Differential diagnosis

Occasionally, before the rash has appeared, the initial pain is taken for an emergency such as acute appendicitis or myocardial infarction. An early painful red plaque may suggest cellulitis until other plaques in the dermatome appear or until vesicles develop on their tops. Otherwise, the dermatomal distribution and the pain allow zoster to be distinguished easily from herpes simplex, eczema and impetigo.

## Investigations

Cultures are of little help as they take 5–7 days, and are only positive in 70% of cases. Biopsy or Tzanck smears show multinucleated giant cells and a ballooning degeneration of keratinocytes, indicative of a herpes infection. Any clinical suspicions about underlying conditions, such as Hodgkin's disease, chronic lymphatic leukaemia or AIDS, require further investigation.

## Treatment

Systemic treatment should be given to all patients if diagnosed in the early stages of the disease. It is essential that this treatment should start within the first 5 days of an attack. Famciclovir and valaciclovir are as effective as aciclovir (Formulary 2, p. 397) and more reliably absorbed; they depend on virus-specific thymidine kinase for their antiviral activity. All three drugs are safe, and using them early cuts down the chance of post-herpetic neuralgia, particularly in the elderly.

If diagnosed late in the course of the disease, systemic treatment is not likely to be effective and treatment should be supportive with rest, analgesics and bland applications such as calamine. Secondary bacterial infection should be treated appropriately.

A trial of systemic carbamazepine, gabapentin or amitriptyline, or 4 weeks of topical capsaicin cream (Formulary 1, p. 392), despite the burning sensation it sometimes causes, may be worthwhile for established post-herpetic neuralgia.

Prevention may be better than cure. Vaccination of elderly patients with a live attenuated vaccine to the varicella-zoster virus has been shown to reduce the incidence of both herpes zoster and post-herpetic neuralgia, but the place for this treatment has not yet been established.

> **Learning points**
> - Post-herpetic neuralgia affects the elderly rather than the young
> - Systemic aciclovir works best if given early in the course of the disease
> - Look for an underlying cause when there is dissemination outside the main affected dermatomes

## Herpes simplex

### Cause

Herpesvirus hominis is the cause of herpes simplex. The virus is ubiquitous and carriers continue to shed virus particles in their saliva or tears. It has been separated into two types. The lesions caused by type II virus occur mainly on the genitals, while those of type I are usually extragenital; however, this distinction is not absolute.

The route of infection is through mucous membranes or abraded skin. After the episode associated with the primary infection, the virus may become latent, possibly within nerve ganglia, but still capable of giving rise to recurrent bouts of vesication (recrudescences).

### Presentation

#### Primary infection

The most common recognizable manifestation of a primary type I infection in children is an acute gingivostomatitis accompanied by malaise, headache, fever and enlarged cervical nodes. Vesicles, soon turning into ulcers, can be seen scattered over the lips and mucous membranes. The illness lasts about 2 weeks.

The virus can also be inoculated directly into the skin (e.g. during wrestling). A herpetic whitlow is one example of this direct inoculation. The uncomfortable pus-filled blisters on a fingertip are seen most often in medical personnel attending patients with unsuspected herpes simplex infections.

Primary type II virus infections, usually transmitted sexually, cause multiple and painful genital or perianal blisters which rapidly ulcerate.

#### Recurrent (recrudescent) infections

These strike in roughly the same place each time. They may be precipitated by respiratory tract infections (cold sores), ultraviolet radiation, menstruation or even stress. Common sites include the face (Fig. 16.29), the lips (type I) and the genitals (type II), but lesions can occur anywhere. Tingling, burning or even pain is followed within a few hours by the development of erythema and clusters of tense

**Fig. 16.29** The grouped vesicles of herpes simplex, here provoked by sunlight. Those in the lower group are beginning to crust.

vesicles. Crusting occurs within 24–48 h and the whole episode lasts about 12 days.

### Complications

● Herpes encephalitis or meningitis can occur without any cutaneous clues.
● Disseminated herpes simplex: widespread vesicles may be part of a severe illness in newborns, debilitated children or immunosuppressed adults.
● Eczema herpeticum: patients with atopic eczema are particularly susceptible to widespread cutaneous herpes simplex infections. Those looking after patients with atopic eczema should stay away if they have cold sores.
● Herpes simplex can cause recurrent dendritic ulcers leading to corneal scarring.
● In some patients, recurrent herpes simplex infections are regularly followed by erythema multiforme (p. 110).

### Investigations

None are usually needed. Doubts over the diagnosis can be dispelled by culturing the virus from vesicle fluid. Antibody titres rise with primary, but not with recurrent infections.

### Treatment

'Old-fashioned' remedies suffice for occasional mild recurrent attacks; sunblock may cut down their frequency. Dabbing with surgical spirit is helpful, and secondary bacterial infection can be reduced by topical bacitracin, mupirocin, framycetin or fusidic acid. Aciclovir cream, applied five or six times a day for the first 4 days of the episode, may cut down the length of attacks. More effective still is oral aciclovir (Formulary 2, p. 397), 200 mg five times daily for 5 days, although this is usually reserved for those with widespread or systemic involvement. Famciclovir and valaciclovir are metabolized by the body into aciclovir and are as effective as aciclovir, having the additional advantage of better absorption and fewer doses per day.

Recurrences in the immunocompromised can usually be prevented by long-term treatment at a lower dosage.

## Molluscum contagiosum

### Cause

This common pox virus infection can be spread by direct contact (e.g. sexually or by sharing a towel at the swimming bath).

### Presentation and course

The incubation period ranges from 2 to 6 weeks. Often, several members of one family are affected. Individual lesions are shiny, white or pink, and hemispherical; they grow slowly up to 0.5 cm in diameter. A central punctum, which may contain a cheesy core, gives the lesions their characteristic umbilicated look.

On close inspection, a mosaic appearance may be seen. Multiple lesions are common (Fig. 16.30) and their distribution depends on the mode of infection. Atopic individuals and the immunocompromised are prone to especially extensive infections, spread by scratching and the use of topical steroids.

Untreated lesions usually clear in 6–9 months, often after a brief local inflammation. Large solitary lesions may take longer. Some leave depressed scars.

### Complications

Eczematous patches often appear around mollusca. Traumatized or overtreated lesions may become secondarily infected.

**Fig. 16.30** An umbilicus surrounded by umbilicated papules of molluscum contagiosum.

### Differential diagnosis

Inflamed lesions can simulate a boil. Large solitary lesions in adults can be confused with a keratocanthoma (p. 305), an intradermal naevus (p. 295) or even a cystic basal cell carcinoma (p. 301). Confusion with warts should not arise as these have a rough surface and no central pore.

### Investigations

None are usually needed, but the diagnosis can be confirmed by looking under the microscope for large swollen epidermal cells, easily seen in unstained preparations of debris expressed from a lesion. Extensive mollusa of the beard area may suggest need for HIV testing.

### Treatment

Many simple destructive measures cause inflammation and then resolution. They include squeezing out the lesions with forceps, piercing them with an orange stick (preferably without phenol) and curettage. Liquid nitrogen, wart paints and topical imiquimod may also be helpful.

These measures are fine for adults, but young children dislike them and as mollusca are self-limiting, doing nothing is often the best option. Sometimes a local anaesthetic cream (EMLA; Formulary 1, p. 392), under polythene occlusion for an hour, will help children to tolerate more attacking treatment. Sparse eyelid lesions can be left alone but patients with numerous lesions may need to be referred to an ophthalmologist for curettage. Common sense measures help to limit spread within the family.

> **Learning points**
>
> ● If you cannot tell mollusca from warts, buy a lens
> ● Do not hurt young children with mollusca. You will not be able to get near them next time something more serious goes wrong

## Orf

### Cause

Contagious pustular dermatitis is common in lambs. Its cause is a parapox virus that can be transmitted to those handling infected animals. The condition is therefore most commonly seen on the hands of shepherds, of their wives who bottle-feed lambs, and of butchers, vets and meat porters.

### Presentation and course

The incubation period is 5–6 days. Lesions, which may be single or multiple, start as small firm papules that change into flat-topped, apparently pustular nodules with a violaceous and erythematous surround (Fig. 16.31). The condition clears up spontaneously in about a month.

**Fig. 16.31** The pseudopustular nodule of orf.

### Complications

● Lymphadenitis and malaise are common.
● Erythema multiforme.
● 'Giant' lesions can appear in the immunosuppressed.

### Differential diagnosis

Diagnosis is usually simple if contact with sheep is recognized. Milker's nodules, a pox virus infection acquired from cow's udders, can look like orf, as can staphylococcal furuncles.

### Investigations

None are usually needed. If there is any doubt, the diagnosis can be confirmed by the distinctive electron microscopic appearance of the virus obtained from crusts.

### Treatment

A topical antibiotic helps to prevent secondary infection; otherwise no active therapy is needed.

## Acquired immunodeficiency syndrome (AIDS)

The human immunodeficiency virus (HIV) can be acquired from contaminated body fluids, particularly semen and blood. In the UK and the USA, most cases have been in homosexual or bisexual men; however, in parts of Africa the disease is most often spread heterosexually. Intravenous drug abusers who share contaminated needles and syringes are also at high risk. Up to half of babies born to infected mothers are infected transplacentally, but this reduces to less than 2% with the use of maternal antiretroviral therapy, elective caesarean section and avoidance of breastfeeding.

The global epidemic is not slackening off although the pattern of transmission in industrialized nations is changing. Heterosexual transmission now accounts for 25–30% of new cases in Europe and the USA. Each year around 4.1 million people are newly infected with HIV worldwide and 2.8 million die from it.

## Pathogenesis

The human immunodeficiency viruses HIV-1 and HIV-2 (mainly in West Africa) are RNA retroviruses containing reverse transcriptase enzymes, which allow the viral DNA copy to be incorporated into the chromosomes of the host cell. Their main target is a subset of T lymphocytes (helper/inducer cells) that express glycoprotein CD4 molecules on their surface (p. 23). These bind to the surface envelope of the HIV. Viral replication within the helper/inducer cells kills them, and their depletion leads to the loss of cell-mediated immunity so characteristic of HIV infection. A variety of opportunistic infections then follow.

## Course

The original infection may be asymptomatic, or followed by a glandular fever-like illness at the time of seroconversion. After a variable latent phase, which may last several years, a persistent generalized lymphadenopathy develops. The term 'AIDS-related complex' refers to the next stage, in which many of the symptoms of AIDS (e.g. fever, weight loss, fatigue or diarrhoea) may be present without the opportunistic infections or tumours characteristic of full-blown AIDS. Not all of those infected with HIV will develop AIDS but, for those who do, the average time from infection to the onset of AIDS is about 10 years without treatment. Once AIDS develops, if untreated, about half will die within 1 year and three-quarters within 4 years. Encouragingly, the use of highly active antiretroviral therapy (HAART) has led to marked reductions in the rates of illness and death in HIV-infected individuals, with life expectancy of treated patients following diagnosis now measured in decades.

## Skin changes in AIDS

Skin conditions are often the first clue to the presence of AIDS. The following are important.

**1** *Kaposi's sarcoma* (Figs 16.32–16.34) is caused by human herpesvirus 8 and is the most common HIV-associated malignancy, although the incidence has dropped markedly since the introduction of antiretroviral therapy. The lesions of classic

**Fig. 16.32** Disseminated Kaposi's sarcoma in AIDS.

**Fig. 16.33** Kaposi's sarcoma in AIDS.

Kaposi's sarcoma are multiple purplish patches or nodules. In AIDS, the lesions may be atypical, sometimes looking like bruises or pyogenic granulomas (p. 316). The diagnosis can easily be missed and the mouth must always be examined.

**2** *Seborrhoeic eczema and folliculitis* (Fig. 16.35) are seen in at least 50% of patients, often starting at an early stage of immunosuppression. The underlying cause may be an overgrowth of *Pityrosporum*

**Fig. 16.34** Kaposi's sarcoma of hard palate, anterior fauces and uvula in AIDS.

**Fig. 16.36** Hairy leukoplakia on the side of the tongue.

**Fig. 16.35** Seborrhoeic dermatitis (otitis externa) and seborrhoeic folliculitis in HIV disease.

yeasts. An itchy folliculitis of the head, neck and trunk, and an eosinophilic folliculitis have also been described.

**3** *Skin infections* – florid, unusually extensive or atypical examples of common infections may be seen with one or more of the following: herpes simplex, herpes zoster, molluscum contagiosum, oral and cutaneous *Candida*, tinea, scabies and staphylococci. Facial and perianal warts are common. Hairy leuko-

plakia (Fig. 16.36), often on the sides of the tongue, may be caused by proliferation of the Epstein–Barr virus. Bacillary angiomatosis may look like Kaposi's sarcoma and is caused by the bacillus that causes cat-scratch fever. Syphilis can coexist with AIDS, as can mycobacterial infections.

**4** *Other manifestations* – dry skin is common in AIDS; so is pruritus. Psoriasis may start or worsen with AIDS. Diffuse alopecia is not uncommon. Drug eruptions are often seen in AIDS patients.

### Management

The clinical diagnosis of HIV infection is confirmed by a positive blood test for antibodies to the virus. Patients should be counselled before and after testing for HIV antibody. Sexual contacts of infected individuals should be traced.

Modern drugs for HIV infections increase life expectancy, but are not 'cures' in the usual sense. They reduce the viral load but are expensive and sometimes toxic. Guidelines on how to use them change constantly, and so the drug treatment of HIV infections should be directed by specialists in the field, who will monitor the plasma viral load and CD4 count regularly (Table 16.1). Difficult decisions to be made include the timing of treatment – the benefits of starting early have to be balanced against the risk of toxicity – and choosing the right drug combination of HAART – usually triple therapy with two nucleoside reverse transcriptase inhibitors plus either a non-nucleoside reverse transcriptase

**Table 16.1** Recommendations for starting highly active antiretroviral treatment (HAART) in the adult.

| Disease stage | Decision |
|---|---|
| Symptomatic | Treat |
| Asymptomatic | |
| CD4 <200 × 10⁶/L | Treat |
| CD4 200–350 × 10⁶/L | Treatment generally offered |
| CD4 >350 × 10⁶/L | Defer treatment unless high viral load |

inhibitor or a protease inhibitor. The regimen will be changed if there is clinical or virological deterioration, or if the patient becomes pregnant.

Treatment otherwise is symptomatic and varies according to the type of opportunistic infection detected. Prophylactic treatment against a number of life-threatening infections is also worthwhile, and prolongs life expectancy. Educating the public to avoid risky behaviour, such as unprotected sexual intercourse, is still hugely important.

## Mucocutaneous lymph node syndrome (Kawasaki's disease)

This acute systemic vasculitis involving medium-sized vessels may be caused by a recent parvovirus infection. The disease affects young children whose erythema, although often generalized, becomes most marked in a glove and stocking distribution; it may be associated with indurated oedema of the palms and soles. Peeling around the fingers and toes is one obvious feature but is not seen at the start. Bilateral conjunctival injection and erythema of the lips, buccal mucosa and tongue ('strawberry tongue') are common.

The episode is accompanied by fever and usually resolves within 2 weeks. Despite its name, not all patients have lymphadenopathy. The danger of this condition lies in the risk of developing pancarditis and coronary artery vasculitis leading on to aneurysms or dilatation. The pathology is close to that of polyarteritis nodosa. Aspirin and intravenous γ globulin are the mainstay of treatment; both should be given early in the disease and reduce the risk of coronary artery involvement.

## Gianotti–Crosti syndrome

This is a rather uncommon reaction to an infection with hepatitis B virus in childhood. Small reddish papules erupt bilaterally over the limbs and face, and fade over the course of a few weeks. Jaundice is uncommon, although tests of liver function give abnormal results.

## Herpangina

This is an acute infectious illness, caused by group A coxsackie viruses. The patient is usually a child with a fever, and a severe sore throat covered in many small vesicles, which rapidly become superficial ulcers. Episodes resolve in about a week.

## Hand, foot and mouth disease

This is usually caused by coxsackie A16. Minor epidemics occur in institutions. The oral vesicles are larger and fewer than those of herpangina. The hand and foot lesions are small greyish vesicles with a narrow rim of redness around (Fig. 16.37). The condition settles within a few days.

**Fig. 16.37** The typical vesicles of hand, foot and mouth disease.

## Measles

An incubation period of 10 days is followed by fever, conjunctival injection, photophobia and upper respiratory tract catarrh. Koplik's spots (pinhead-sized white spots with a bright red margin) are seen at this stage on the buccal mucosa. The characteristic 'net-like' rash starts after a few days, on the brow and behind the ears, and soon becomes extensive before fading with much desquamation. Prevention is by immunization with the combined MMR (measles–mumps–rubella) vaccine.

## Rubella

After an incubation period of about 18 days, lymphadenopathy occurs a few days before the evanescent pink macular rash, which fades, first on the trunk, over the course of a few days. Rubella during the first trimester of pregnancy carries a risk of damage to the unborn child. Prevention is by immunization with the combined MMR vaccine.

## Erythema infectiosum (fifth disease)

This is caused by the human parvovirus B19 and occurs in outbreaks, often in the spring. A slapped cheek erythema is quickly followed by a reticulate erythema of the shoulders. The affected child feels well, and the rash clears over the course of a few days. Other features, sometimes not accompanied by a rash, include transient anaemia and arthritis.

## Fungal infections

### Dermatophyte infections (ringworm)

#### Cause

Three genera of dermatophyte fungi cause tinea infections (ringworm).
- *Trichophyton* – skin, hair and nail infections.
- *Microsporum* – skin and hair.
- *Epidermophyton* – skin and nails.

Dermatophytes invade only into the stratum corneum, and the inflammation they cause is a result of metabolic products of the fungus or delayed hypersensitivity. In general, zoophilic fungi (those transmitted to humans by animals) cause a more severe inflammation than anthropophilic ones (spread from person to person).

#### Presentation and course

This depends upon the site and on the strain of fungus involved.

#### Tinea pedis (athlete's foot)

This is the most common type of fungal infection in humans. The sharing of wash places (e.g. in showers) and of swimming pools predisposes to infection; spores in occlusive footwear encourage relapses.

Most cases are caused by one of three organisms: *Trichophyton rubrum* (the most common and the most stubborn), *Trichophyton mentagrophytes* var. *interdigitale* and *Epidermophyton floccosum*.

There are three common clinical patterns.
**1** Soggy interdigital scaling, particularly in the fourth and fifth interspace (all three organisms; Fig. 16.38).
**2** A diffuse dry scaling of the soles (usually *T. rubrum*; Fig. 16.39).
**3** Recurrent episodes of vesication (usually *T. mentagrophytes* var. *interdigitale* or *E. floccosum*).

#### Tinea of the nails

Toe nail infection is usually associated with tinea pedis. The initial changes occur at the free edge of the nail, which becomes yellow and crumbly (Fig. 16.40). Subungual hyperkeratosis, separation

**Fig. 16.38** Tinea pedis. Scaly area spreading to the sole from the toe webs.

**Fig. 16.39** Powdery scaling, most obvious in the skin creases, caused by a *Trichophyton rubrum* infection.

**Fig. 16.40** Chronic tinea of the big toe nail. Starting distally, the thickness and discoloration are spreading proximally.

of the nail from its bed and thickening may then follow. Usually, only a few nails are infected but rarely all are. Finger nail lesions are similar, but less common, and are seldom seen without a chronic *T. rubrum* infection of the skin of the same hand.

### Tinea of the hands

This is usually asymmetrical and associated with tinea pedis and unilateral onychomycosis. *Trichophyton*

*rubrum* may cause a barely perceptible erythema of one palm with a characteristic powdery scale in the creases.

### Tinea of the groin

This is common and affects men more often than women. The eruption is sometimes unilateral or asymmetrical. The upper inner thigh is involved and lesions expand slowly to form sharply demarcated plaques with peripheral scaling (Fig. 16.41). In contrast to candidiasis of the groin area, the scrotum is usually spared. A few vesicles or pustules may be seen within the lesions. The organisms are the same as those causing tinea pedis.

### Tinea of the trunk and limbs

Tinea corporis is characterized by plaques with scaling and erythema most pronounced at the periphery. A few small vesicles and pustules may be seen within them. The lesions expand slowly and healing in the centre leaves a typical ring-like

**Fig. 16.41** A very gross example of tinea of the groin. The *Trichophyton rubrum* infection has spread on to the abdomen and thighs, aided by the use of topical steroids.

**Fig. 16.42** Animal ringworm of the beard area showing boggy inflamed swellings (kerion).

pattern. In some patients the fungus elicits almost no inflammation, in which case the infection is a marginated patch of rough scaling skin.

*Tinea of the scalp* (*tinea capitis*; see also p. 210, Fig. 14.8)

This is usually a disease of children. The causative organism varies from country to country. Fungi coming from human sources (anthropophilic organisms) cause bald and scaly areas, with minimal inflammation and hairs broken off 3–4 mm from the scalp.

Fungi coming from animal sources (zoophilic fungi) induce a more intense inflammation than those spread from person to person. In ringworm acquired from cattle, for example, the boggy swelling, with inflammation, pustulation and lymphadenopathy, is often so fierce that a bacterial infection is suspected; such a lesion is called a kerion and the hair loss associated with it may be permanent. Tinea of the beard area is usually caused by zoophilic species and shows the same features (Fig. 16.42). In favus, caused by *Trichophyton schoenleini*, the picture is dominated by foul-smelling yellowish crusts surrounding many scalp hairs, and sometimes leading to scarring alopecia. The scalp and hair of black children are especially prone to infection with *Trichophyton tonsurans* (p. 210).

### Complications

**1** Fierce animal ringworm of the scalp (Fig. 16.43) can lead to a permanent scarring alopecia.
**2** A florid fungal infection anywhere can induce

**Fig. 16.43** Animal ringworm of a child's scalp: not truly a kerion as flat and non-pustular.

**Fig. 16.44** 'Tinea incognito'. Topical steroid applications have thinned the skin and altered much of the morphology. A recognizable active spreading edge is still visible.

vesication on the sides of the fingers and palms (a trichophytid or 'id reaction').
**3** Epidemics of ringworm occur in schools.
**4** The usual appearance of a fungal infection can be masked by mistreatment with topical steroids (tinea incognito; Fig. 16.44).

### Differential diagnosis

This varies with the site. Some of the more common problems are listed in Table 16.2.

**Table 16.2** Common problems in the differential diagnosis of dermatophyte infections.

| Area | Differential diagnosis |
|------|------------------------|
| Scalp | Alopecia areata, psoriasis, seborrhoeic eczema, carbuncle, abscess, trichotillomania |
| Feet | Erythrasma, interdigital intertrigo, eczema |
| Trunk | Discoid eczema, psoriasis, candidiasis, pityriasis rosea |
| Groin | Candidiasis, erythrasma, intertrigo, irritant and allergic contact dermatitis, psoriasis, neurodermatitis |
| Nails | Psoriasis, paronychia, trauma, ageing changes |
| Hand | Chronic eczema, granuloma annulare, xerosis, dyshidrotic eczema |

## Investigations

The microscopic examination of a skin scraping, nail clipping or plucked hair is a simple procedure. The scraping should be taken from the scaly margin of a lesion, with a small curette or a scalpel blade, and clippings or scrapings from the most crumbly part of a nail. Broken hairs should be plucked with tweezers. Specimens are cleared in potassium hydroxide (p. 40). Branching hyphae can easily be seen (see Fig. 3.7) using a scanning (×10) or low-power (×25) objective lens, with the iris diaphragm almost closed and the condenser racked down. Hyphae may also be seen within a cleared hair shaft, or spores may be noted around it.

*Cultures* should be carried out in a mycology or bacteriology laboratory. Transport medium is not necessary, and specimens can be sent in folded black paper or a dry Petri dish. The report may take as long as a month; microscopy is much quicker.

*Wood's light* (ultraviolet light) examination of the scalp usually reveals a green fluorescence of the hairs in *Microsporum audouini* and *M. canis* infections. The technique is useful for screening children in institutions where outbreaks of tinea capitis still sometimes occur, but the most common fungus causing tinea capitis (*Trichophyton tonsurans*) does not fluoresce.

## Treatment

### Local

This is all that is needed for minor skin infections. The more recent imidazole preparations (e.g. miconazole and clotrimazole) and the allylamines such as terbinafine (Formulary 1, p. 388) have largely superseded time-honoured remedies such as benzoic acid ointment (Whitfield's ointment) and tolnaftate. They should be applied twice daily. Magenta paint (Castellani's paint), although highly coloured, is helpful for exudative or macerated areas in body folds or toe webs. Occasional dusting with an antifungal powder is useful to prevent relapses.

*Topical nail preparations* Many patients now prefer to avoid systemic treatment. For them a nail lacquer containing amorolfine is worth a trial. It should be applied once or twice a week for 6 months; it is effective against stubborn moulds such as *Hendersonula* and *Scopulariopsis*. Ciclopirox is an alternative topical treatment available in the USA. Both amorolfine and tioconazole nail solutions (Formulary 1, p. 388) can be used as adjuncts to systemic therapy (p. 395).

### Systemic

This is needed for tinea of the scalp or of the nails, and for widespread or chronic infections of the skin that have not responded to local measures.

*Terbinafine* (Formulary 2, p. 395) has now largely superseded griseofulvin. It acts by inhibiting fungal squalene epoxidase and does not interact with the cytochrome P-450 system. It is fungicidal and so cures chronic dermatophyte infections more quickly and more reliably than griseofulvin. For tinea capitis in children, for example, a 4-week course of terbinafine is as effective as an 8-week course of griseofulvin. Cure rates of 70–90% can be expected for infected finger nails after a 6-week course of terbinafine, and for infected toe nails after a 3-month course. It is not effective in pityriasis versicolor or *Candida* infections.

*Itraconazole* (Formulary 2, p. 396) is now preferred to ketoconazole, which occasionally damages the liver, and is a reasonable alternative to terbinafine if this is contraindicated. It is effective in tinea corporis, cruris and pedis and also in nail infections. Fungistatic rather than fungicidal, it interferes with the cytochrome P-450 system, so a review of any other medication being taken is needed before a prescription is issued. Its wide spectrum makes it useful also in pityriasis versicolor and candidiasis.

*Griseofulvin* (Formulary 2, p. 395) was for many years the drug of choice for chronic dermatophyte infections, but is now largely reserved for the treatment of tinea capitis. It has proved to be a safe drug, but treatment may have to be stopped because of persistent headache, nausea, vomiting or skin eruptions. The drug should not be given in pregnancy or to patients with liver failure or porphyria. It interacts with coumarin anticoagulants, the dosage of which may have to be increased.

## Candidiasis

### Cause

*Candida albicans* is a classic opportunistic pathogen. Even in transient and trivial local infections in the apparently fit, one or more predisposing factors such as obesity, moisture and maceration, immobility, diabetes, pregnancy, the use of broad-spectrum antibiotics, or perhaps the use of the contraceptive pill, will often be found to be playing some part. Opportunism is even more obvious in the overwhelming systemic infections of the immunocompromised (Fig. 16.45).

---

**Learning points**

- Do not prescribe terbinafine or itraconazole for psoriasis of the nails or chronic paronychia. Get mycological proof first
- Your patient's asymmetrical 'eczema' is spreading despite local steroids – think of a dermatophyte infection
- Consider tinea in acute inflammatory and purulent reactions of the scalp and beard

---

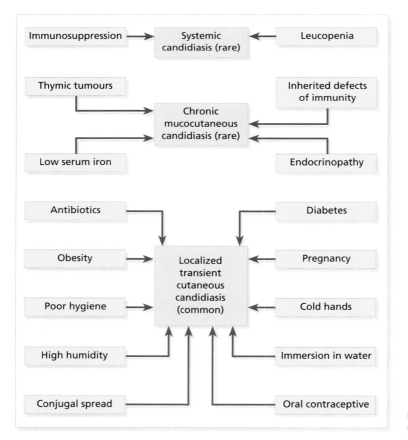

**Fig. 16.45** Factors predisposing to the different types of candidiasis.

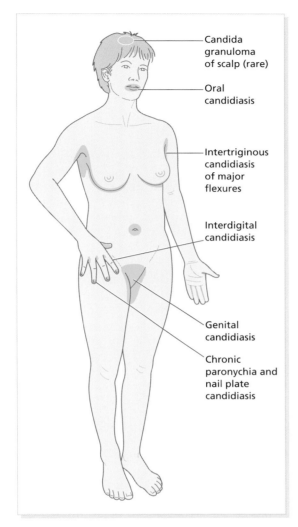

**Fig. 16.46** Sites susceptible to *Candida* infection.

**Fig. 16.47** Candidal angular stomatitis associated with severe candidiasis of the tongue.

### *Candida intertrigo*

A moist glazed area of erythema and maceration appears in a body fold; the edge shows soggy scaling, and outlying satellite papulopustules. These changes are most common under the breasts, and in the armpits and groin, but can also occur between the fingers of those whose hands are often in water.

### *Genital candidiasis*

Most commonly presents as a sore itchy vulvovaginitis, with white curdy plaques adherent to the inflamed mucous membranes and a whitish discharge. The eruption may extend to the groin folds. Conjugal spread is common; in males, similar changes occur under the foreskin (Fig. 16.48) and in the groin.

Diabetes, pregnancy and antibiotic therapy are common predisposing factors.

### *Paronychia*

Acute paronychia is usually bacterial, but in chronic paronychia *Candida* may be the sole pathogen, or be found with other opportunists such as *Proteus* or *Pseudomonas* sp. The proximal and sometimes the lateral nail folds of one or more fingers become bolstered and red (see Fig. 13.28). The cuticles are lost and small amounts of pus can be expressed. The adjacent nail plate becomes ridged and discoloured. Predisposing factors include wet work, poor peripheral circulation and vulval candidiasis.

### *Presentation*

This varies with the site (Fig. 16.46).

### *Oral candidiasis* (see also Chapter 13)

One or more whitish adherent plaques (like bread sauce) appear on the mucous membranes. If wiped off they leave an erythematous base. Under dentures, candidiasis will produce sore red areas. Angular stomatitis, usually in denture wearers (Fig. 16.47), may be candidal.

**Fig. 16.48** Pink circinate areas with only a little scaling. Consider Reiter's syndrome or candidiasis.

### Chronic mucocutaneous candidiasis

Persistent candidiasis, affecting most or all of the areas described above, can start in infancy. Sometimes the nail plates as well as the nail folds are involved. *Candida* granulomas may appear on the scalp. Several different forms have been described including those with autosomal recessive and dominant inheritance patterns. In the *Candida* endocrinopathy syndrome, chronic candidiasis occurs with one or more endocrine defects, the most common of which are hypoparathyroidism and Addison's disease. A few late-onset cases have underlying thymic tumours.

### Systemic candidiasis

This is seen against a background of severe illness, leucopenia and immunosuppression. The skin lesions are firm red nodules, which can be shown by biopsy to contain yeasts and pseudohyphae.

### Investigations

Swabs from suspected areas should be sent for culture. The urine can be tested for sugar. In chronic mucocutaneous candidiasis, a detailed immunological work-up will be needed, focusing on troubles associated with cell-mediated immunity.

### Treatment

Predisposing factors should be sought and eliminated (e.g. denture hygiene may be important). Infected skin folds should be separated and kept dry. Those with chronic paronychia should keep their hands warm and dry.

Amphotericin, nystatin and the imidazole group of compounds are all effective topically. For the mouth, these are available as oral suspensions, lozenges and oral gels (Formulary 1, p. 388). False teeth should be removed at night, washed and steeped in antiseptic or a nystatin solution. For other areas of candidiasis, creams, ointment and pessaries are available (Formulary 1, p. 396). Magenta paint is also a useful but messy remedy for the skin flexures. In chronic paronychia, the nail folds can be packed with an imidazole cream or drenched in an imidazole solution several times a day. Genital candidiasis responds well to a single day's treatment with either itraconazole and fluconazole (Formulary 2, p. 281). Both are also valuable for recurrent oral candidiasis of the immunocompromised, and for the various types of chronic mucocutaneous candidiasis.

> **Learning points**
>
> - Something else is often amiss in patients with cutaneous candidiasis
> - Remember that terbinafine has little action against *Candida*

## Pityriasis versicolor

### Cause

The old name, tinea versicolor, should be dropped as the disorder is caused by commensal yeasts (*Pityrosporum orbiculare*) and not by dermatophyte fungi. Overgrowth of these yeasts, particularly in hot humid conditions, is responsible for the clinical lesions.

Carboxylic acids released by the organisms inhibit the increase in pigment production by melanocytes

**Fig. 16.49** Pityriasis versicolor: fawn areas stand out against the untanned background.

**Fig. 16.50** This patient's holiday was spoilt by versicolor ruining her expensive tan.

that occurs normally after exposure to sunlight. The term 'versicolor' refers to the way in which the superficial scaly patches, fawn or pink on non-tanned skin (Fig. 16.49), become paler than the surrounding skin after exposure to sunlight (Fig. 16.50). The condition should be regarded as non-infectious.

### Presentation and course

The fawn or depigmented areas, with their slightly branny scaling and fine wrinkling, look ugly. Otherwise they are symptom-free or only slightly itchy. Lesions are most common on the upper trunk but can become widespread. Untreated lesions persist, and depigmented areas – even after adequate treatment – are slow to regain their former colour. Recurrences are common.

### Differential diagnosis

In vitiligo (p. 281), the border is clearly defined, scaling is absent, lesions are larger, the limbs and face are often affected and depigmentation is more complete; however, it may sometimes be hard to

distinguish vitiligo from the pale non-scaly areas of treated versicolor. Seborrhoeic eczema of the trunk tends to be more erythematous, and is often confined to the presternal or interscapular areas. Pityriasis alba often affects the cheeks. Pityriasis rosea, tinea corporis, secondary syphilis, leprosy and erythrasma seldom cause real confusion.

### Investigations

Scrapings, prepared and examined as for a dermatophyte infection (p. 40), show a mixture of short branched hyphae and spores (a 'spaghetti and meatballs' appearance). Culture is not helpful because the organism does not grow on Sabouraud's medium.

---

**Learning points**

- This is not a dermatophyte infection, so do not try griseofulvin or terbinafine
- Patients think the treatment has not worked if their pale patches do not disappear straight away – warn them about this in advance

## Treatment

A topical preparation of one of the imidazole group of antifungal drugs (Formulary 1, p. 388) can be applied at night to all affected areas for 2–4 weeks. Equally effective and cheaper, but messier and more irritant, is a 2.5% selenium sulphide mixture in a detergent base (Selsun shampoo). This should be lathered on to the patches after an evening bath, and allowed to dry. Next morning it should be washed off. Three applications at weekly intervals are adequate. A shampoo containing ketoconazole is now available (Formulary 1, p. 382), and is less messy but just as effective as the selenium ones. Alternatively, selenium sulphide lotion (USA) can be applied for 10 min, rinsed off and re-applied daily for 1 week. For widespread or stubborn infections, systemic itraconazole (200 mg/day for 7 days), fluconazole or ketoconazole may be curative, but interactions with other drugs must be avoided (Formulary 2, p. 396). Recurrence is common after any treatment.

## Deep fungal infections

### Histoplasmosis

*Histoplasma capsulatum* is found in soil and in the droppings of some animals (e.g. bats). Airborne spores are inhaled and cause lung lesions, which are in many ways like those of tuberculosis. Later, granulomatous mouth or skin lesions may appear, particularly in the immunocompromised. Amphotericin B or itraconazole, given systemically, is often helpful.

### Coccidioidomycosis

The causative organism, *Coccidioides immitis*, is present in the soil in arid areas in the USA. Its spores are inhaled, and the pulmonary infection may be accompanied by a fever and reactive plaques. As cell-mediated immunity develops, erythema nodosum (p. 112) may be seen. In a few patients the infection becomes disseminated, with ulcers or deep abscesses in the skin. Treatment is usually not needed; the disorder is typically self-limiting. Fluconazole is used for progressing cavitations of the lungs, for the immunosuppressed and for severe cases.

### Blastomycosis

Infections with *Blastomyces dermatitidis* are virtually confined to rural areas of the USA. Rarely, the organism is inoculated into the skin; more often it is inhaled and then spreads systemically from the pulmonary focus to other organs including the skin. There the lesions are wart-like hyperkeratotic nodules, which spread peripherally with a verrucose edge, suggesting squamous cell carcinomas. They tend to clear and scar centrally. Treatment is with systemic amphotericin B or itraconazole.

### Sporotrichosis

The causative fungus, *Sporotrichum schencki*, lives saprophytically in soil or on wood in warm humid countries.

Infection is through a wound, where later an indolent nodule arises. Later still, nodules appear in succession along the draining lymphatics (Fig. 16.15). Itraconazole (200–400 mg/day for 3–6 months) is the treatment of choice. Potassium iodide is also effective and much cheaper.

### Actinomycosis

The causative organism, *Actinomyces israeli*, is bacterial but traditionally considered with the fungi. It has long branching hyphae and is part of the normal flora of the mouth and bowel. In actinomycosis, a lumpy induration and scarring coexist with multiple sinuses discharging pus-containing 'sulphur granules', made up of tangled filaments. Favourite sites are the jaw, and the chest and abdominal walls. Long-term penicillin is the treatment of choice.

### Mycetoma (Madura foot)

Various species of fungus or actinomycetes may be involved. They gain access to the subcutaneous tissues, usually of the feet or legs, via a penetrating wound. The area becomes lumpy and distorted, later enlarging and developing multiple sinuses. Pus exuding from these shows tiny diagnostic granules. Surgery may be a valuable alternative to the often poor results of medical treatment, which is with systemic antibiotics or antifungal drugs, depending on the organism isolated.

## Further reading

Angus JS, Langan M, Stanway A, *et al.* (2006) The many faces of secondary syphilis: a re-emergence of an old disease. *Clinical and Experimental Dermatology* **31**, 741–745.

Deeks SG. (2006) Antiretroviral treatment of HIV infected adults. *British Medical Journal* **332**, 1489.

Diven DG. (2001) An overview of poxviruses. *Journal of the American Academy of Dermatology* **44**, 1–14.

Grundmann H, Aires-de-Sousa M, Boyce J, *et al.* (2006) Emergence and resurgence of meticillin-resistant *Staphylococcus aureus* as a public-health threat. *Lancet* **368**, 874–885.

Gupta AK, Bluhm R & Summerbell R. (2002) Pityriasis versicolor. *Journal of the European Academy of Dermatology and Venereology* **16**, 19–33.

Hart CA & Thomson AP. (2006) Meningococcal disease and its management in children. *British Medical Journal* **333**, 685–690.

Higgins EM, Fuller LC & Smith CH. (2000) Guidelines for the management of tinea capitis. *British Journal of Dermatology* **143**, 53–58.

Kyle AA & Dahl MV. (2004) Topical therapy for fungal infections. *American Journal of Clinical Dermatology* **5**, 443–451.

Lesher JL Jr. (2000) *An Atlas of Microbiology of the Skin.* Parthenon, London.

Manders M. (1998) Toxin-mediated streptococcal and staphylococcal disease. *Journal of the American Academy of Dermatology* **39**, 383–398.

Oxman MN, Levin MJ, Johnson GR, *et al.* (2005) A vaccine to prevent herpes zoster and postherpetic neuralgia in older adults. *New England Journal of Medicine* **352**, 2271–2284.

Roberts DT. (1999) Onychomycosis: current treatment and future challenges. *British Journal of Dermatology* **141** (Supplement 56), 1–4.

Sterling JC, Handfield-Jones S & Hudson P. (2001) Guidelines for the treatment of cutaneous warts. *British Journal of Dermatology* **144**, 4–11.

Tyring SK, McCrary ML & Severson J. (1999) Varicella zoster virus. *Journal of the American Academy of Dermatology* **41**, 1–14.

# **17** Infestations

Infestation, the presence of animal parasites on or in the body, is common in tropical countries and less so in temperate ones. Infestations fall into two main groups:
1 those caused by arthropods; and
2 those caused by worms.

## Arthropods

Table 17.1 lists some of the ways in which arthropods affect the skin. Only a few can be discussed here.

**Table 17.1** Arthropods and their effects on the skin.

| Type of arthropod | Manifestations |
| --- | --- |
| *Insects* | |
| Hymenoptera | Bee and wasp stings |
| | Ant bites |
| Lepidoptera | Caterpillar dermatitis |
| Coleoptera | Blisters from cantharidin |
| Diptera | Mosquito and midge bites |
| | Myiasis |
| Aphaniptera | Human and animal fleas |
| Hemiptera | Bed bugs |
| Anoplura | Lice infestations |
| | |
| *Mites* | |
| *Demodex folliculorum* | Normal inhabitant of facial hair follicles |
| *Sarcoptes scabiei* | Human and animal scabies |
| Food mites | Grain itch, grocer's itch, etc. |
| Harvest mites | Harvest itch |
| Feather mites | In pet birds, nests and sometimes feather pillows |
| House dust mite | Possible role in atopic eczema |
| *Cheyletiella* | Papular urticaria |
| Ticks | Tick bites. Vector of rickettsial infections and erythema migrans (p. 228) |

## Lice infestations (pediculosis)

Lice are flattened wingless insects that suck blood. Their eggs, attached to hairs or clothing, are known as nits. The main feature of all lice infestations is severe itching, followed by scratching and secondary infection.

Two species are obligate parasites in humans: *Pediculus humanus* (with its two varieties: *P. humanus capitis*, the head louse, and *P. humanus corporis*, the body louse) and *Phthirus pubis* (the pubic louse).

### *Head lice*

#### *Cause*

Head lice are still common: up to 10% of children have them, even in the smartest schools. Many of these children have few or no symptoms. Infestations peak between the ages of 4 and 11 years, and are more common in girls than boys. A typical infested scalp will carry about 10 adult lice, which measure some 3–4 mm in length, are greyish and often rather hard to find (Fig. 17.1). However, egg cases (nits) can be seen easily enough, firmly stuck to the hair shafts. Spread from person to person is achieved by head-to-head contact, and perhaps by shared combs or hats.

#### *Presentation and course*

The main symptom is itching, although this may take several months to develop. At first the itching is mainly around the sides and back of the scalp: later it spreads generally over the scalp. Scratching and secondary infection soon follow and, in heavy infestations, the hair becomes matted and smelly. Draining lymph nodes often enlarge.

**Fig. 17.1** Head louse. Blood from a recent meal can be seen in the gut of this adult louse.

## Complications

Secondary bacterial infection may be severe enough to make the child listless and feverish.

## Differential diagnosis

All patients with recurrent impetigo or crusted eczema on their scalps should be carefully examined for the presence of nits.

## Investigations

None are usually required.

## Treatment

The finding of living moving lice means that the infestation is current and active, and needs treatment. Empty egg cases signify only that there has been an infestation in the past, but suggest the need for periodic re-inspection.

Malathion, carbaryl and synthetic pyrethroids (phenothrin and permethrin) (Formulary 1, p. 389) are the treatments of choice now. They are equally effective at killing lice and eggs; malathion has the extra virtue of sticking to the hair and so protecting against re-infection for 6 weeks.

Lotions should remain on the scalp for at least 12 h, and are more effective than shampoos. The application should be repeated after 1 week so that any lice that survive the first application and hatch out in that interval can be killed. A toothcomb helps to remove nits but occasionally matting is so severe that the hair has to be clipped short. A systemic antibiotic may be needed to deal with severe secondary infection. If live lice are found on follow-up, a pediculicide from another chemical class should be used. Pillow cases, towels, hats and scarves should be laundered or dry cleaned. Other members of the family and school mates should be checked.

Some recommend, as an alternative to the treatments mentioned above, that the hair should be combed repeatedly with a special 'detection comb'; however, the use of a pediculicide is more effective than physical methods. Systemic ivermectin therapy is reserved for infestations resisting the treatments listed above.

> **Learning point**
>
> - Always look for signs of head lice before attributing enlarged cervical lymph nodes to anything more sinister.

## Body lice

### Cause

Body louse infestations are now uncommon except in the unhygienic and socially deprived. Morphologically, the body louse looks just like the head louse, but lays its eggs in the seams of clothing in contact with the skin. Transmission is via infested bedding or clothing.

### Presentation and course

Self-neglect is usually obvious; against this background there is severe and widespread itching, especially on the trunk. The bites themselves are soon obscured by excoriations and crusts of dried blood or serum. In chronic untreated cases ('vagabond's disease'), the skin becomes generally thickened, eczematized and pigmented; lymphadenopathy is common.

*Differential diagnosis*

In scabies, characteristic burrows are seen (p. 263). Other causes of chronic itchy erythroderma include eczema and lymphomas, but these are ruled out by the finding of lice and nits.

*Investigations*

Clothing should be examined for the presence of eggs in the inner seams.

*Treatment*

First and foremost, treat the infested clothing and bedding. Lice and their eggs can be killed by high temperature laundering, dry cleaning and tumble-drying. Less competent patients will need help here. Once this has been achieved, 5% permethrin cream rinse or 1% lindane lotion (USA only) (Formulary 1, p. 389) can be used on the patient's skin.

**Pubic lice**

*Cause*

Pubic lice (crabs) are broader than scalp and body lice, and their second and third pairs of legs are well adapted to cling on to hair. They are usually spread by sexual contact, and most commonly infest young adults.

*Presentation*

Severe itching in the pubic area is followed by eczematization and secondary infection. Among the excoriations will be seen small blue–grey macules of altered blood at the site of bites. The shiny translucent nits are less obvious than those of head lice (Fig. 17.2). Pubic lice spread most extensively in hairy males and may even affect the eyelashes.

*Differential diagnosis*

Eczema of the pubic area gives similar symptoms but lice and nits are not seen.

**Fig. 17.2** Pediculosis pubis. Numerous eggs (nits) can be seen on the plucked pubic hairs.

*Investigations*

The possibility of coexisting sexually transmitted diseases should be kept in mind.

*Treatment*

Carbaryl, permethrin and malathion are all effective treatments. Aqueous solutions are less irritant than alcoholic ones. They should be applied for 12 h or overnight – and not just to the pubic area, but to all surfaces of the body, including the perianal area, limbs, scalp, neck, ears and face (especially the eyebrows and the beard, if present). Treatment should be repeated after 1 week, and infected sexual partners should also be treated. Shaving the area is not necessary.

Infestation of the eyelashes is particularly hard to treat, as this area is so sensitive that the mechanical removal of lice and eggs can be painful. Applying a thick layer of petrolatum twice a day for 2 weeks has been recommended. Aqueous malathion is effective for eyelash infestations but does not have a product licence for this purpose.

Patients should avoid close bodily contact until they and their partners have been treated and completed their follow-up.

## Insect bites

Insects inject venoms to kill prey and defend themselves. These stings cause painful inflammatory reactions soon after the attack. Insects also inject chemicals as they feed, usually to anticoagulate the blood. These chemicals and some toxins may cause purpuric and allergic reactions characterized by itching papules or wheals.

Different people can react differently, depending upon the type of immunological reaction. Nothing happens after the first bite because there has been no previous exposure and hence no chance for induction of an immune response. With continued biting over time, many individuals develop a cell-mediated immune response that produces itchy red bumps 1–4 days after bites. These last for up to 2 weeks. Others develop immediate IgE-mediated reactions that cause wheals within minutes after a bite and that can cause anaphylaxis. Some develop both types. In this situation, a wheal may appear within a few minutes and then disappear, to be followed hours later by a firm itchy persistent papule, often with a central haemorrhagic punctum. Bullous reactions are common on the legs of children.

The diagnosis of insect bites is usually obvious; when it is not, the term papular urticaria is sometimes used.

### Papular urticaria

#### Cause

This term, with its hint that the condition is a variant of ordinary urticaria, is a misnomer. Papular urticaria is nothing more than an excessive, possibly allergic, reaction to insect bites. The source of the bites may be simple garden pests but more often is a parasite on a domestic pet. Often the source cannot be traced.

#### Presentation

Lesions are usually most common on the arms or legs. They consist of groups or lines of small itchy excoriated smooth pink papules (Fig. 17.3)

**Fig. 17.3** Florid insect bites on the leg. Note the tendency of the lesions to lie in lines and groups.

of a uniform size that may become bullous and infected. Some clear to leave small scars or pigmented macules.

#### Course

An affected child will usually 'grow out' of the problem in a few years, even if the source of the bites is not dealt with. Individual lesions last for 1–2 weeks and recur in distinct crops, especially in the summer – hence the lay term 'heat bumps'. The lesions will disappear with any change of environment (e.g. by going on holiday). Surprisingly often only one member of a family is affected, perhaps because the others have developed immunological tolerance after repeated bites.

#### Complications

Itching leads to much discomfort and loss of sleep. Impetiginization is common.

#### Differential diagnosis

The grouped excoriated papules of papular urticaria are quite different from the skin changes of scabies, in which burrows are the diagnostic feature. Atopic prurigo may be more difficult to distinguish but here there is usually a family history of atopy and frankly eczematous plaques in a typical distribution.

*Investigations*

The parents should be encouraged to act as detectives in their own environment, but some resist the idea that the lesions are caused by bites, asking why the other family members are not affected. This attitude is often supported by veterinarians who, after a superficial look at infested animals, pronounce them clear. In such cases the animal should be brushed vigorously while standing on a polythene sheet. Enough dandruff-like material can then be obtained to send to a reliable veterinary laboratory. Often the cause is a *Cheyletiella* mite infestation.

*Treatment*

Local treatment with a topical corticosteroid or calamine lotion, and the regular use of insect repellents, may be of some help but the ultimate solution is to trace the source of the bites or await spontaneous remission.

Infested animals should be treated by a veterinarian, and insecticidal powders should be used for soft furnishings in the home. Sometimes professional exterminators are needed, but even measures such as these can meet with little success.

## Bed bugs (Hemiptera)

Bed bugs are once again prevalent in hotels, houses and hostels. During the day, bed bugs hide in crevices in walls and furniture; at night they can travel considerable distances to reach a sleeping person. Burning wheals, turning into firm papules, occur in groups wherever the crawling bugs have easy access to the skin – the face, neck and hands being the most common sites. Often bites appear in groups of three, recalling the bug's breakfast, lunch and dinner. Treatment should be based on the application of insecticides to walls and furniture where the bugs hide.

## Myiasis

The larvae of several species of fly develop only if deposited in living flesh; humans are one of several possible hosts. The skin lesions look like boils, but movement may be detected within them.

The diagnosis is proved by incising the nodule and extracting the larva.

### *Scabies*

*Cause*

Scabies is caused by the mite *Sarcoptes scabiei* var. *hominis* (Fig. 17.4). Adult mites are 0.3–0.4 mm long and therefore just visible, although hard to see except through a lens. It is now well established that the mites are transferred from person to person by close bodily contact and not via inanimate objects.

Once on the skin, fertilized female mites can move over the surface at up to 2 cm/min, but can burrow through the stratum corneum at only about 2 mm/day. They produce two or three oval eggs each day, which turn into sexually mature mites in 2–3 weeks. The number of adult mites varies from case to case – from less than 10 in a clean adult to many more in an unwashed child. The generalized eruption of scabies, and its itchiness, are thought to be caused by a sensitization to the mites or their products.

*Epidemiology*

Scabies is endemic in many developing countries, and high levels of prevalence go with poverty, overcrowding and poor hygiene. In other populations,

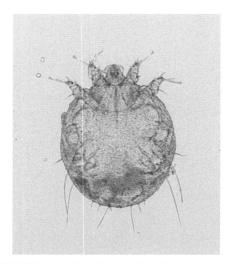

**Fig. 17.4** The adult female acarus (scabies mite).

scabies rises and falls cyclically, peaking every 15–25 years. The idea of 'herd immunity' has been put forward to explain this, spread being most easy when a new generation of susceptible individuals has arisen. Scabies is most common in the autumn and winter.

## Presentation

For 4–6 weeks after a first infestation there may be no itching, but thereafter it dominates the picture, often being particularly bad at night and affecting several people. In contrast, in a second attack of scabies, itching starts within a day or two, because these victims already have immunity to produce the itchy allergic reactions.

The most dramatic part of the eruption – excoriated, eczematized or urticarial papules – is usually on the trunk, and marks feeding spots where the mites were a day or two ago. Do not search for the mite here. Do not search for a moving mite either; they are too small to see. Look instead for burrows where female mites lay their eggs (Fig. 17.5).

Most burrows lie on the sides of the fingers, finger webs, sides of the hand and on the flexural aspects of the wrists. Other favourite sites include

**Fig. 17.6** The characteristic plantar lesions of scabies in infancy.

the elbows, ankles and feet (especially in infants; Fig. 17.6), nipples and genitals (Fig. 17.7). Only in infancy does scabies affect the face. Burrows are easily missed, grey–white, slightly scaly tortuous lines of up to 1 cm in length. The acarus may be seen through a lens as a small dark dot at the most recent least scaly end of the burrow. With experience it can be removed for microscopic confirmation (p. 40). On the genitals, burrows are associated with erythematous rubbery nodules (Fig. 17.8).

## Course

Scabies persists indefinitely unless treated. In the chronic stage, the number of mites may be small and diagnosis is correspondingly difficult. Relapses after apparently adequate treatment are common and can be put down to re-infestation from undetected and untreated contacts.

## Complications

- Secondary infection, with pustulation, is common (Fig. 17.9). Rarely, glomerulonephritis follows this.
- Repeated applications of scabicides can cause skin irritation and eczema.
- Persistent itchy red nodules may remain on the genitals or armpits of children for some months after adequate treatment.
- Venereal disease may be acquired at the same time as scabies.

**Fig. 17.5** Typical burrows seen on the side of the thumb.

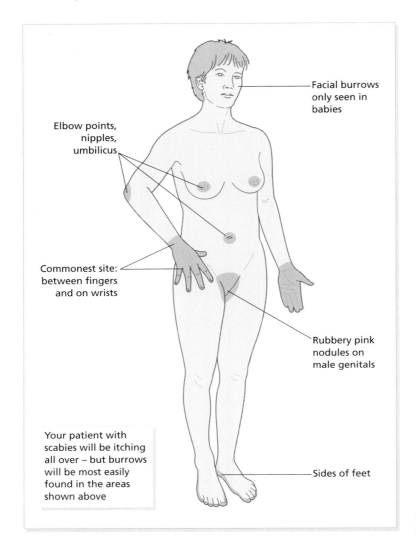

Facial burrows only seen in babies

Elbow points, nipples, umbilicus

Commonest site: between fingers and on wrists

Rubbery pink nodules on male genitals

Your patient with scabies will be itching all over – but burrows will be most easily found in the areas shown above

Sides of feet

**Fig. 17.7** Common sites of burrows in scabies.

● Crusted (Norwegian) scabies, which may not be itchy, is a widespread crusted eruption in which vast numbers of mites are found. It affects people with mental retardation or immunosuppression, and can be the unsuspected source of epidemics of ordinary scabies (e.g. in nursing homes).

### Differential diagnosis

Only scabies shows characteristic burrows. Animal scabies from pets induces an itchy rash in humans but this lacks burrows. The lesions of papular urticaria (p. 261) are excoriated papules, in groups, mainly on the legs. Late-onset atopic eczema (p. 91), cholinergic urticaria (p. 105), lichen planus (p. 72), neurotic excoriations (p. 345) and dermatitis herpetiformis (p. 125) have their own distinctive features.

### Investigations

With practice an acarus can be picked neatly with a needle from the end of its burrow and identified microscopically; failing this, eggs and mites can be

**Fig. 17.8** Unmistakable rubbery nodules on the penis, diagnostic of scabies.

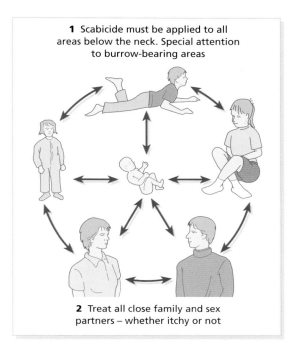

**1** Scabicide must be applied to all areas below the neck. Special attention to burrow-bearing areas

**2** Treat all close family and sex partners – whether itchy or not

**Fig. 17.10** The treatment of scabies.

**Fig. 17.9** Scabies with bacterial superinfection.

seen microscopically in burrow scrapings mounted in potassium hydroxide (p. 40) or mineral oil. Some find dermatoscopy (p. 39) a quick and reliable way to find the mite.

### Treatment

Treatment should be started if the diagnosis seems likely on clinical grounds, even if the presence of mites cannot be confirmed microscopically. Do not treat just the patient; treat all members of the family and sexual contacts too, whether they are itching or not (Fig. 17.10).

Use an effective scabicide: there are many on the market now (Formulary 1, p. 389). In the UK, the preferred treatment is with permethrin, with malathion as the second choice. Topical treatment plus ivermectin (on a named patient basis in the UK), in a single dose of 200 µg/kg by mouth, is effective for Norwegian scabies and scabies that does not respond to topical measures alone.

A convenient way to apply scabicides to the skin is with a 5 cm (2 in) paintbrush. The number of applications recommended varies from dermatologist to dermatologist. There is no doubt that some preparations, such as malathion, disappear quickly from the skin, leaving it vulnerable to any mites hatching out from eggs that have survived. A second application, a week after the first, is then essential. With permethrin this may be less important. Another good reason for recommending a second application is that it will cover areas left out during an inefficient first application.

Most now recommend that the treatment should be applied to the scalp, neck, face and ears as well as to the rest of the skin. Areas which must be included are the genitals, soles of the feet, gluteal fold, and the skin under the free edge of the nails. The scabicide should be re-applied if the hands are washed. A hot bath before treatment is no longer recommended.

Residual itching may last for several days, or even a few weeks, but this does not need further applications of the scabicide. Rely instead on calamine lotion or crotamiton.

For babies, toddlers and children up to 2 years old we advise special care with treatment. Permethrin is licensed for infants over the age of 2 months, although needs to be used with caution. 6% Precipitated sulphur in petrolatum has been used in children for many years without adverse effects. In any case, aqueous preparations are best for children as alcoholic ones can sting.

Permethrin is probably safe in pregnancy and in nursing mothers as little is absorbed, and any that is absorbed is rapidly detoxified and eliminated.

Have a printed sheet (see 'Further Reading' at the end of this chapter) to give to the patient and go through it with them – scabies victims are notoriously confused.

Ordinary laundering deals satisfactorily with clothing and sheets. Mites die in clothing unworn for 1 week.

**Fig. 17.11** Larva migrans – a red serpiginous line on the instep.

## Larva migrans (creeping eruption)

The larvae of hookworms that go through their full life cycle only in cats or dogs can penetrate human skin when it is in contact with soil or sand contaminated by the faeces of these animals. Larva migrans is most frequently found in the tropics and subtropics, and is the most common parasitic infection of the skin seen in travellers, typically returning from beach holidays in the Caribbean, Central America or Africa. It is now also being acquired in the UK.

The larvae move under the skin creating tortuous red itchy lines (Fig. 17.11) which advance at the rate of a few millimetres a day. As humans are a dead-end host for the larvae they do eventually die, but this can be speeded up by either local treatment with 15% thiabendazole cream applied twice daily or a single oral dose of ivermectin or albendazole. Freezing the larva in its estimated position just ahead of the track is traditionally recommended but rarely effective, probably because it is missed.

> **Learning points**
>
> - Paravenereal diseases hunt in packs: does your patient with scabies also have pubic lice, genital mollusca or something even worse?
> - Look for mites in the burrows, where they are laying their eggs, not in the widespread itchy red papular lesions
> - Never forget to treat the contacts – itchy or not – as, if you do not, they will re-infect your patient and waste everybody's time

> **Learning point**
>
> - Do not think that cutaneous larva migrans is a tropical disease. Recent reports document the first cases acquired in the UK.

## Parasitic worms

A textbook of tropical medicine should be consulted for more details on this subject.

## Onchocerciasis

This is endemic in much of Central America and Africa where it is an important cause of blindness. The buffalo gnat (*Simulium* species) carries the filarial worm to humans. Infested humans become itchy with an excoriated papular eruption. Later the skin may thicken and become hyper- or hypopigmented. Dermal nodules are found, mainly near bony prominences, and contain both mature worms and microfilariae. It is the latter that invade the eye, leading to blindness. The diagnosis is confirmed by detecting active microfilariae in skin snips teased out in saline and examined microscopically. Ivermectin is now the treatment of choice. A single dose produces a prolonged reduction of microfilarial levels, and should be repeated every year until the adult worms die out. Diethylcarbamazine and suramin are now obsolete.

## Filariasis

This is endemic throughout much of the tropics. The adult filarial worms, usually *Wucheria bancrofti*, inhabit the lymphatics where they excite an inflammatory reaction with episodes of lymphangitis and fever, gradually leading to lymphatic obstruction and lymphoedema, usually of the legs or scrotum. Such swellings can be massive (elephantiasis). There is an eosinophilia and microfilariae are found in the peripheral blood, mainly at night; their vector from human to human is the mosquito, in which the larvae mature. Diethylcarbamazine or ivermectin is the treatment of choice.

## Other worm infestations

● Threadworm (pinworm) infestation in children can cause severe anal and vulval pruritus. The small worms are seen best at night-time when the itch is worst. Treatment is with a single dose of mebendazole 100 mg, or piperazine.

● Swimmer's itch, in tropical and lake waters, may be caused by the penetration through the skin of the cercariae of schistosomes of non-human origin. These cause itching red papules on exposed areas, especially the legs. The skin should be towelled off immediately after swimming to prevent the schistosomes penetrating the skin as it dries. Schistosomes dip in human hosts. No systemic treatments are needed.

● The larval stages of the pork tapeworm (cysticercosis) can present as multiple firm nodules in the skin.

● Larger fluctuant cysts may be caused by hydatid disease.

## Further reading

Dodds CS. (2003) Interventions for treating head lice (Cochrane review) In: *The Cochrane library* Issue 1. Oxford Update software.

Frankowski BL. (2004) American Academy of Paediatrics' guidelines for the prevention and treatment of head lice infestation. *American Journal of Management Care* **10** (Supplement 9), S269–272.

Mehlhorn H. (2001) *Encyclopedic Reference of Parasitology*. Springer, Berlin.

*A patient information leaflet* on scabies is available through the British Association of Dermatologists at www.bad.org.uk

*Guidelines for scabies* have been prepared by the Association of Genitourinary Medicine and are available at www.bashh.org/guidelines/2002/scabies_0901b.pdf

# **18** Skin reactions to light

Ultraviolet radiation (UVR) can be helpful when used to treat diseases such as psoriasis, but it can also be harmful (Fig. 18.1). It causes photoageing, is the leading cause of skin cancers and causes or worsens several skin disorders. UVR is non-ionizing, but changes the skin by reacting with endogenous light-absorbing chemicals (chromophores), which include DNA, RNA, urocanic acid and melanin. Different types of skin (now conventionally divided into six types; Table 18.1) react differently to UVR, and require different degrees of protection against the sun.

The UVR spectrum is divided into three parts (Fig. 18.2), each having different effects on the skin, although ultraviolet C (UVC) does not penetrate the ozone layer of the atmosphere and is therefore currently irrelevant to skin disease. Virtually all of the UVB is absorbed in the epidermis, whereas some 30% of the ultraviolet A (UVA) reaches the dermis. The B wavelengths (UVB: 290–320 nm) cause sunburn and are effectively screened out by window glass. UVA is longwave ultraviolet light, from 320 nm to the most violet colour perceptible to the eye (about 400 nm). It ages and tans the skin. The differences between the wavelengths can be recorded conveniently in the form of action spectra, which show how effective each is at producing different biological effects, such as clearing psoriasis or causing erythema.

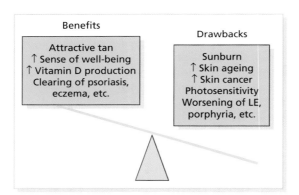

**Fig. 18.1** The balance between the benefits and drawbacks of sun exposure.

> **Learning point**
>
> Do not let your patients be hoodwinked. The drawbacks of artificial tanning far outweigh the advantages

## Sunburn

### Cause

UVB penetrates the epidermis and superficial dermis, stimulating the production and release of prostaglandins, leukotrienes, histamine, interleukin 1 (IL-1) and tumour necrosis factor α (TNF-α). These cause

| Type | Definition | Description |
|------|-----------|-------------|
| I | Always burns but never tans | Pale skin, red hair, freckles |
| II | Usually burns, sometimes tans | Fair skin |
| III | May burn, usually tans | Darker skin |
| IV | Rarely burns, always tans | Mediterranean |
| V | Moderate constitutional pigmentation | Latin American, Middle Eastern |
| VI | Marked constitutional pigmentation | Black |

**Table 18.1** Skin types classified by their reactions to ultraviolet radiation (UVR).

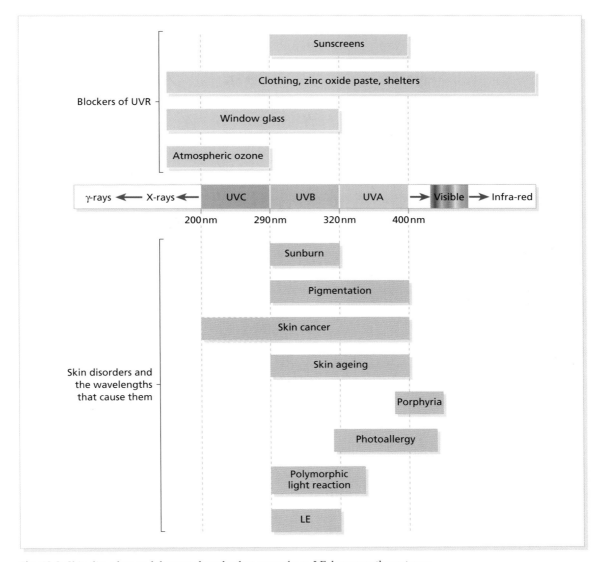

**Fig. 18.2** Skin disorders and the wavelengths that cause them. LE, lupus erythematosus.

pain and stimulate the production of the inducible nitric oxide synthase (iNOS) enzyme. This generates high concentrations of nitric oxide which cause the characteristic dermal vasodilatation and redness.

## Presentation and course

Skin exposed to too much UVB smarts and becomes red several hours later. Severe sunburn is painful and may blister. The redness is maximal after 1 day,

contemparaneously with peak levels of the iNOS enzyme, and then settles over the next 2–3 days, leaving sheet-like desquamation (Fig. 18.3), diffuse pigmentation (a 'tan') and, sometimes, discrete lentigines.

## Differential diagnosis

Phototoxic reactions caused by drugs are like an exaggerated sunburn.

**Fig. 18.3** Peeling after acute sunburn. This doctor's son should have known better.

## Investigations

None are required.

## Treatment

The treatment is symptomatic. Baths may be cooling and oily shake lotions (e.g. oily calamine lotion), oil-in-water lotions or creams are comforting. Potent topical corticosteroids (Formulary 1, p. 385) help if used early and briefly. Oral aspirin (a prostaglandin synthesis inhibitor) relieves the pain. Sprays containing benzocaine also relieve pain, but occasionally sensitize.

## Phototoxicity

Basic photochemical laws require a drug to absorb UVR to cause such a reaction. Most drugs listed in Table 18.2 absorb UVA as well as UVB, and so window glass, protective against sunburn, does not protect against most phototoxic drug reactions.

## Presentation and course

Tenderness and redness occur only in areas ex-

**Table 18.2** Drugs commonly causing photosensitivity.

Amiodarone
Chlorpropamide
Nalidixic acid
Oral contraceptives
Phenothiazines
Psoralens
Quinidine
Sulphonamides
Tetracyclines
Thiazides

**Fig. 18.4** Extreme photosensitivity of a patient taking griseofulvin. Note sparing of the area covered by the watch strap and ring.

posed both to sufficient drug and to sufficient UVR (Fig. 18.4). The signs and symptoms are those of sunburn. The skin may later develop a deep tan.

## Cause

These reactions are not immunological. Everyone exposed to enough of the drug, and to enough UVR, will develop the reaction. Some drugs that can cause phototoxic reactions are listed in Table 18.2. In addition, contact with psoralens in plants (Fig. 18.5) can cause a localized phototoxic dermatitis (phyto-photodermatitis; Fig. 18.6). These areas burn and may blister, leaving pigmentation in linear streaks and bizarre patterns.

## Differential diagnosis

Photoallergic reactions are difficult to distinguish, the more so as the same drugs can often cause both

**Fig. 18.5** Cow parsley contains psoralens and is a common cause of photodermatitis.

**Fig. 18.6** Severe bullous eruption in areas in contact with giant hogweed (contains psoralens) and then exposed to sunlight (phytophotodermatitis).

photoallergic and phototoxic reactions. The main differences between phototoxicity and photoallergy are shown in Table 18.3.

## Investigations

None are usually required. In difficult cases, photo-patch testing can be carried out in special centres. The action spectrum (the wavelengths that cause the reaction) may incriminate a particular drug.

## Treatment

This is the same as for sunburn. Drugs should be stopped if further exposure to ultraviolet light is likely.

> **Learning points**
>
> If the skin reacts badly to light through glass then:
> - sunscreens are usually ineffective
> - think of drugs or porphyria

## Photoallergy

Drugs, topical or systemic, and chemicals on the skin can interact with UVR and cause immunological reactions.

## Cause

UVR converts an immunologically inactive form of a drug into an antigenic molecule. An immunological reaction, analogous to allergic contact dermatitis (p. 86), is induced if the antigen remains in the skin or is formed there on subsequent exposure to the drug and UVR. Many of the same drugs that cause phototoxic reactions can also cause photoallergic ones.

## Presentation

Photoallergy is often similar to phototoxicity. The areas exposed to UVR become inflamed, but the

**Table 18.3** Features distinguishing phototoxicity from photoallergy.

| Phototoxicity | Photoallergy |
|---|---|
| Erythematous and smooth (may blister) | Eczematous and rough (may weep) |
| Immediate onset | Delayed onset (when immunity develops; may not occur on first exposure) |
| Hurts | Itches |
| Photopatch testing negative | Photopatch testing positive |
| Lasts 3–5 days | Lasts 3–14 days |

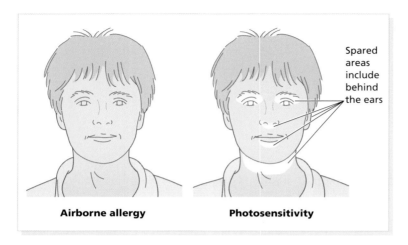

**Fig. 18.7** Features distinguishing airborne allergy from photosensitivity.

reaction usually becomes eczematous, appears later and lasts longer. The eruption will be on exposed areas such as the hands, the V of the neck, the nose, the chin and the forehead. There is also a tendency to spare the upper lip under the nose, the eyelids and the submental region (Fig. 18.7). Often, the eruption does not occur on the first exposure to ultraviolet, but only after a second or further exposures. A lag phase of one or more weeks is needed to induce an immune response.

## Course

The original lesions are red patches, plaques, vesicles or bullae, which usually become eczematous. They tend to resolve when either the drug or the exposure to UVR is stopped, but this may take several weeks.

## Complications

Some drugs, such as the sulphonamides, can cause chronic actinic dermatitis.

## Investigations

Photopatch testing by an expert can confirm the diagnosis. The chemical is applied for 24 h and the skin is then irradiated with UVA. An acute photoallergic contact dermatitis is then elicited. A control patch, not irradiated, rules out ordinary allergic contact dermatitis.

## Treatment

The drug should be stopped and the patient protected from further ultraviolet exposure (avoidance, clothing and sunscreens). Potent topical corticosteroids or a short course of a systemic corticosteroid will hasten resolution and provide symptomatic relief.

## Chronic actinic dermatitis (actinic reticuloid)

Some patients with a photoallergic reaction never get over it and go on developing sun-induced eczematous areas long after the drug has been stopped.

## Cause

This is not clear but some believe minute amounts of the drug persist in the skin indefinitely.

## Presentation

This is the same as a photoallergic reaction to a drug. The patient goes on to develop a chronic dermatitis, with thick plaques on sun-exposed areas.

## Course

These patients may be exquisitely sensitive to UVR. They are usually middle-aged or elderly men who react after the slightest exposure, even through window glass or from fluorescent lights. Affected individuals also are or become allergic to a range of contact allergens, especially oleoresins in some plants (e.g. chrysanthemums).

## Complications

None, but the persistent severe pruritic eruption can lead to depression and even suicide.

## Differential diagnosis

Airborne allergic contact dermatitis may be confused, but does not require sunlight. Sometimes the diagnosis is difficult, as exposure both to sunlight and to the airborne allergen occurs only out of doors. Airborne allergic contact dermatitis also affects sites that sunlight is less likely to reach, such as eyelids and under the chin (Fig. 18.7). A continuing drug photoallergy, a polymorphic light eruption (see below) or eczema as a result of some other cause must also be considered.

Histology shows a dense lymphocytic infiltrate and sometimes atypical activated lymphocytes suggestive of a lymphoma, but the disorder seldom becomes malignant.

## Investigations

Persistent light reaction can be confirmed experimentally by exposing uninvolved skin to UVA or UVB. Patch tests and photopatch tests help to distinguish between photoallergy and airborne allergic contact dermatitis, and the action spectrum may point to a certain drug. This sort of testing is difficult, and should be carried out only in specialist centres.

## Treatment

Usually cared for by specialists, these patients need extreme measures to protect their skin from UVR. These include protective clothing and frequent applications of combined UVA and UVB blocking agents (Formulary 1, p. 383). Patients must protect themselves from UVR coming through windows or from fluorescent lights. Some can only go out at night. As even the most potent topical steroids

are often ineffective, systemic steroids or immunosuppressants (e.g. azathioprine) may be needed for long periods.

## Polymorphic light eruption

This is the most frequent cause of a so-called 'sun allergy'.

### Cause

It is speculated that UVR causes a natural body chemical to change into an allergen. Mechanisms are similar to those in drug photoallergy. Some people seem genetically predisposed, because other family members may also be affected.

### Presentation

Small itchy red papules, papulovesicles or eczematous plaques arise from 2 h to 5 days, most commonly at 24 h, after exposure to UVR. The eruption is itchy and usually confined to sun-exposed areas (Fig. 18.8), remembering that some UVR passes through thin clothing. Not all exposed skin develops disease so there are papules and plaques rather than generalized redness.

**Fig. 18.8** Polymorphic light eruption: eczematous plaques on the face of a sad freckly boy. Persists throughout the summer but fades in the winter.

## Course

The disorder tends to recur each spring after UVR exposure. Tanning protects some patients so that if the initial exposures are limited, few or no symptoms occur later. Such patients can still enjoy sun exposure and outdoor activities. Others are so sensitive, or their skin pigments so poorly that fresh exposures continue to induce reactions throughout the summer. These patients require photoprotection, and must limit their sun exposure and outdoor activities. The rash disappears during the winter.

## Differential diagnosis

Phototoxic reactions, photoallergic reactions, miliaria rubra, chronic actinic dermatitis, ordinary eczemas, allergic reactions to sunscreens and airborne allergic contact dermatitis should be considered.

## Investigations

It may be possible to reproduce the dermatitis by testing non-sun-exposed skin with UVB and UVA.

## Treatment

If normal tanning does not confer protection, sunscreens (Formulary 1, p. 383) should be used. Protective clothing, such as wide-brimmed hats, long-sleeved shirts and long trousers, is helpful. In some patients, a 4-week course of psoralen with UVA (PUVA; p. 66) in the late spring can create enough tan to confer protection for the rest of the season. Moderately potent topical steroids (Formulary 1, p. 385) usually improve the eruption. A tapering course of systemic steroids may tide people over during severe or early spring outbreaks. Hydroxychloroquine (Formulary 2, p. 405) may be effective when used over the sunny season.

## Actinic prurigo

This is clinically distinct from a polymorphic light eruption although its unknown cause may be the same. Papules, crusts and excoriations arise on sun-exposed areas and sometimes also on other sites. Lesions may persist through the winter. It is common among North American Indians and may resemble excoriated acne, bites, eczema, erythropoietic protoporphyria or neurotic excoriations. It may be associated with atopy.

## Solar urticaria

This is discussed in Chapter 8. Wheals occur in the sun-exposed areas, within minutes. Some patients are reacting to UVB, others to UVA, and still others to visible light. Some patients have erythropoietic protoporphyria (p. 382) and this should be considered particularly if solar urticaria starts in infancy.

## Actinic keratoses

These are discussed in Chapter 20.

## Actinic cheilitis

This is discussed in Chapter 13 and see Fig. 27.14.

## Lupus erythematosus

Many patients with lupus erythematosus (p. 131) become worse after exposure to UVR, especially to UVB. This is particularly true of the subacute cutaneous variant associated with antibodies to SS-A and SS-B. They should be warned about this, and protect themselves from the sun (avoidance, clothing and sunscreens).

## Carcinomas

The sun's rays can cause basal cell carcinomas, squamous cell carcinomas and malignant melanomas. These are discussed in Chapter 20. People with more than five episodes of sunburn double their risk of developing a melanoma.

## Exacerbated diseases

UVR is useful in the treatment of many skin diseases, but it can also make some worse (Table 18.4).

## Porphyria cutanea tarda

This is described in Chapter 21.

**Table 18.4** The effect of sunlight on some skin diseases.

| Helps | Worsens |
|---|---|
| Atopic eczema | Darier's disease |
| Cutaneous T-cell lymphoma | Herpes simplex |
| Parapsoriasis | Lupus erythematosus |
| Pityriasis lichenoides | Pellagra |
| Pityriasis rosea | Photoallergy/toxicity |
| Pruritus of renal failure, liver disease | Porphyrias (excluding acute intermittent) |
| AIDS | Xeroderma pigmentosum |
| Psoriasis | |

## Cutaneous ageing

The trouble with old skin is the way it looks rather than the way it behaves. Skin chronically damaged by UVR during childhood thereafter looks old. This 'photoageing' effect causes the skin to become thin on the extremities, so that it bruises (Bateman's purpura) and tears easily (Fig. 18.9). The elastic fibres become clumped and amorphous, leading clinically to a yellow pebbly look called actinic elastosis (Fig. 18.10). Chronic exposure to sunlight, or to UVR in tanning parlours, also causes lentigines, freckles, roughness and, of course, skin cancers. The bronzed young skins of today will become the wrinkled, spotted, rough, prune-like ones of tomorrow. About 25% of our lifetime dose of sun exposure occurs in childhood.

Wrinkles occur when the dermis loses its elastic recoil, failing to snap back properly into shape. UVR damages elastic tissue and hastens this pro-

**Fig. 18.10** 'Sailor's skin' (cutis rhomboidalis nuchae): the deep creases on the back of the neck contain many comedones.

cess. Although cosmetic procedures (Ch. 22) can smooth wrinkles out, there is no way to reverse the damage fully; however, tretinoin cream (Formulary 1, p. 389) seems to help some patients. Use of lasers, peels, radiotherapy and intense pulsed light have advocates, particularly for reducing redness, telangiectases and lentigines. Surgical 'face lifts' remove redundant skin and pull the rest tighter (Chapter 27). Fillers can be injected into deep wrinkles (p. 337). Prevention (reducing exposure to UVR) is better than any 'cure', and is especially important in sunny climates (Table 18.5).

Skin ages even in sun-protected areas, but much more slowly. Compare the buttock skin with skin on the face, forearms or back to be convinced. The dermis thins, skin collagen falls by about 1% per year throughout adult life and becomes more stable (less elastic). Fibroblasts become sparser in the dermis, accounting for reduced collagen synthesis and slower wound healing.

**Fig. 18.9** Thin skin on the back of the hand. The whitish areas are stellate pseudoscars, the skin having never been broken. The pseudoscars follow the dispersion of senile (Bateman's) purpura.

**Table 18.5** Tips to avoid skin damage for those living in a sunny climate.

1 Apply sunscreen daily to all exposed parts – rain or shine; reapply after 20 min
2 Reapply sunscreen often when outdoors
3 Do not skimp. SPF calculations are based on 2 mg/cm$^2$ coverage. Most people underuse
4 Use a sunscreen with a protective factor (SPF) of at least 15, preferably 30
5 Choose a sunscreen that screens out both UVA and UVB
6 Wear wide-brimmed hats
7 Wear dense-weave clothing. If you can see through it, it's not completely protective
8 Target outdoor activities for early morning or late afternoon
9 Seek the shade
10 Avoid tanning salons
11 Do not sunbathe
12 Wear cosmetics, including lipstick
13 Help your children to protect themselves

---

**Learning point**

If your family or patients have type I or II skin tell them that it is never too late to protect themselves from excessive sun exposure. You might be one of the few able to persuade them to think of the future

## Further reading

Alam M, Hsu TS, Dover JS, Wrone DA & Arndt KA. (2003) Nonablative laser and light treatments: histology and tissue effects: a review. *Lasers in Surgery and Medicine* **33**, 30–39.

Berneburg M, Plettenberg H & Krutmann J. (2000) Photoaging of human skin. *Photodermatology, Photoimmunology and Photomedicine* **16**, 239–244.

Das D, Lloyd JJ, Walshaw D, *et al.* (2004) Provocation testing in polymorphous light eruption using fluorescent ultraviolet (UV) A and UVB lamps. *British Journal of Dermatology* **151**, 1066–1070.

Epstein JH. (1999) Phototoxicity and photoallergy. *Seminars in Cutaneous Medicine and Surgery* **18**, 274–284.

Ferguson J & Dover J. (2006) *Photodermatology*. Blackwell Publishing, Oxford.

Gonzalez E & Gonzalez S. (1996) Drug photosensitivity, idiopathic photodermatitis, and sunscreens. *Journal of the American Academy of Dermatology* **35**, 871–875.

Hawk J. (1998) *Photodermatology*. Hodder Arnold, London.

Krutman J, Hönigsmann H, Elmets CA & Bergstresser PR. (2001) *Dermatological Phototherapy and Photodiagnostic Methods*. Springer, Berlin.

Ling TC, Gibbs NK & Rhodes LE. (2003) Treatment of polymorphic light eruption. *Photodermatology, Photoimmunology and Photomedicine* **19**, 217–227.

Murphy GM. (2004) Investigation of photosensitive disorders. *Photodermatology, Photoimmunology and Photomedicine* **20**, 305–311.

Poblete-Gutierrez P, Wiederholt T, Merk HF & Frank J. (2006) The porphyrias: clinical presentation, diagnosis and treatment. *European Journal of Dermatology* **16**, 230–240.

Rabe JH, Mamelak AJ, McElguun PJ, *et al.* (2006) Photoaging: mechanisms and repair. *Journal of the American Academy of Dermatology* **55**, 1–19.

Railan D & Kilmer S. (2005) Ablative treatment of photoaging. *Dermatologic Therapy* **18**, 227–241.

# **19** Disorders of pigmentation

## Normal skin colour

The colour of normal skin comes from a mixture of pigments. Untanned Caucasoid skin is pink, tinted from white by oxyhaemoglobin in the blood within the dermis. Melanin (see below) blends with this colour, and may be increased (e.g. after a suntan). Melanin is also responsible for the shades of brown seen not only in Congoid (Negroid) skin, but also in the other races. Various hues are caused by the addition to these pigments of yellow from carotene, found mainly in subcutaneous fat and in the horny layer of the epidermis. There is no natural blue pigment; when blue is seen, it is either because of an optical effect from normal pigment (usually melanin) in the dermis, or the presence of an abnormal pigment. Skin pigmentation (measured by skin reflectance) is darkest near the equator and correlates with latitude and ultraviolet radiation (UVR). Skin colour seems to have evolved as a compromise between being dark enough to block the damage to DNA caused by ultraviolet radiation and photolysis of the essential metabolite, folate, and light enough to allow vitamin D to be synthesized in the skin (p. 15).

Hair colour is determined by the relative amounts of the different types of melanin. Eumelanin predominates in black hair and phaeomelanin in red.

## Melanogenesis

Melanin is formed from the essential aminoacid phenylalanine through a series of enzymatic steps in the liver and skin. Tyrosine, formed in the liver by hydroxylation of the essential amino acid pheny-lalanine under the influence of phenylalanine hydro-xylase, is the substrate for the reactions that occur in melanocytes (Fig. 19.1). These are the only cells in the epidermis to contain tyrosinase (dopa oxidase), the rate-limiting enzyme in melanogenesis. Phaeo-melanins and trichochromes, the pigments in red hair, are synthesized in a similar way, except that cysteine reacts with dopaquinone and is incorpor-ated into the subsequent polymers. Phaeomelanins and eumelanins may intermesh to form mixed melanin polymers.

Eumelanins and phaeomelanins differ from neuromelanins, the pigments found in the sub-stantia nigra and in cells of the chromaffin system (e.g. adrenal medulla, sympathetic ganglia). The latter are derived from tyrosine using a different enzyme, tyrosine hydroxylase, which is not found in melanocytes.

Melanin is made within melanosomes (see Fig. 2.6), tiny particles measuring about $0.1 \times 0.7\ \mu m$, shaped either like American footballs (eumelanosomes, containing eumelanin) or British soccer balls (phaeomelanosomes, containing phaeomelanin). Eventually, fully melanized melanosomes pass into the dendritic processes of the melanocyte to be injected into neighbouring keratinocytes. Once there, the melanosomes are engulfed in lysosomal packages (melanosome complexes) and distributed throughout the cytoplasm. Such secretory lysosomes are common to various haematopoietic cells and melanocytes. This explains why some genetic dis-orders of pigmentation (e.g. rare forms of albinism such as the Hermansky–Pudlak and Chediak–Higashi syndromes) are linked with abnormal immune function.

Negroids/Congoids are not black because they have more melanocytes than Caucasoids, but because their melanocytes produce more and larger mel-anosomes, which are broken down less rapidly in the melanosome complexes. Melanins protect against UVR damage by absorbing and scattering the rays, and by scavenging free radicals.

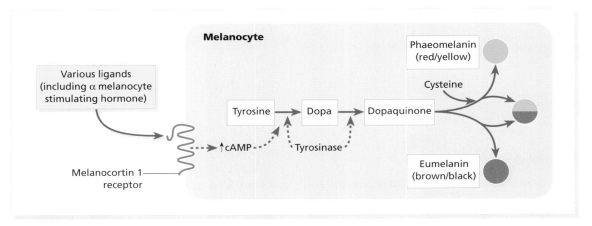

**Fig. 19.1** The control of melanogenesis. Melanocortin 1 receptor (MC1R) activity is both constitutive and rate limiting when promoting melanogenesis, via cyclic adenosine monophosphate (cAMP) production and tyrosinase stimulation. The MC1R is activated by ligands such as α-melanocyte stimulating hormone (α-MSH) and other pituitary peptides. In the absence of such ligands or the MC1R itself (knockout animals), and with loss-of-function mutations of the MC1R, phaeomelanin is produced. The precise mechanism by which ultraviolet radiation stimulates melanogenesis remains uncertain.

## Control of melanogenesis

Melanogenesis can be increased by several stimuli, the most important of which is UVR. Tanning involves two distinct reactions.

**1** Immediate pigment darkening (IPD) following exposure to longwave ultraviolet (UVA 320–400 nm). This pigment darkening occurs over minutes to days, dependent on UV dose and constitutive skin colour, and is responsible for the well-known phenomenon of a 'false tan'. It is not brought about by melanin synthesis but oxidation of preformed melanin and redistribution of melanin from perinuclear melanosomes to peripheral dendrites.

**2** Delayed tanning (DT): the production of *new* pigment occurs some 3–4 days after exposure to medium-wave ultraviolet (UVB: 290–320 nm) and UVA and is maximal at 7 days. It depends on the proliferation of melanocytes, an increase in tyrosinase activity and melanosome production, and an increased transfer of new melanosomes to their surrounding keratinocytes.

A neat control mechanism involving glutathione has been postulated. Reduced glutathione in the epidermis, produced by the action of glutathione reductase on glutathione, inhibits tyrosinase. UVR and some inflammatory skin conditions may induce pigmentation by oxidizing glutathione and so blocking its inhibition of melanogenesis.

Melanocytes are also influenced by melanocyte-stimulating hormone (MSH) peptides from the pituitary and other areas of the brain (Fig. 19.1). Their melanocyte-stimulating activity is caused by a common heptapeptide sequence, cleaved from the precursor protein, pro-opiomelanocortin, as a result of two proconvertase enzymes. However, these MSH peptides may play little part in the physiological control of pigmentation. Hypophysectomy will not cause a black skin to lighten and only large doses of adrenocorticotrophic hormone (ACTH), in pathological states (p. 287), will increase skin pigmentation. It is now known that UVR induces both keratinocytes and melanocytes in the skin to secrete pro-opiomelanocortin and MSH peptides and so MSH may have a paracrine or autocrine function. In the skin, α-MSH also acts as an anti-inflammatory agent by antagonizing the effects of interleukin 1 (IL-1) in inducing IL-2 receptors on lymphocytes (p. 23) and in inducing pyrexia. Oestrogens and progestogens (and possibly testosterone too) may, in some circumstances, stimulate melanogenesis, either directly (by acting on oestrogen and progestogen receptors in the melanocyte) or by increasing the release of MSH peptides from the pituitary.

## Genetics and skin pigmentation

Genetic differences determine the pigmentation of the different races (Chapter 14, p. 205). A black person living in Britain and a white person living in Africa will remain black and white, respectively. None the less, there is some phenotypic variation in skin colour (e.g. tanning after sun exposure). Red hair is the result of genetic variations in the amino acid sequence of the melanocortin 1 receptor (MC1R) (Fig. 19.1). Some genodermatoses with abnormal pigmentation are described in Chapter 24.

**Table 19.1** Some abnormal pigments.

**Endogenous**

*Haemoglobin-derived*

| | |
|---|---|
| Methaemoglobin ⎫ | Blue colour in vessels, |
| Sulphaemoglobin ⎬ | cyanosis |
| Carboxyhaemoglobin | Pink |
| Bilirubin ⎫ | |
| Biliverdin ⎭ | Yellow–green |
| Haemosiderin | Brown |

*Drugs*

| | |
|---|---|
| Gold | Blue-grey (chrysiasis) |
| Silver | Blue-grey (argyria) |
| Bismuth | Grey |
| Mepacrine | Yellow |
| Clofazamine | Red |
| Phenothiazines | Slate-grey |
| Amiodarone | Blue-grey |

*Diet*

| | |
|---|---|
| Carotene | Orange |

**Exogenous**

*Tattoo pigments*

| | |
|---|---|
| Carbon | Blue-black |
| Coal dust | Blue-black |
| Cobalt | Blue |
| Chrome | Green |
| Cadmium | Yellow |
| Mercury | Red |
| Iron | Brown |

*Local medications*

| | |
|---|---|
| Silver nitrate | Black |
| Magenta paint | Magenta |
| Gentian violet | Violet |
| Eosin | Pink |
| Potassium permanganate | Brown |
| Dithranol (anthralin) | Purple |
| Tar | Brown |
| Iodine | Yellow |

## Abnormal skin colours

These may be caused by an imbalance of the normal pigments mentioned above (e.g. in cyanosis, chloasma and carotenaemia) or by the presence of abnormal pigments (Table 19.1). Sometimes it is difficult to distinguish between the colours of these pigments (e.g. the gingery brown colour of haemosiderin is readily confused with melanin). Histological stains may be needed to settle the issue. In practice though, apart from tattoos, most pigmentary problems are caused by too much or too little melanin.

### Decreased melanin pigmentation

Some conditions in which there is a lack of melanin are listed in Table 19.2. A few of the more important, and the mechanisms involved, are summarized in Fig. 19.2.

**Table 19.2** Some causes of hypopigmentation.

| | |
|---|---|
| Genetic | Albinism |
| | Piebaldism |
| | Phenylketonuria |
| | Waardenburg's syndrome |
| | (p. 281) |
| | Chediak–Higashi syndrome: |
| | (autosomal recessive lysosomal |
| | defect p. 281) |
| | Tuberous sclerosis (p. 351) |
| Endocrine | Hypopituitarism |
| Chemical | Contact with substituted phenols |
| | (in rubber industry) |
| | Chloroquine and |
| | hydroxychloroquine |
| Post-inflammatory | Eczema |
| | Pityriasis alba |
| | Psoriasis |
| | Sarcoidosis |
| | Lupus erythematosus |
| | Lichen sclerosus et atrophicus |
| | Cryotherapy |
| Infections | Leprosy |
| | Pityriasis versicolor |
| | Syphilis, yaws and pinta |
| Tumours | Halo naevus |
| | Malignant melanoma |
| Miscellaneous | Vitiligo |
| | Idiopathic guttate hypomelanosis |

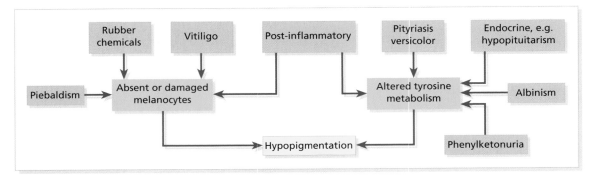

**Fig. 19.2** The mechanisms involved in some types of hypopigmentation.

## Oculocutaneous albinism

Various genetic conditions exist in which there is a defect in the synthesis or packaging of melanin in the melanocyte, or a defective transfer of melanosomes to surrounding keratinocytes (Chapter 2). In the most common type, little or no melanin is made in the skin and eyes (oculocutaneous albinism) or in the eyes alone (ocular albinism – not discussed further here). The prevalence of albinism of all types ranges from 1 in 20 000 in the USA and UK to 5% in some communities.

### Cause

The hair bulb test (see 'Investigations' below) separates oculocutaneous albinism into two main types: tyrosinase negative and tyrosinase positive. Roughly equal numbers of the two types are found in most communities, both being inherited as autosomal recessive traits. This explains how children with two albino parents can sometimes themselves be normally pigmented, the genes being complementary in the double heterozygote (Fig. 19.2).

The tyrosinase gene lies on chromosome 11q14-q21. More than 20 allelic variations have been found there in patients with tyrosinase-negative albinism. The gene for tyrosinase-positive human albinism has been mapped to chromosome 15q11-q13. It probably encodes for an ion channel protein in the melanosome involved in the transport of tyrosine.

**Fig. 19.3** Oculocutaneous albinism. An albino baby born to a normally pigmented African family (autosomal recessive inheritance).

### Presentation and course

The whole epidermis is white and pigment is also lacking in the hair, iris and retina (Fig. 19.3). Albinos have poor sight, photophobia and a rotatory nystagmus. As they grow older, tyrosinase-positive albinos gain a little pigment in their skin, iris and hair. Negroid skin becomes yellow–brown and the hair becomes yellow. Tyrosinase-positive albinos may also develop freckles. Sunburn is common on unprotected skin. As melanocytes are present, albinos have non-pigmented melanocytic naevi and may develop amelanotic malignant melanomas.

## Complications

In the tropics these unfortunate individuals develop numerous sun-induced skin cancers even when they are young, confirming the protective role of melanin.

## Differential diagnosis

Piebaldism and vitiligo are described below.

## Investigations

Prenatal diagnosis of albinism is now possible but may not be justifiable in view of the good prognosis. Nowadays, DNA-based diagnostic screening of amniotic fluid cells or chorionic villi sampling is favoured.

The hair bulb test, in which plucked hairs are incubated in dihydroxyphenylalanine, distinguishes tyrosinase-positive from tyrosinase-negative types.

## Treatment

Avoidance of sun exposure and protection with opaque clothing, wide-brimmed hats and sunscreen creams (Formulary 1, p. 383) are essential and allow albinos in temperate climates to live a relatively normal life. Early diagnosis and treatment of skin tumours is critical. In the tropics, the outlook is less good and the termination of affected pregnancies may be considered.

## Other types of albinism

There are several syndromes of albinism. They include the rare autosomal recessive Hermansky–Pudlak syndrome (oculocutaneous albinism and platelet storage disease, prolonged bleeding, neutropenia occasionally accompanied by pulmonary fibrosis and granulomatous colitis) and the equally uncommon Chediak–Higashi syndrome (oculocutaneous albinism with marked susceptibility to infections, caused by abnormal inclusions in phagocytic leucocytes).

## Piebaldism

These patients often have a white forelock of hair and patches of depigmentation lying symmetrically on the limbs, trunk and central part of the face, especially the chin. The condition is present at birth and is inherited as an autosomal dominant trait. The *KIT* proto-oncogene encodes the tyrosine kinase transmembrane cellular receptor on certain stem cells; without this they cannot respond to normal signals for development and migration. Melanocytes are absent from the hypopigmented areas. The depigmentation, often mistaken for vitiligo, may improve with age. There is no effective treatment. Waardenburg's syndrome includes piebaldism (with a white forelock in 20% of cases), hypertelorism, a prominent inner third of the eyebrows, irides of different colour and deafness.

## Phenylketonuria

This rare metabolic cause of hypopigmentation has a prevalence of about 1 in 25 000. It is described in Chapter 21.

## Hypopituitarism

The skin changes here may alert an astute physician to the diagnosis. The complexion has a pale, yellow tinge; there is thinning or loss of the sexual hair; the skin itself is atrophic. The hypopigmentation is caused by a decreased production of pituitary melanotrophic hormones (p. 278).

## Vitiligo

The word vitiligo comes from the Latin word *vitellus* meaning 'veal' (pale, pink flesh). It is an acquired circumscribed depigmentation, found in all races; its prevalence may be as high as 0.5–1%; its inheritance is polygenic.

## Cause and types

There is a complete loss of melanocytes from affected areas. There are two main patterns: a common generalized one and a rare segmental type. *Generalized vitiligo*, including the acrofacial variant, usually starts after the second decade. There is a family history in 30% of patients and this type is most frequent in those with autoimmune diseases such as diabetes, thyroid disorders and pernicious anaemia.

It is postulated that, in this type, melanocytes are the target of a cell-mediated autoimmune attack or self-destruct because of an inability to remove toxic melanin precursors. *Segmental vitiligo* is restricted to one part of the body, but not necessarily to a dermatome. It occurs earlier than generalized vitiligo, and is not associated with autoimmune diseases. Trauma and sunburn can precipitate both types.

### Clinical course

*Generalized type* The sharply defined, usually symmetrical (Figs. 19.4, 14.3–5), white patches are especially common on the backs of the hands, wrists, fronts of knees, neck and around body orifices. The hair of the scalp and beard may depigment too. In Caucasoids, the surrounding skin is sometimes partially depigmented or hyperpigmented (trichrome vitiligo). The course is unpredictable: lesions may remain static or spread, sometimes following minor trauma (Köbner phenomenon); occasionally, they repigment spontaneously from the hair follicles.

*Segmental type* The individual areas look like the generalized type but their segmental distribution

**Fig. 19.4** Striking patchy vitiligo on the knees.

**Fig. 19.5** Vitiligo: patchy repigmentation is caused by the migration of melanocytes from the depths of the hair follicles.

is striking. Spontaneous repigmentation occurs more often in this type than in generalized vitiligo (Fig. 19.5).

### Differential diagnosis

Contact with depigmenting chemicals, such as hydroquinones and substituted phenols in the rubber industry, should be excluded. Pityriasis versicolor (p. 254) must be considered; its fine scaling and less complete pigment loss separate it from vitiligo. Post-inflammatory depigmentation (p. 283) may look very like vitiligo but is less white and improves spontaneously. The patches of piebaldism are present at birth. Sometimes leprosy must be excluded – by sensory testing and a general examination. Other tropical diseases that cause patchy hypopigmentation are leishmaniasis (p. 234), yaws (p. 228) and pinta.

### Treatment

The cosmetic disfigurement from vitiligo can be devastating to affected paients. Treatment is unsatisfactory. In the white patches pigment cells are only present deep in the hair follicles and treatments mostly try to get melanocytes to divide and migrate into affected skin. Repigmentation is thus often heralded by freckling at follicles within patches Recent patches may respond to a potent or very potent topical corticosteroid, applied for 1–2 months.

After this, the strength should be gradually tapered to a mildly potent steroid for maintenance treatment. Alternatively, calcineurin inhibitors, such as 0.1% tacrolimus ointment, may work, but responses generally seem no better than those to topical corticosteroids. Some patients improve with psoralens (trimethylpsoralen or 8-methoxypsoralen, in a dosage of 0.4–0.6 mg/kg body weight), taken 1–2 h before graduated exposure to natural sunshine or to artificial UVA (PUVA; p. 66). Narrow-band (311 nm) UVB may also be effective. Therapy is given 2–3 times weekly for at least 6 months; new lesions seem to respond best.

Less reliable treatments include irradiating skin with a 308-nm excimer laser and antioxidant therapy with Ginkgo biloba extract or catalase. Where pigment is absent in hair follicles or in skin without hair follicles, autologous skin grafts are becoming popular, although they remain experimental. The two most common procedures transplant either minigraft implants of 1 mm cylinders or epidermal roofs of suction-raised blisters from unaffected skin. Melanocyte and stem cell transplants, in which single cell suspensions are made from unaffected skin and applied to dermabraded vitiliginous skin, are also being investigated.

As a general rule, established vitiligo is best left untreated in most white people, although advice about suitable camouflage preparations (Formulary 1, p. 383) to cover unsightly patches should be given. These include staining with dihydroxyacetone self-tanning lotions, or covering with theatrical make-up. Sun avoidance and screening preparations (Formulary 1, p. 383) are needed to avoid sunburn of the affected areas and a heightened contrast between the pale and dark areas. Black patients with extensive vitiligo can be completely and irreversibly depigmented by creams containing the monobenzyl ether of hydroquinone. The social implications must be discussed and carefully considered, and written consent given, before such treatment is undertaken.

> **Learning points**
>
> - Vitiligo looks ugly and sunburns easily. Treat with cosmetic cover and sunscreens or sun avoidance
> - Do not promise a cure

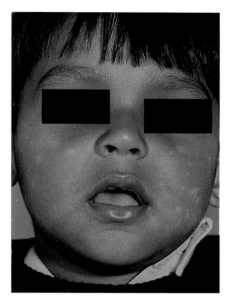

**Fig. 19.6** Pityriasis alba.

### Post-inflammatory depigmentation

This may follow eczema, psoriasis, sarcoidosis, lupus erythematosus and, rarely, lichen planus. It may also result from cryotherapy or a burn. In general, the more severe the inflammation, the more likely pigment is to decrease rather than increase in its wake. These problems are most significant in Negroids and Asians (see Ch. 14). With time, the skin usually repigments. Pityriasis alba is common on the faces of children. The initial lesion is probably a variant of eczema (pinkish with fine scaling), which fades leaving one or more pale, slightly scaly, areas (Fig. 19.6 and 14.2). Exposure to the sun makes the patches more obvious.

### Sun damage

Confetti-like white macules occur amongst the mottled hyperpigmentation of severe sun damage in a condition called idiopathic guttate hypomelanosis.

### White hair

Melanocytes in hair bulbs become less active with age and white hair (canities) is a universal sign of ageing (p. 220). Early greying of the hair is seen in the rare premature ageing syndromes, such as Werner's syndrome, and in autoimmune conditions such as pernicious anaemia, thyroid disorders and Addison's disease.

## Disorders with increased pigmentation (hypermelanosis)

Some of these disorders are listed in Table 19.3. The most common are described below and the mechanisms involved are summarized in Fig. 19.7.

**Table 19.3** Some causes of hyperpigmentation.

| | |
|---|---|
| Genetic | Freckles |
| | Lentigines |
| | *Café au lait* macules |
| | Peutz–Jeghers syndrome |
| | Xeroderma pigmentosum (Chapter 24) |
| | Albright's syndrome: segmental hyperpigmentation, fibrous dysplasia of bones, precocious puberty |
| Endocrine | Addison's disease |
| | Cushing's syndrome |
| | Pregnancy |
| | Renal failure |
| Metabolic | Biliary cirrhosis |
| | Haemochromatosis |
| | Porphyria |
| Nutritional | Malabsorption |
| | Carcinomatosis |
| | Kwashiorkor |
| | Pellagra |
| Drugs | Photosensitizing drugs |
| | ACTH and synthetic analogues |
| | Oestrogens and progestogens |
| | Psoralens |
| | Arsenic |
| | Busulfan |
| | Minocycline |
| Post-inflammatory | Lichen planus |
| | Eczema |
| | Secondary syphilis |
| | Systemic sclerosis |
| | Lichen and macular amyloidosis |
| | Cryotherapy |
| Poikiloderma | |
| Tumours | Acanthosis nigricans (p. 323) |
| | Pigmented naevi (p. 294) |
| | Malignant melanoma (p. 306) |
| | Mastocytosis (p. 317) |

ACTH, adenocorticotrophic hormone.

### Freckles (ephelides)

Freckles are so common that to describe them seems unnecessary. They are seen most often in the red-haired or blond person as sharply demarcated, light brown–ginger macules, usually less than 5 mm in diameter. They multiply and become darker with sun exposure.

Increased melanin is seen in the basal layer of the epidermis without any increase in the number of melanocytes, and without elongation of the rete ridges (Fig. 19.8). No treatment is necessary.

### Melanotic macule of the lip

This common lesion (Fig. 19.9) worries doctors but is benign. Its histology is similar to that of a freckle (Fig. 19.8).

### Lentigo

Simple and senile lentigines look alike. They are light or dark brown macules, ranging from 1 mm to 1 cm across. Although usually discrete, they may have an irregular outline. Simple lentigines arise most often in childhood as a few scattered lesions, often on areas not exposed to sun, including the mucous membranes. Senile or solar lentigines are common after middle age on the backs of the hands ('age spots', 'liver spots'; Fig. 19.10) and on the face (Fig. 19.11). In contrast to freckles, lentigines have increased numbers of melanocytes. They should be distinguished from freckles, from junctional melanocytic naevi (p. 294) and from a lentigo maligna (p. 307). Treatment is usually unnecessary and prevention, by sun avoidance and the use of sunscreens, is the best approach. Careful cryotherapy has stood the test of time and fares well when compared with modern treatments mentioned below. Melanin-specific high energy lasers (e.g. pigmented lesion dye laser, 510 nm; Q-switched ruby laser, 694 nm; Q-switched alexandrite laser, 755 nm) are extremely effective for treating ugly lesions. Liver spots associated with actinic damage lighten or clear with the daily application of 0.1% tretinoin cream (Formulary 1, p. 389) or 2–4% hydroquinone (Formulary 1, p. 383) or a combination of these with or without a retinoid, α-hydroxy acid, or topical corticosteroid (Formulary 1, p. 385).

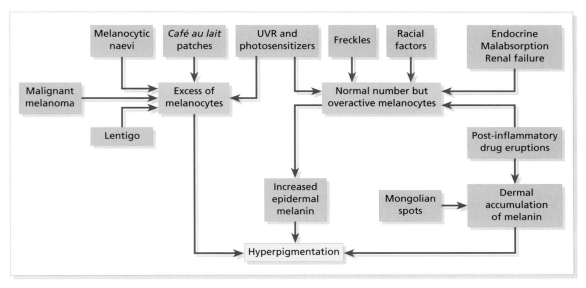

**Fig. 19.7** The mechanisms of some types of hyperpigmentation. UVR, ultraviolet radiation.

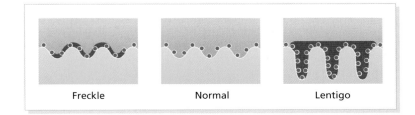

**Fig. 19.8** Histology of a freckle and a lentigo.

**Fig. 19.9** Melanotic macule of the lip: slow to evolve and benign, as suggested by its even colour and sharp margin.

**Fig. 19.10** Senile lentigines on the back of an elderly hand ('liver spots'). Note accompanying atrophy.

**Fig. 19.11** A simple lentigo showing a sharp edge and an even distribution of pigment.

### Conditions associated with multiple lentigines

Three rare but striking syndromes feature multiple lentigines.

#### Peutz–Jeghers syndrome

Profuse lentigines are seen on and around the lips in this autosomal dominant condition (Fig. 19.12). Scattered lentigines also occur on the buccal mucosa, gums, hard palate, hands and feet. The syndrome is important because of its association with polyposis of the small intestine, which may lead to recurrent intussusception and, rarely, to malignant transformation of the polyps. Ten per cent of affected women have ovarian tumours.

**Fig. 19.12** Profuse lentigines on and around the lips in the Peutz–Jeghers syndrome.

#### Cronkhite–Canada syndrome

This consists of multiple lentigines on the backs of the hands and a more diffuse pigmentation of the palms and volar aspects of the fingers. It may also be associated with gastrointestinal polyposis. Alopecia and nail abnormalities complete the rare but characteristic clinical picture.

#### LEOPARD syndrome

This is an acronym for generalized **l**entiginosis associated with cardiac abnormalities demonstrated by **E**CG, **o**cular hypertelorism, **p**ulmonary stenosis, **a**bnormal genitalia, **r**etardation of growth and **dea**fness.

### Melasma (chloasma)

Melasma is an acquired, symmetrical hypermelanosis occurring on sun-exposed skin, especially the face. The areas of increased pigmentation are well defined and their edges may be scalloped. The condition is much more common in women, affects all races but is most prevalent in dark-skinnned individuals with skin types IV–VI (see Table 18.1). The hypermelanosis becomes darker after exposure to the sun. There are many causes including sunlight, pregnancy 'the mask of pregnancy' (Fig 19.13), oestrogens and oral contraceptives, scented cosmetics, thyroid dysfunction and photosensitizing drugs (see Table 18.2). The placenta may secrete sex hormones that stimulate melanocytes. Recently, over-expression of α-MSH (p. 278) has been demonstrated in lesional skin. Most of the extra melanin lies in the epidermis, but there is some in the dermis too, making treatment difficult.

#### Treatment

This is unsatisfactory. A sunscreen will make the pigmentation less obvious during the summer and minimize the chance of spread.

Some find bleaching agents that contain hydroquinone helpful. The optimal effect is achieved with preparations containing 2–5% hydroquinone (Formulary 1, p. 383), applied for 6–10 weeks. After this, maintenance treatment should be with

**Fig. 19.13** Chloasma worsened by sun exposure.

preparations containing no more than 2% hydroquinone. In stubborn cases, the hydroquinone may be combined with a topical steroid and a retinoid for short-term use. Chemical peels have become popular. α-Hydroxy acids, especially glycolic acid, are the most versatile but require expertise for proper application. Small test sites should be treated and assessed before formal, more widespread, treatment with any modality.

## Endocrine hyperpigmentation

### Addison's disease

Hyperpigmentation caused by the overproduction of ACTH is often striking. It may be generalized or limited to the skin folds, creases of the palms, scars and the buccal mucosa.

### Cushing's syndrome

Increased ACTH production may cause a picture like that of Addison's disease. The hyperpigmentation may become even more marked after adrenalectomy (Nelson's syndrome).

### Pregnancy

There is a generalized increase in pigmentation during pregnancy, especially of the nipples and areolae, and of the linea alba. Melasma (p. 286) may also occur. The nipples and areolae may remain pigmented for a while after parturition.

### Chronic renal failure

The hyperpigmentation of chronic renal failure and of patients on haemodialysis is caused by an increase in levels of pituitary melanotrophic peptides, normally cleared by the kidney.

### Porphyria

Formed porphyrins, especially uroporphyrins, are produced in excess in cutaneous hepatic porphyria and congenital erythropoietic porphyria (p. 328). These endogenous photosensitizers induce hyperpigmentation on exposed areas; skin fragility, blistering, milia and hypertrichosis are equally important clues to the diagnosis.

## Nutritional hyperpigmentation

Any severe wasting disease, such as malabsorption, AIDS, tuberculosis or cancer, may be accompanied by diffuse hyperpigmentation. Kwashiorkor presents a mixed picture of generalized hypopigmentation and patchy post-inflammatory hyperpigmentation, and in this condition the hair is red–brown or grey.

## Chemicals causing hyperpigmentation

Table 18.2 lists drugs that commonly photosensitize. All can cause hyperpigmentation of the exposed skin. Psoralens are used in the photochemotherapy of psoriasis (Chapter 5) and, more rarely, of vitiligo.

The term 'berloque dermatitis' (Fig. 19.14) refers to a 'pendant' of hyperpigmentation, often on the side of the neck, where cosmetics have been applied which contain the photosensitizing 5-methoxypsoralen. Cosmetics for men (e.g. pre- and aftershaves) are a thriving source of these.

**Fig. 19.14** A drop of psoralen-containing perfume on the chest photosensitized this pendant-shaped area. It became pigmented after exposure to the sun.

---

**Learning point**

Don't forget that photosensitizing cosmetics can cause facial hyperpigmentation, even in men

---

Arsenic is not used medically nowadays. Once it caused 'raindrop' depigmentation within a diffuse bronzed hyperpigmentation.

Busulfan and bleomycin, used to treat some forms of leukaemia, frequently cause diffuse hyperpigmentation but may also cause brown streaks (flagellate hyperpigmentation). Minocycline can leave blue–black drug deposits in inflamed acne spots on the shins or on the mucosae. They can be removed with Q-switched ruby laser (694 nm) treatment.

## Post-inflammatory hyperpigmentation

This is common after lichen planus (p. 72). It is also a feature of systemic sclerosis (p. 138) and some types of cutaneous amyloidosis, and is often an unwelcome sequel of cryotherapy.

## Poikiloderma

Poikiloderma is the name given to a triad of signs: reticulate pigmentation, atrophy and telangiectasia. It is not a disease but a reaction pattern with many causes including X-irradiation, photocontact reactions, and connective tissue and lymphoreticular disorders. Congenital variants (Rothmund–Thomson syndrome, Bloom's syndrome and Cockayne's syndrome) associated with photosensitivity dwarfism and mental retardation also occur.

## Further reading

Hann SK & Nordlund JJ. (2000) *Vitiligo*. Blackwell Publishing, Oxford.

Nordlund JJ, Boissy RE, Hearing VJ, King RA, Oetting WS & Ortonne JP. (2006) *The Pigmentary System*, 2nd edn. Blackwell Publishing, Oxford.

Ortonne JP & Passeron T. (2005) Melanin pigmentary disorders: treatment update. *Dermatology Clinics* 23, 209–226.

Taylor SC. (2002) Skin of color: biology, structure, function and implications for dermatologic disease. *Journal of the American Academy of Dermatology* **46** (Supplement 2), 41–62.

# **20** Skin tumours

This chapter deals with skin tumours arising from both the epidermis and its appendages, and from the dermis (Table 20.1).

## Prevention

Many skin tumours (e.g. actinic keratoses, lentigines, keratoacanthomas, basal cell carcinomas, squamous cell carcinomas, malignant melanomas and, arguably, acquired melanocytic naevi) would all become less common if Caucasoids, especially those with a fair skin, protected themselves adequately against sunlight. The education of those living in sunny climates or holidaying in the sun has already reaped great rewards here (Fig. 20.1). Successful campaigns have focused on regular self-examination and on reducing sun exposure by avoidance, clothing and sunscreen preparations (Figs 20.2 and 20.3). Public compliance has been encouraged by imaginative slogans like the Australian 'sun smart' and 'slip, slap, slop' advice (slip on the shirt, slap on the hat and slop on the sunscreen), the American Academy of Dermatology 'ABCs' (away, block, cover up, shade) leaflet and that lovable American creature Joel Mole.

**Table 20.1** Skin tumours.

| Derived from | Benign | Premalignant/ carcinoma *in situ* | Malignant |
|---|---|---|---|
| Epidermis and appendages | Viral wart<br>Cutaneous horn<br>Seborrhoeic keratosis<br>Skin tag<br>Linear epidermal naevus<br>Melanocytic naevus<br>Sebaceous naevus<br>Epidermal/pilar cyst<br>Milium<br>Chondrodermatitis<br>  nodularis helicis | Actinic keratosis | Basal cell carcinoma<br>Squamous cell carcinoma<br>Malignant melanoma<br>Paget's disease of the nipple<br>  (although strictly a breast tumour) |
| Dermis | Haemangioma<br>Lymphangioma<br>Glomus tumour<br>Pyogenic granuloma<br>Dermatofibroma<br>Neurofibroma<br>Neuroma<br>Keloid<br>Lipoma<br>Lymphocytoma cutis<br>Mastocytosis | | Kaposi's sarcoma<br>Lymphoma<br>Dermatofibrosarcoma protuberans<br>Metastases |

**Fig. 20.1** This family lived in the tropics. No prizes for guessing which of them avoided the sun.

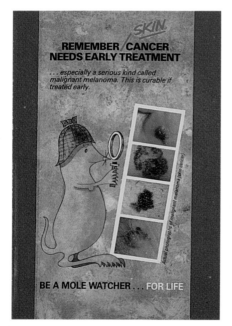

**Fig. 20.2** An eye-catching and effective way of teaching the public how to look at their moles. A pamphlet produced by the Cancer Research Campaign in the UK.

## Tumours of the epidermis and its appendages

### Benign

### *Viral warts*

These are discussed in Chapter 16, but are mentioned here for three reasons.

**Fig. 20.3** These Australian schoolchildren are wearing legionnaire's caps with large peaks and flaps. These are fashionable after several clever campaigns, and the 'no hat, no play' rule has become an accepted way of life.

**1** Solitary warts are sometimes misdiagnosed on the face or hands of the elderly.
**2** A wart is one of the few benign tumours in humans that is, without doubt, caused by a virus, the human papilloma virus.
**3** Some human papilloma viruses are prime players in the pathogenesis of malignant tumours.

Seventy per cent of transplant patients who have been immunosuppressed for over 5 years have multiple viral warts and there is growing evidence that immunosuppression, some types of human papilloma virus and ultraviolet radiation interact in this setting to cause squamous cell carcinoma (p. 303).

### *Cutaneous horn*

This common horn-shaped excrescence (Fig. 20.4), arising from keratinocytes, may resemble a viral wart clinically. Excision, or curettage with cautery to the base, is the treatment of choice. The histology should be checked.

**Fig. 20.5** Typical multiple seborrhoeic warts on the shoulder. Each individual lesion might look worryingly like a malignant melanoma but, in the numbers seen here, the lesions must be benign.

**Fig. 20.4** Cutaneous horn with a bulbous fleshy base.

### Seborrhoeic keratosis (basal cell papilloma, seborrhoeic wart)

This is a common benign epidermal tumour, unrelated to sebaceous glands. The term 'senile wart' should be avoided as it offends many patients.

**Fig. 20.6** Numerous unsightly seborrhoeic warts of the face.

#### Cause

Usually unexplained but:
- multiple lesions may be inherited (autosomal dominant);
- occasionally follow an inflammatory dermatosis;
- very rarely, the sudden eruption of hundreds of itchy lesions is associated with an internal neoplasm (Leser–Trélat sign).

#### Presentation

Seborrhoeic keratoses usually arise after the age of 50 years, but flat inconspicuous lesions are often visible earlier. They are often multiple (Figs 20.5 and 20.6) but may be single. Lesions are most common on the face and trunk. The sexes are equally affected.

#### Physical signs

- A distinctive 'stuck-on' appearance due to 'tucked under' shoulders, as chewed chewing gum might appear.
- May be flat, raised, filiform or pedunculated.
- Surface may be smooth or verrucous.
- Colour varies from yellow–white to dark brown–black.
- Surface may have greasy scaling and scattered keratin plugs ('currant bun' appearance).
- If oval, long axis parallels skin lines.

#### Clinical course

Lesions may multiply with age but remain benign.

**Fig. 20.7** Dermatosis papulosa nigra.

**Fig. 20.8** Stucco keratoses. Numerous small dry white/grey stuck-on lesions on the lower leg.

### Differential diagnosis

Seborrhoeic keratoses are easily recognized. Occasionally, they can be confused with a pigmented cellular naevus, a pigmented basal cell carcinoma and, most importantly, with a malignant melanoma. *Dermatosis papulosa nigra* (Fig. 20.7 and p. 208) is a long-winded name for a common variant of seborrhoeic keratoses affecting black adults. Multiple pigmented papules, just raised or filiform, appear on the face and neck but may extend to the trunk. The lesions may be unsightly and catch on jewellery. Histologically, they are like seborrhoeic warts. The condition may run in families, being inherited as an autosomal dominant trait.

*Stucco keratoses* are another variant of seborrhoeic keratoses and are seen most often around the ankles after the age of 50 years (Fig. 20.8). They have a similar 'stuck on' appearance to seborrhoeic warts and are small (1–2 mm) white keratotic papules that are easily lifted off the skin with a finger nail, without bleeding.

### Investigations

Biopsy is needed only in rare dubious cases. The histology is diagnostic (Fig. 20.9): the lesion lies above the general level of the surrounding epidermis and consists of proliferating basal cells and horn cysts. Stucco keratoses have a slightly different histology with loose lamellated hyperkeratosis overlying regular papillomatosis.

### Treatment

Seborrhoeic keratoses can safely be left alone, but ugly or easily traumatized ones can be removed

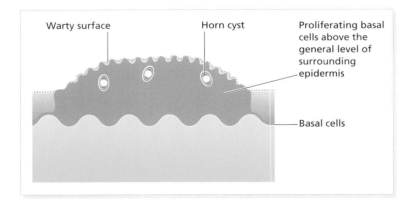

**Fig. 20.9** Histology of a seborrhoeic keratosis.

with a curette under local anaesthetic (this has the advantage of providing histology), or by cryotherapy. If treatment is requested for dermatosis papulosa nigra, gentle electrodessication or snipping of a few trial lesions initially is the best approach. Cryotherapy should be avoided as hypo- or hyperpigmentation may result.

---

**Learning point**

If you cannot tell most seborrhoeic warts from a melanoma you will send too many elderly people unnecessarily to the pigmented lesion clinic

---

### Skin tags (acrochordon)

These common benign outgrowths of skin affect mainly the middle-aged and elderly.

### Cause

This is unknown but the trait is sometimes familial. Skin tags are most common in obese women, and rarely are associated with tuberous sclerosis (p. 351), acanthosis nigricans (p. 323) or acromegaly, and diabetes.

### Presentation and clinical course

Skin tags occur around the neck and within the major flexures. They look unsightly and may catch on clothing and jewellery. They are soft skin-coloured or pigmented pedunculated papules (Fig. 20.10).

### Differential diagnosis

The appearance is unmistakable. Tags are rarely confused with small melanocytic naevi.

### Treatment

Small lesions can be snipped off with fine scissors, frozen with liquid nitrogen or destroyed with a hyfrecator without local anaesthesia. There is no way of preventing new ones from developing.

## Naevi

The term naevus refers to a skin lesion that has a localized excess of one or more types of cell in a normal cell site. It is the name used for a cutaneous hamartoma. Histologically, the cells are identical to or closely resemble normal cells. Naevi may be composed mostly of keratinocytes (e.g. in epidermal naevi), melanocytes (e.g. in congenital melanocytic naevi), connective tissue elements (e.g. in connective tissue naevi) or a mixture of epithelial and connective tissue elements (e.g. in sebaceous naevi).

### Linear epidermal naevus

This lesion is an example of cutaneous mosaicism (p. 348) and so tends to follow Blaschko's lines (Fig. 20.11). Keratinocytes in these lines of wart-like growth are genetically different from their normal appearing neighbours. Keratolytics (Formulary 1,

**Fig. 20.10** Numerous axillary skin tags.

**Fig. 20.11** Linear warty epidermal naevus.

**Table 20.2** Classification of melanocytic naevi.

Congenital melanocytic naevi
Acquired melanocytic naevi
   Junctional naevus
   Compound naevus
   Intradermal naevus
   Spitz naevus
   Blue naevus
   Atypical melanocytic naevus

p. 384) lessen the roughness of some and small epidermal naevi may be excised. Alternatively, a trial area may be destroyed with a carbon dioxide laser and the subsequent scar assessed before extending treatment .

### Melanocytic naevi

Melanocytic naevi (moles) are localized benign tumours of melanocytes. Their classification (Table 20.2) is based on the site of the aggregations of the abnormal melanocytes (Fig. 20.12).

#### Cause and evolution

The cause is unknown. A genetic factor is likely in many families, working together with excessive sun exposure during childhood.

With the exception of congenital melanocytic naevi, most appear in early childhood, often with a sharp increase in numbers during adolescence and after severe sunburns. Further crops may appear during pregnancy, oestrogen therapy, flare-ups of lupus erythematosus or, rarely, after cytotoxic chemotherapy and immunosuppression. New melanocytic naevi appear less often after the age of 20 years.

Melanocytic naevi in childhood are usually of the 'junctional' type, with proliferating melanocytes in clumps at the dermo-epidermal junction. Later, the melanocytes round off and 'drop' into the dermis. A 'compound' naevus has both dermal and junctional components. With maturation the junctional component disappears so that the melanocytes in an 'intradermal' naevus are all in the dermis (Fig. 20.12).

#### Presentation

*Congenital melanocytic naevi* (Figs 20.13 and 20.14) These are present at birth or appear in the neonatal period and are seldom less than 1 cm in diameter. Their colour varies from brown to black or blue–black. With maturity some become protuberant and hairy, with a cerebriform surface. Such lesions can be disfiguring (e.g. a 'bathing trunk' naevus). Congenital melanocytic naevi carry an increased risk of malignant transformation, depending on their size (up to 10% in those with a diameter greater than 40 cm and less than 0.5% in those with a diameter less than 1.5 cm). This risk of developing melanoma appears to be maximum in childhood and adolescence.

*Junctional melanocytic naevi* (Fig. 20.15) These are roughly circular macules. Their colour ranges from mid brown to black and may vary even within a single lesion. Most melanocytic naevi of the palms, soles, mucous membranes and genitals are of this type.

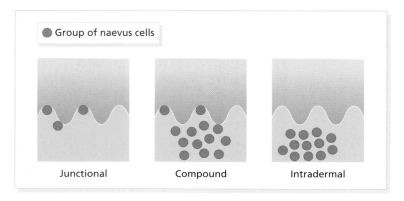

**Fig. 20.12** Types of acquired melanocytic naevi.

**Fig. 20.13** Congenital melanocytic naevus.

**Fig. 20.15** Junctional melanocytic naevus.

**Fig. 20.14** A large hairy congenital melanocytic naevus.

**Fig. 20.16** Compound melanocytic naevus. No recent change.

*Compound melanocytic naevi* (Fig. 20.16) These are domed pigmented nodules of up to 1 cm in diameter. They arise from junctional naevi as melanocytes 'drop off' from the epidermis to form collections of cells in the dermis. They may be light or dark brown but their colour is more even than that of junctional naevi. Most are smooth, but larger ones may be cerebriform, or even hyperkeratotic and papillomatous; many bear hairs.

*Intradermal melanocytic naevi* (Fig. 20.17) These look like compound naevi but are less pigmented and often skin-coloured.

*Spitz naevi* (in the past misleadingly called juvenile melanomas; Fig. 20.18) These are seen most often

**Fig. 20.17** Intradermal melanocytic naevus with numerous shaved hairs.

**Fig. 20.18** Spitz naevus.

in children. They develop over a month or two as solitary pink or red nodules of up to 1 cm in diameter and are most common on the face and legs. Although benign, they are often excised because of their rapid growth.

*Blue naevi* (Fig. 20.19) So-called because of their striking slate grey–blue colour, blue naevi usually appear in childhood and adolescence, on the limbs, buttocks and lower back. They are usually solitary.

**Fig. 20.19** The blue ink matches the blue naevus.

*Mongolian spots* Pigment in dermal melanocytes is responsible for these bruise-like greyish areas seen on the lumbosacral area of most Down's syndrome and many Asian and black babies (Fig. 15.1). They usually fade during childhood.

*Atypical naevus/mole syndrome* (dysplastic naevus syndrome; Fig. 20.20). Clinically atypical melanocytic naevi can occur sporadically or run in families as an autosomal dominant trait, with incomplete penetrance, affecting several generations. Some families

**Fig. 20.20** Atypical moles in a 12-year-old girl. Note the malignant melanoma lying between the scapulae.

with atypical naevi are melanoma prone and in 20% of these, mutations in the cell cycle regulating gene *CDKN2A* on chromosome 9p21 are found. The many large irregularly pigmented naevi are most obvious on the trunk but some may be present on the scalp. Their edges are irregular and they vary greatly in size – many being over 1 cm in diameter. Some are pinkish and an inflamed halo may surround them. Some have a mammillated surface. Patients with multiple atypical melanocytic or dysplastic naevi with a positive family history of malignant melanoma should be followed up 6-monthly for life. Melanomas develop in almost all patients with atypical mole syndrome who have both a parent and sibling with the syndrome and a history of melanoma.

> **Learning point**
>
> Even if you think it is harmless, don't be afraid to refer to a dermatologist a patient with a mole that has changed

## Differential diagnosis of melanocytic naevi

● *Malignant melanomas* This is the most important part of the differential diagnosis. Melanomas are very rare before puberty, single and more variably pigmented and irregularly shaped (other features are listed below under 'Complications').
● *Seborrhoeic keratoses* These can cause confusion in adults but have a stuck-on appearance and are warty. Tell-tale keratin plugs and horny cysts may be seen with the help of a lens or dermatoscope.
● *Lentigines* These may be found on any part of the skin and mucous membranes. More profuse than junctional naevi, they are usually grey–brown rather than black, and develop more often after adolescence.
● *Ephelides* (freckles) These are tan macules less than 5 mm in diameter. They are confined to sun-exposed areas, being most common in blond or red-haired people.
● *Haemangiomas* Benign proliferations of blood vessels, including haemangiomas and pyogenic granulomas, may be confused with a vascular Spitz naevus or an amelanotic melanoma. Dermatoscopy is most helpful in distinguishing from a naevus or melanoma.

## Histology

Most acquired lesions fit into the scheme given in Fig. 20.12: orderly nests of abnormal melanocytes are seen in the junctional region, in the dermis, or in both. However, some types of melanocytic naevi have their own distinguishing features. In congenital naevi, the abnormal melanocytes may extend to the subcutaneous fat, and hyperplasia of other skin components (e.g. hair follicles) may be seen. A Spitz naevus has a histology worryingly similar to that of a melanoma. It shows dermal oedema and dilated capillaries, and is composed of large epithelioid and spindle-shaped melanocytes, some of which may be in mitosis.

In a blue naevus, the abnormal melanocytes are seen in the mid and deep dermis.

The main features of clinically atypical ('dysplastic') naevi are lengthening and bridging of rete ridges, and the presence of junctional nests showing melanocytic dysplasia (nuclear pleomorphism and hyperchromatism). Fibrosis of the papillary dermis and a lymphocytic inflammatory response are also seen.

## Complications

*Inflammation* Pain and swelling are common but are not features of malignant transformation. They are caused by trauma, bacterial folliculitis or a foreign body reaction to hair after shaving or plucking.

*Depigmented halo* (Fig. 20.21) So-called 'halo naevi' are uncommon but benign. There may be vitiligo elsewhere. The naevus in the centre often involutes spontaneously before the halo repigments.

*Malignant change* This is extremely rare except in congenital melanocytic naevi, where the risk has been estimated at 0.5–10% depending on their size (Fig. 20.22 and see above), and in the atypical naevi of melanoma-prone families. It should be considered if the following changes occur in a melanocytic naevus:
● enlargement;
● increased or decreased pigmentation;
● altered shape;
● altered contour;

**Fig. 20.21** Halo naevus.

**Fig. 20.22** Malignant melanoma developing within a congenital melanocytic naevus.

- inflammation;
- ulceration;
- itch; or
- bleeding.

If *changing* lesions are examined carefully, remembering the 'ABCDE' features of malignant melanoma (Table 20.3), few malignant melanomas will be missed.

### Treatment

Excision is needed when:

**Table 20.3** The ABCDE of malignant melanoma.

**A**symmetry
**B**order irregularity
**C**olour variability
**D**iameter greater than 0.5 cm
**E**volution (change)

**Fig. 20.23** Sebaceous naevus of the scalp.

**1** a naevus is unsightly;
**2** malignancy is suspected or is a known risk (e.g. in a large congenital melanocytic naevus); or
**3** a naevus is repeatedly inflamed or traumatized.

### Sebaceous naevus (Fig. 20.23)

A flat hairless area at birth, usually in the scalp, these naevi become more yellow and more raised at puberty. Basal cell carcinomas appear on some in adult life.

### Epidermoid and pilar cysts

Often incorrectly called 'sebaceous cysts', these are common and can occur on the scalp, face, behind the ears and on the trunk. They often have a central punctum; when they rupture or are squeezed, foul-smelling cheesy material comes out. Histologically, the lining of a cyst resembles normal epidermis (an epidermoid cyst) or the outer root sheath of the hair follicle (a pilar cyst). Occasionally, an adjacent foreign body reaction is noted. Treatment is by excision, or by incision followed by expression of the contents and removal of the cyst wall.

**Fig. 20.24** Milia.

**Fig. 20.25** Chondrodermatitis nodularis helicis. The inflammation of the underlying cartilage is painful enough to wake up patients repeatedly at night.

## Milia

Milia are small subepidermal keratin cysts (Fig. 20.24). They are common on the face in all age groups and appear as tiny white millet seed-like papules of 0.5–2 mm in diameter. They are occasionally seen at the site of a previous subepidermal blister (e.g. in epidermolysis bullosa and porphyria cutanea tarda). The contents of milia can be picked out with a sterile needle or pointed scalpel blade (No. 11) without local anaesthesia.

## Chondrodermatitis nodularis helicis (painful nodule of the ear, ear corn; Fig. 20.25)

This terminological mouthful is strictly not a neoplasm but a chronic inflammation. A painful nodule develops on the helix or antehelix of the ear, most often in men. It looks like a small corn, is tender and prevents sleep if that side of the head touches the pillow. Histologically, a thickened epidermis overlies inflamed cartilage. Wedge resection under local anaesthetic is effective if cryotherapy or intralesional triamcinolone injection fails.

## Premalignant tumours

### Actinic keratoses

These discrete rough-surfaced lesions crop up on sun-damaged skin. They are best considered as premalignant. Pathologically there is a case for classifying them as squamous cell carcinomas *in situ* but very few progress to invasive squamous cell carcinomas.

### Cause

The effects of sun exposure are cumulative. Those with fair complexions living near the equator are most at risk and invariably develop these 'sun warts'. A recent UK survey showed that one-third of men over 70 years had actinic keratoses. Melanin protects, and actinic keratoses are not seen in black skin. Conversely, albinos are especially prone to develop them.

### Presentation

They affect the middle-aged and elderly in temperate climates, but younger people in the tropics. The pink or grey rough scaling macules or papules seldom exceed 1 cm in diameter (Fig. 20.26). Their rough surface is sometimes better felt than seen.

### Complications

Transition to an invasive squamous cell carcinoma, although rare, should be suspected if a lesion enlarges, becomes nodular, ulcerates or bleeds. Luckily,

**Fig. 20.26** Typical rough-surfaced actinic keratoses on the scalp.

such tumours seldom metastasize. A 'cutaneous horn' is a hard keratotic protrusion based on an actinic keratosis, a squamous cell papilloma or a viral wart (Fig. 20.4).

### Differential diagnosis

There is usually no difficulty in telling an actinic keratosis from a seborrhoeic wart, a viral wart (p. 235), a keratoacanthoma, an intra-epidermal carcinoma or an invasive squamous cell carcinoma.

### Investigations

A biopsy is needed if there is concern over invasive change.

### Histology

Alternating zones of hyper- and parakeratosis overlie a thickened or atrophic epidermis. The normal maturation pattern of the epidermis may be lost and occasional pleomorphic keratinocytes may be seen. Solar elastosis is seen in the superficial dermis.

### Treatment

Freezing with liquid nitrogen or carbon dioxide snow is simple and effective. Shave removal or curettage is best for large lesions and cutaneous horns. Multiple lesions, including subclinical ones, can be treated with 5-fluorouracil cream (Formulary 1, p. 392) after specialist advice. The cream is applied once or twice daily until there is a marked inflammatory response in the treated area. This takes about 3 weeks and only then should the applications be stopped. Healing is rapid. Most patients dislike the pain and appearance of their faces during treatment but are pleased with their 'new' smooth skin afterwards. Severe discomfort from the treatment may be alleviated by the short-term application of a local steroid. 5-Fluorouracil cream is more effective for keratoses on the face than on the arms. Alternatively, less effective but causing less inflammation, 5-fluorouracil cream can be applied on just 1 or 2 days a week for 8 weeks.

Recently, encouraging results have also been seen with imiquimod, a modulator of innate immunity. It activates Toll-like receptors, causing an immune reaction that destroys abnormal cells. Applied as a cream 2–3 times weekly for 16 weeks, the response is similar to that following 5-fluorouracil, described above. Multiple lesions and even subclinical ones respond to the treatment. 3% Sodium diclofenac made up in a hyaluronate gel creates less havoc but also lower cure rates. Photo-dynamic therapy (p. 377), using aminolaevulinic acid hydrochloride followed by blue light, is effective but requires specialist facilities. Lesions that do not respond should be regarded with suspicion, and biopsied. None of these topical therapies is effective against established malignancy.

> **Learning points**
>
> - Catch lesions early: small ones are easy to get rid of; larger ones can eat into cartilage or bone
> - Don't sit and watch doubtful lesions near the eye

## Malignant epidermal tumours

### Basal cell carcinoma (rodent ulcer)

This is the most common form of skin cancer. It crops up most commonly on the faces of the middle-aged or elderly. Lesions invade locally but, for practical purposes, never metastasize.

## Cause

Prolonged sun exposure is the main factor so these tumours are most common in white people who have lived in sunny areas, high latitudes, or near the equator. They may also occur in scars caused by X-rays, vaccination or trauma. Photosensitizing pitch, tar and oils can act as cocarcinogens with ultraviolet radiation. Previous treatment with arsenic, once present in many 'tonics', predisposes to multiple basal cell carcinomas, often after a lag of many years.

Multiple basal cell carcinomas are found in the naevoid basal cell carcinoma syndrome (Gorlin's syndrome) where they may be associated with palmoplantar pits, jaw cysts and abnormalities of the skull, vertebrae and ribs. The syndrome is inherited as an autosomal dominant trait and is caused by a mutation of the Patched gene, involved in embryonic tissue growth and organization.

## Presentation

*Nodulo-ulcerative* This is the most common type. An early lesion is a small glistening translucent, sometimes umbilicated, skin-coloured papule that slowly enlarges. Central necrosis, although not invariable, leaves an ulcer with an adherent crust and a rolled pearly edge (Fig. 20.27). Coarse telangiectatic vessels often run across the tumour's surface (Fig. 20.28). Without treatment such lesions may reach 1–2 cm in diameter in 5–10 years.

**Fig. 20.28** Basal cell carcinoma with marked telangiectasia and ulceration.

*Cystic* The lesion is at first like the nodular type, but later cystic changes predominate and the nodule becomes tense and more translucent, with marked telangiectasia.

*Cicatricial (morphoeic)* These are slowly expanding yellow or white waxy plaques with an ill-defined edge. Ulceration and crusting, followed by fibrosis, are common, and the lesion may look like an enlarging scar (Fig. 20.29).

*Superficial (multicentric)* These arise most often on the trunk. Several lesions may be present, each expanding slowly as a red, pink or brown scaly irregular thin plaque with a fine 'whipcord' edge (Fig. 20.30). Such lesions can grow to more than 10 cm in diameter.

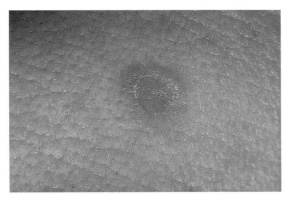

**Fig. 20.27** Early basal cell carcinoma with rolled opalescent edge and central crusting.

**Fig. 20.29** Cicatricial basal cell carcinoma.

**Fig. 20.30** Persistent scaly plaque – the whipcord edge gives away the diagnosis of a superficial basal cell carcinoma.

**Fig. 20.31** A pigmented tumour on the temple. The opalescent rim points to the diagnosis of a basal cell carcinoma.

*Pigmented* Pigment may be present in all types of basal cell carcinoma, causing all or part of the tumour to be brown or have specks of brown or black within it (Fig. 20.31).

**Fig. 20.32** A grossly neglected basal cell carcinoma invading underlying bone.

### Clinical course

The slow but relentless growth destroys tissue locally. Untreated, a basal cell carcinoma can invade underlying cartilage or bone (Fig. 20.32) or damage important structures such as the tear ducts.

### Histology

Small, darkly blue staining basal cells grow in well-defined aggregates which invade the dermis (Fig. 20.33). The outer layer of cells is arranged in a palisade. Numerous mitoses and apoptotic bodies

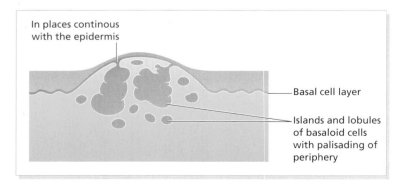

In places continous with the epidermis

Basal cell layer

Islands and lobules of basaloid cells with palisading of periphery

**Fig. 20.33** Histology of nodular basal cell carcinoma.

are seen. In the cicatricial type, the islands of tumour are surrounded by fibrous tissue.

## Differential diagnosis

A nodular basal cell carcinoma may be confused with an intradermal melanocytic naevus, a squamous cell carcinoma, a giant molluscum contagiosum (p. 243), a traumatized benign papule or a keratoacanthomatous squamous cell carcinoma. Pigmented basal cell carcinomas should be distinguished from seborrhoeic warts and malignant melanomas. A cicatricial basal cell carcinoma may mimic morphoea (p. 141) or a scar. A superficial basal cell carcinoma may be confused with an intra-epidermal carcinoma, with psoriasis (Chapter 5) or with nummular eczema (p. 99).

## Treatment

There is no single treatment of choice for all basal cell carcinomas. Treatment should be tailored to the type of tumour, its site and the age and general health of the patient. Surgical wounds closed with sutures generally heal with less apparent scar than those left to heal by secondary intention, and this may be a consideration in the choice of treatment, particularly for tumours on the face and keloid-prone areas. Published guidelines are very useful (see Further reading).

In general, excision, with 0.5 cm of surrounding normal skin, is the treatment of choice for discrete nodular and cystic tumours in patients under 60 years. This can be performed by excising an ellipse of skin containing the tumour and normal margins.

Cicatricial tumours, with their ill-defined edges, and lesions near vital structures should be excised by specialist surgeons. Mohs' micrographic surgery is highly effective; it includes careful histological checks in all planes of tissue excised during the operation (p. 373). Mohs' surgery is also becoming the treatment of choice for large (greater than 1 cm) tumours, and for tumours on cosmetically important sites such as the nose, and for tumours in certain anatomical areas such as the inner canthus or the nasolabial folds.

Radiotherapy is also effective; it is seldom used now for biopsy-proven lesions in patients under 70 years, but is helpful when surgery is contra-

indicated. Cryotherapy, curettage and cautery and photodynamic therapy are sometimes useful for superficial lesions (p. 373). Sometimes treatment with curettage and cautery may be preferable to aggressive treatment for selected tumours and for elderly patients; there is seldom justification for doing nothing. The 5-year cure rate for all types of basal cell carcinoma is over 95% but regular follow-up is advisable to detect local recurrences when they are small and remediable.

## Squamous cell carcinoma

This is a common tumour in which malignant keratinocytes show a variable capacity to form keratin.

## Cause

These tumours often arise in skin damaged by ultraviolet radiation and also by X-rays and chronic inflammation. The majority of squamous cell skin cancers carry typical ultraviolet-induced mutations in the p53 tumour suppressor gene, emphasizing the significant part ultraviolet radiation plays in the development of this cancer. Other carcinogens include pitch, tar, mineral oils and inorganic arsenic (p. 301). Certain rare genetic disorders, with defective DNA repair mechanisms, such as xeroderma pigmentosum (p. 352), lead to multiple squamous and basal cell carcinomas, and to malignant melanoma. The DNA of some types of human papilloma virus (p. 235) can be integrated into the nuclear DNA of keratinocytes and cause malignant transformation. Immunosuppression and ultraviolet radiation predispose to this.

Multiple self-healing squamous cell carcinomas are found in the autosomal dominant trait described by Ferguson-Smith. The abnormal gene lies on chromosome 9q.

## Clinical presentation and course

Tumours may arise as thickenings in an actinic keratosis or, *de novo*, as small scaling nodules; rapidly growing anaplastic lesions may start as ulcers with a granulating base and an indurated edge (Fig. 20.34). Squamous cell carcinomas are common on the lower lip (Fig. 13.36) and in the mouth. Tumours

**Fig. 20.34** Squamous cell carcinoma. Not a venous ulcer – too high up the leg, too raised and no signs of venous insufficiency.

arising in chronic draining sinuses, chronic ulcers, areas of previous X-radiation or thermal injury, or chronic inflammation are the most likely to metastasize. Tumours arising in non-exposed sites, such as the perineum and sole of foot and on the ear and lip may metastasize. Squamous cell carcinomas arising in sun-exposed areas and in actinic keratoses seldom metastasize except in immunosuppressed patients. Tumours more than 2 cm in diameter are twice as likely to recur and metastasize compared with smaller tumours. Metastatic potential is also high in tumours greater than 4 mm in depth or invading to the subcutaneous tissue, in poorly differentiated tumours; in tumours with perineural involvement; and in those arising in the immunosuppressed, such as recipients of solid organ transplants.

### Histology

Keratinocytes disrupt the dermo-epidermal junction and proliferate irregularly into the dermis. Malignant cells usually retain the capacity to produce keratin (Fig. 20.35).

### Treatment

After the diagnosis has been confirmed by biopsy, low-risk tumours should be excised with a 0.5-cm border of normal skin. Wider excision (6 mm or more) or Mohs' micrographic surgery is recommended for high-risk tumours. Sometimes keratin stains are used to help track perineural spread. Sentinel lymph node examination is usually not recommended, but palpation of regional nodes is important in work-up and follow-up. Radiotherapy is effective but should be reserved for the frail and elderly and special situations. Follow-up for up to 5 years is recommended for patients with recurrent disease and for those with high-risk tumours.

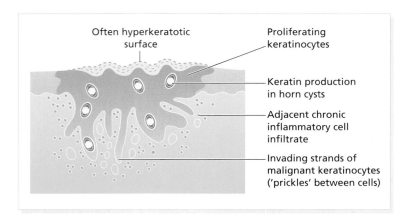

Often hyperkeratotic surface

Proliferating keratinocytes

Keratin production in horn cysts

Adjacent chronic inflammatory cell infiltrate

Invading strands of malignant keratinocytes ('prickles' between cells)

**Fig. 20.35** The histology of a squamous cell carcinoma.

**Fig. 20.36** Intra-epidermal carcinoma: a slowly expanding warty plaque. Note the reniform projections and notches so suggestive of an *in situ* malignancy.

## Other types of squamous cell carcinoma

### Intra-epidermal squamous cell carcinoma (Bowen's disease)

Usually single, these slowly expanding pink scaly plaques (Fig. 20.36) take years to reach a diameter of a few centimetres. Their border is sharply defined, with reniform projections and notches giving them an amoeboid shape. About 3% progress into an invasive squamous cell carcinoma. The presence of several may be a clue to previous exposure to carcinogens (e.g. excessive sun exposure, arsenic in a tonic when young).

### Differential diagnosis

An intra-epidermal squamous cell carcinoma is often mistaken for psoriasis (Chapter 5), discoid eczema (p. 99), superficial basal cell carcinoma (p. 301) or for Paget's disease in the perianal region.

### Treatment

These lesions are unaffected by local steroids. Small lesions may occasionally be left under observation in the frail and elderly. Cryotherapy or curettage are the treatments of choice for small lesions on a site where healing should be good (e.g. face or trunk); excision is an alternative. Photodynamic therapy (p. 377) is useful for large lesions on a poorly healing site (e.g. the lower legs of the elderly). Topical 5-fluorouracil or imiquimod is helpful for multiple lesions (see Guidelines in Further reading).

### Keratoacanthomatous squamous cell carcinoma

These rapidly growing squamous cell tumours do not invade and occasionally resolve spontaneously.

### Cause

Photosensitizing chemicals such as tar and mineral oils can act as cocarcinogens with ultraviolet radiation. They may also follow therapeutic immunosuppression.

### Clinical features

They occur mainly on the exposed skin of fair individuals. More than two-thirds are on the face and most of the rest are on the arms. The lesion starts as a pink papule that rapidly enlarges; it may reach a diameter of 1 cm in a month or two. After 5–6 weeks the centre of the nodule forms either a keratinous plug or a crater (Fig. 20.37). If left, the lesion may resolve spontaneously over 6–12 months leaving an ugly depressed scar.

**Fig. 20.37** Keratoacanthomatous squamous cell carcinoma with its epidermal shoulders and central plug of keratin.

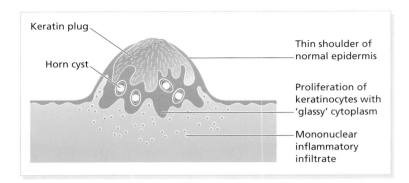

**Fig. 20.38** Histology of keratoacanthomatous squamous cell carcinoma.

Labels in figure: Keratin plug; Horn cyst; Thin shoulder of normal epidermis; Proliferation of keratinocytes with 'glassy' cytoplasm; Mononuclear inflammatory infiltrate

## Histology

It is not possible to diagnose a keratoacanthomatous squamous cell carcinoma histologically unless the architecture of the whole lesion can be assessed, including its base (Fig. 20.38). A typical lesion is symmetrical and composed of proliferating fronds of epidermis that show mitotic activity but retain a well-differentiated squamous appearance with the production of much 'glassy' keratin. The centre of the cup-shaped mass is filled with keratin, and invasion of the malignant cells into the deeper dermis does not occur.

## Treatment

Excision or curettage and cautery are both effective. Occasionally, a further curetting may be needed but this should be performed only once; if this is still ineffective, the lesion must be excised with a narrow margin of surrounding skin.

## Malignant melanoma

Malignant melanoma attracts a huge amount of publicity because it is so often lethal. However, still too many members of the public are unaware of its increasing incidence and dangers.

## Incidence

The incidence in white people in the UK and USA is doubling every 10 years. In Scotland and northern parts of the USA the incidence is now about 10 per 100 000 per year, with females being affected more often than males. There is a higher incidence in white people living near the equator than in temperate zones and there the female preponderance is lost. The highest incidence, more than 40 per 100 000 per year, is seen in white people living in Australia and New Zealand. The tumour is rare before puberty and in black people, Asians and Orientals and when it does occur in these races it is most often on the palms, soles or mucous membranes.

## Cause

### Genetic

● *Susceptibility genes* Rarely (around 6%), melanomas are familial, occurring in families where two or more first-degree relatives have a melanoma. Molecular defects in both tumour suppressor genes and oncogenes have been linked to these melanomas; the one attracting most interest at present lies on chromosome 9p and encodes a tumour suppressor gene designated p16, also known as *CDKN2A*. Mutations in *CDKN2A* confer on carriers a risk of melanoma of 20% by the age of 40 years and 40% by 60 years. Other high-risk susceptibility genes include *CDK4* and an unidentified one on a locus on chromosome 1p22. The more melanomas there are in a single family, the more likely they are brought about by a high-risk susceptibility gene. If just two members in a family have a melanoma then they are more likely to be caused by low-risk susceptibility genes interacting with phenotypic (e.g. red hair and freckles) and environmental factors (e.g. sunlight).

● *Susceptible phenotypes* Malignant melanomas are most common in white people with blond or red hair, many freckles and a fair skin that tans poorly.

Those of Celtic origin are especially susceptible. Melanoma can affect several members of a single family in association with atypical (dysplastic) naevi (p. 296).

*Sunlight* Both the incidence and mortality increase with decreasing latitude. Tumours occur most often, but not exclusively, on exposed skin. Episodic exposure of fair-skinned individuals to intense sunlight is thought to be the main cause of the steadily increasing incidence of melanoma worldwide. For melanomas, the number of sunburns seems more relevant than cumulative ultraviolet radiation dose.

*Pre-existing melanocytic naevi* The risk of developing a malignant melanoma is highest in those with atypical naevi, congenital melanocytic naevi or many banal melanocytic naevi. A pre-existing naevus is seen histologically in about 30% of malignant melanomas.

## Prevention and early diagnosis

Every photon of sunlight that hits the skin has a chance to provoke a cancer-causing mutation so protection of skin from ultraviolet radiation is critical. This is best done by avoiding exposure of skin to sunlight and tanning booths. Dermatologists joke that the best sunscreen is a house. Tight-weave clothing, hats and sunscreens reduce exposure but may provide a false sense of security. Although sunscreens help, avoidance of excessive sun exposure is better. The skin protection factor (SPF) of a sunscreen or sunblock is the ratio of the time it takes to sunburn skin protected by sunscreen divided by the time it takes to sunburn adjacent unprotected skin. The amount of sunscreen applied to get these ratios is the volume of a golf ball. Most sunscreen users apply much less, and apply sunscreen only when outdoor activities are planned. If every photon counts, sunscreen should be applied to sun-exposed skin every day. When golf, tennis, sailing or other outdoor activity beckons, a sunscreen of SPF 15 or more should be used and reapplied after 20 min to add a second coat and to catch missed areas. The sunscreen should be reapplied during the day, by those living in sunny climates especially because it washes off with swimming or sweating. Ideally, sunscreens should block both UVA and UVB.

Early diagnosis is critical and there is now ample evidence that melanoma publicity campaigns, regular self-examination and the education of primary care physicians have all played their part in reducing the mortality rate from melanoma.

## Clinical features

Eighty per cent of invasive melanomas are preceded by a superficial and radial growth phase, shown clinically as the expansion of an irregularly pigmented macule or plaque (Fig. 20.39). Most are multicoloured mixtures of black, brown, blue, tan and pink. Their margins are irregular with reniform projections and notches. Malignant cells are at first usually confined to the epidermis and uppermost dermis, but eventually invade more deeply and may metastasize (Fig. 20.39).

There are four main types of malignant melanoma.
1 *Lentigo maligna melanoma* occurs on the exposed skin of the elderly. An irregularly pigmented, irregularly shaped macule (a lentigo maligna) may have been enlarging slowly for many years as an *in situ* melanoma before an invasive nodule (the lentigo maligna melanoma) appears (Fig. 20.40).
2 *Superficial spreading melanoma* is the most common type in Caucasoids. Its radial growth phase shows varied colours and is often palpable (Figs 20.41 and 20.42). A nodule coming up within such a plaque signifies deep dermal invasion and a poor prognosis (Table 20.4).
3 *Acral lentiginous melanoma* (Fig. 14.12) occurs on the palms and soles and, although rare in Caucasoids, is the most common type in Chinese and Japanese people. The invasive phase is again signalled by a nodule coming up within an irregularly pigmented macule or patch.
4 *Nodular melanoma* (Fig. 20.43) appears as a pigmented nodule with no preceding *in situ* phase. It is the most rapidly growing and aggressive type.

Melanomas can also described by their colour, site and degree of spread.
● *Totally amelanotic melanomas* (Fig. 20.44) are rare and occur especially on the soles of the feet. Flecks of pigment can usually be seen with a lens. Desmoplastic melanomas are rare. They are seen most often on the head, neck, palms and soles. They are sometimes amelanotic.

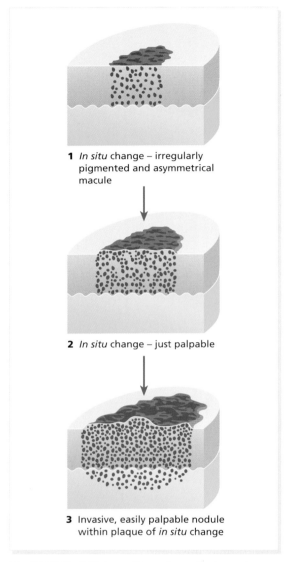

**1** *In situ* change – irregularly pigmented and asymmetrical macule

**2** *In situ* change – just palpable

**3** Invasive, easily palpable nodule within plaque of *in situ* change

**Fig. 20.39** Radial intra-epidermal growth phase of melanoma (1 and 2) precedes vertical and invasive dermal growth phase (3).

**Fig. 20.40** This elderly patient, her friends and family doctor had ignored for too long the slowly spreading macule of a lentigo maligna: now she has a frankly invasive melanoma within it (the darker area).

**Fig. 20.41** Superficial spreading melanoma of the jawline. Small, and still curable at this stage.

• *Subungual melanomas* are painless areas of pigmentation expanding under the nail and onto the nail fold (Hutchinson's sign Fig. 14.13).
• *Metastatic melanoma* has spread to surrounding skin, regional lymph nodes or to other organs. At this stage it can rarely be cured.

## Staging

The most popular staging systems for melanoma are the TNM classification (tumour, node, metastasis; Europe) and the American Joint Committee on Cancer (AJCC) system in the USA (Table 20.4). Both

**Table 20.4** Staging systems for melanoma.

| TNM stage | AJCC stage | Breslow thickness (mm) | 5-year survival (%) |
|---|---|---|---|
| I | Ia | Up to 0.75 | 95 |
| | Ib | 0.76–1.5 | 85 |
| II | IIa | 1.51–4.0 | 65 |
| III | IIb | >4.0 | 45 |
| | III | Nodal disease | 40 |
| IV | IV | Metastatic disease | <10 |

AJCC, American Joint Committee on Cancer; TNM, tumour, node, metastasis.

**Fig. 20.42** This shows the hallmarks of a malignant melanoma with its asymmetry, irregular borders and variations in colour. The pink amelanotic nodule signifies deep dermal invasion.

**Fig. 20.43** A nodular malignant melanoma: just beginning to ulcerate.

**Fig. 20.44** An amelanotic malignant melanoma on the heel of an elderly person. Always obtain histology even if you think it is just a pyogenic granuloma or an atypical wart.

have been refined recently to include ulceration of the tumour and micrometastases in nodes but Table 20.4 gives an idea of the broad categories of each classification. The systems provide a useful guide to prognosis (Table 20.5).

*Histology*

- *Lentigo maligna* Numerous atypical melanocytes, many in groups, are seen along the basal layer extending downwards in the walls of hair follicles.
- *Lentigo maligna melanoma* Dermal invasion occurs, with a breach of the basement membrane region. *In situ* changes are seen in the adjacent epidermis.
- *Superficial spreading melanoma in situ* Large epithelioid melanoma cells permeate the epidermis.
- *Superficial spreading melanoma* The dermal nodule

**Table 20.5** Prognostic indicators in malignant melanoma.

| Indicator | Significance |
| --- | --- |
| Depth of primary tumour | Breslow<br><0.75 mm, 5-year survival 95%<br>0.76–1.5 mm, 5-year survival 85%<br>1.51–4.0 mm, 5-year survival 65%<br>>4.0 mm, 5-year survival 45% |
| Sex | Females do better than males |
| Age | Prognosis worsens after 50 years of age, especially in males |
| Site | The prognosis is poor for tumours on trunk, upper arms, neck and scalp |
| Ulceration | Signifies a poor prognosis |
| Sentinel node | Prognosis worsens with tumour-positive sentinel node |
| Clinical stage | Prognosis worsens with advancing stage (see Table 20.4) |

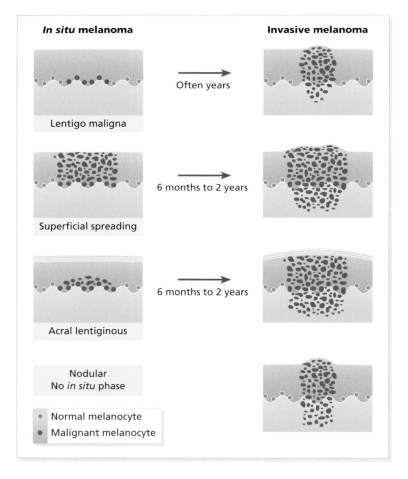

**Fig. 20.45** Histology of the different types of melanoma.

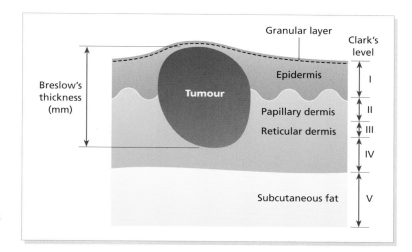

**Fig. 20.46** Schematic representation of Breslow's and Clark's methods of microstaging malignant melanoma.

may be composed of epithelioid cells, spindle cells or naevus-like cells. *In situ* changes are seen in the adjacent epidermis.

- *Acral lentiginous melanoma in situ* Atypical melanocytes are seen in the base of the epidermis and permeating the mid epidermis.
- *Acral lentiginous melanoma* Melanoma cells invade the dermis. *In situ* changes are seen in the adjacent epidermis.
- *Nodular melanoma* The tumour comprises epithelioid, spindle and naevoid cells and there is no *in situ* melanoma in the adjacent epidermis.
- *Desmoplastic melanoma* Melanoma cells are seen amongst a dense fibrous stroma. The overlying epidermis may show signs of a preceding lentigo maligna or acral lentiginous melanoma *in situ*.

## Microstaging

The histology (Fig. 20.45) can be used to assess prognosis. Breslow's method is to measure, with an ocular micrometer, the vertical distance from the granular cell layer to the deepest part of the tumour. Clark's method, used less frequently nowadays, is to assess the depth of penetration of the melanoma in relation to the different layers of the dermis (Fig. 20.46). The thicker and more penetrating a lesion, the worse is its prognosis (see below).

## Differential diagnosis

This includes a melanocytic naevus, seborrhoeic keratosis, pigmented actinic keratosis, lentigo, pigmented basal cell carcinoma and sclerosing haemangioma; all are discussed in this chapter. A malignant melanoma can also be confused with a subungual or periungual haematoma (see Fig. 13.21). A history of trauma helps here, as may paring. 'Talon noir' (Fig. 20.47) is a pigmented petechial area on the heel following minor trauma from ill-fitting training shoes. An amelanotic melanoma is most often confused with a pyogenic granuloma and with a squamous cell carcinoma. Dermatoscopy (p. 39), in experienced hands, helps to distinguish the above but doubtful lesions should be removed without delay for histological examination.

## Prognosis

The prognostic indicators, and their significance, are listed in Table 20.5. They have been established by following up large numbers of patients who have undergone appropriate surgical treatment (p. 312). As a general rule, the prognosis for those patients with non-ulcerated superficial melanomas, less than 1 mm in thickness, is excellent.

**Fig. 20.47** Talon noir.

**Fig. 20.48** Such a wide excision and unsightly graft is no longer acceptable for a thin good-prognosis melanoma. Note the many atypical moles.

## Treatment

*Surgery* Surgical excision, with minimal delay, is required. An excision biopsy, with a 2–5 mm margin of clearance laterally and down to the subcutaneous fat, is recommended for all suspicious lesions. Shave and punch biopsies are not recommended, but can be performed if the lesion is in a cosmetically sensitive site. Punch biopies can lead to a sampling error, and rob the pathologist of the chance to evaluate architecture and malignant changes elsewhere in the tumour. They do not provoke metastasis. Shave biopsies may not include the deep margin, making it difficult to gauge prognosis, and superficial shave biopsies may be misdiagnosed. If the histology confirms the diagnosis of malignant melanoma then wider excision, including the wound of the excision biopsy, should be performed as soon as possible. A minimum of 0.5 cm clearance for melanomas *in situ* and 1 cm clearance is required for all invasive melanomas. Nowadays many surgeons excise 1 cm of normal skin around the tumour (or wound) for every millimetre of tumour thickness, up to 3 mm (Fig. 20.48). The maximum clearance is thus 3 cm of normal skin and, depending on the site, primary closure – without grafting – is often possible. There is no convincing evidence that excision margins wider than 3 cm confer any greater survival advantage. Tissue is removed down to but not including the deep fascia. The guidelines of the British Association of Dermatologists (see Further Reading at the end of this chapter) differ minimally from this simple advice.

If lymph node involvement is suspected clinically then the initial investigation should be with fine needle aspiration. If involvement is confirmed then formal block dissection of the involved group of nodes should be carried out.

The role of sentinel node biopsy in detecting occult nodal metastases remains under investigation. The aim is to carry out elective dissection of the local nodes in positive cases, but avoid this significant procedure when the sentinel node is not involved. The sentinel node, the first and often nearest local node in the lymphatic drainage of the tumour, is detected by a blue dye and a radiolabelled colloid injected intradermally around the tumour before excision. This node is excised and examined histologically for metastases including micrometastases.

If metastases are found, the entire lymph node basin is removed. Although knowing the sentinel lymph node status of a patient helps define prognosis, it offers little if any clinical benefit in terms of enhanced survival. There is little evidence to support elective regional node dissection in the management of clinically node-negative patients with tumours of intermediate thickness (1.5–4.0 mm).

*Adjunctive therapies*  Surgery cures most patients with early melanoma, but its effect on survival lessens as the disease advances. The results of ongoing controlled trials, investigating the role of immunotherapy (e.g. with melanoma-specific antigen vacccines) as an adjunct to surgery in patients with poor prognostic (e.g. TNM stages II and III) melanomas, are awaited with interest. The role of α-interferon as adjuvant treatment remains controversial.

*Chemotherapy*  Although rarely curative, chemotherapy may be palliative in 25% of patients with stage III melanoma. Dacarbazine is often the drug of choice.

## Follow-up care

Patients who have had melanoma should be screened for recurrence and for metastases. Recurrence usually appears as a growth or pigmentation at the original site. In transit melanomas are satellite nodules nearby but not connected to the original tumour. The regional nodal basins should be palpated, but chest X-rays and special scans are not routinely necessary unless there are suspicious symptoms. Desmoplastic melanomas tend to skip the nodes and metastasize directly to the lungs. Eighty percent of recurrent and/or metastatic melanomas occur within 3 years of definitive surgery. Unfortunately, a 5-year melanoma-free follow-up is not a guarantee of cure; 5–8% of metastatic melanoma are discovered after 5 years. A second primary melanoma is not unusual, so general examination of the skin is recommended at follow-up.

*Oral contraceptives and hormone replacement therapy*  These are not contraindicated in patients who have had a melanoma. The risk of subsequent pregnancy on the outcome of melanoma is not known.

> ### Learning points
>
> - Prevention of a malignant melanoma is better than cure. Remember avoidance of sun exposure and 'sun smart' advice to patients
> - Everyone, and especially those with many moles, should be encouraged to examine their own skin regularly
> - Take any change in a mole seriously
> - Don't forget the ABCDE rules when querying a melanoma (Table 20.3)
> - Excise all doubtful lesions and check their histology
> - If excision biopsy shows that an invasive melanoma is less than 1 mm thick, the only question to be asked is whether it has been excised with 1 cm clearance in all directions
> - Support campaigns to educate doctors and the public to recognize melanoma early, in its superficial and curable phase

## Paget's disease of the nipple (apocrine ductal carcinoma) (Fig. 20.49)

A well-defined red scaly plaque spreads slowly over and around the nipple. It is caused by the invasion of the epidermis by cells from an underlying intraductal carcinoma of the breast (Paget cells). The condition is sharply marginated and unilateral, whereas eczemas are usually poorly marginated and affect both nipples. A skin biopsy should be carried out first and if the diagnosis is confirmed mastectomy will be necessary. Extramammary Paget's disease affects other sites bearing apocrine glands (p. 176) and is caused by an underlying ductal

**Fig. 20.49** Be alert to the possibility of Paget's disease if a red plaque affects only one nipple, and alters its normal architecture.

carcinoma of these. The perineum is the next most common site after the breast.

## Tumours of the dermis

### Benign dermal tumours

#### *Developmental abnormalities of blood vessels*

These are either present at birth or appear soon after. They can be classified clinically (Table 20.6) but there is no good clinico-histological correlation. A capillary malformation is composed of a network of capillaries in the upper and mid dermis. A capillary cavernous haemangioma has multiple ectatic channels of varying calibre distributed throughout the dermis and even the subcutaneous fat.

#### *Malformations*

*'Salmon' patches ('stork bites')* These common malformations, present in about 50% of all babies, are caused by dilatated capillaries in the superficial dermis. They are dull red, often telangiectatic macules, most commonly on the nape of the neck ('erythema nuchae'), the forehead and the upper eyelids. Nuchal lesions may remain unchanged, but patches in other areas usually disappear within a year.

*'Port-wine' stains* These are also present at birth and are caused by dilatated dermal capillaries. They are

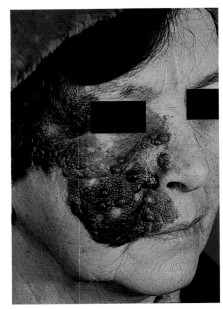

**Fig. 20.50** Lifelong capillary malformation of the cheek showing no tendency to resolve. Note port-wine appearance of the upper pole, contrasting with the nodular elements elsewhere.

pale, pink–purple macules, and vary from the barely noticeable to the grossly disfiguring. Most occur on the face or trunk. They persist, and in middle age may darken and become studded with angiomatous nodules (Fig. 20.50). Occasionally, a port-wine stain of the trigeminal area (Fig. 20.51) is associated with a vascular malformation of the leptomeninges on the same side, which may cause epilepsy or hemiparesis (the Sturge–Weber syndrome), or with glaucoma.

Excellent results have been obtained with careful – and time-consuming – treatment with a 585 nm flashlamp-pumped pulsed dye laser (p. 379). Treatment sessions can begin in babies and anaesthesia is not always necessary. If a trial patch is satisfactory, 40–50 pulses can be delivered in a session and the procedure can be repeated at monthly intervals. Alternatively, some adults become very adept at using cosmetic camouflage (see Fig. 1.6).

*Combined vascular malformations of the limbs* A large port-wine stain of a limb may be associated with overgrowth of all the soft tissues of that limb with or

**Table 20.6** Common vascular naevi.

*Malformations*
Present at birth. Do not involute ('salmon' patch is exception)
1 Capillary ('salmon' patch and 'port-wine' stain)
2 Arterial
3 Venous
4 Combined

*Haemangiomas* (sometimes called angiomatous naevi)
Usually appear after birth. More common in females, 50–60% on head and neck. Involute by 5–9 years after initial proliferation
1 Superficial (capillary)
2 Deep (cavernous)
3 Mixed

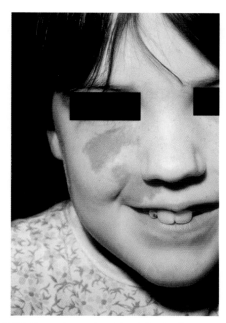

**Fig. 20.51** Port-wine stain of the right cheek. No neurological problems in this patient.

**Fig. 20.52** Classic strawberry naevus, occurred and enlarged rapidly shortly after birth.

**Fig. 20.53** The same strawberry naevus as shown in Fig. 20.52, showing the whitening of the surface which is a sign of spontaneous remission.

without bony hypertrophy. There may be underlying venous malformations (Klippel–Trenaunay syndrome), arteriovenous fistulae (Parkes Weber syndrome) or mixed venous–lymphatic malformations.

### Haemangiomas

*Capillary cavernous haemangioma (strawberry naevus)*
Strawberry naevi appear within a few weeks of birth and grow for a few months, forming a raised compressible swelling with a bright red surface (Fig. 20.52). Spontaneous regression then follows; the surface whitens centrally (Fig. 20.53) and regression is complete by the age of 5 years in 50% of children and in 90% by the age of 9 years, leaving only an area of slight atrophy. Bleeding may follow trauma, and ulceration is common in the napkin (diaper) area.

Observation and encouragement is the management of choice for the great majority. Serial photographs of the way they clear up in other children help parents to accept this. Firm pressure may be needed to stop bleeding. If lesions ulcerate, bleed repeatedly, interfere with feeding or with vision, or

if giant lesions sequestrate platelets (the Kasabach–Merritt syndrome), high doses of systemic steroids should be considered; they are most successful in the proliferative phase. Prednisolone (2–4 mg/kg/day) is given as a single dose in the morning and the dosage tapered to zero after 1 month. Corticosteroid treatment is covered with a H2 blocker such as ranitidine. Ophthalmological help should be sought for all growing periocular haemangiomas; intralesional steroids have proved effective. Sometimes pulsed tuneable dye lasers are used for treating large lesions in infancy. Rarely, plastic surgery is necessary for a few large and unsightly haemangiomas that fail to improve spontaneously or to regress with the above measures.

**Fig. 20.54** Campbell de Morgan spots (cherry angiomas) of the chest.

**Fig. 20.55** Pyogenic granuloma of the palm: soggy after Elastoplast dressing and bleeding easily.

*Campbell de Morgan spots (cherry angiomas)* These benign angiomas are common on the trunks of the middle-aged and elderly. They are small bright red papules and of no consequence (Fig. 20.54).

*Lymphangiomas* The most common type is lymphangioma circumscriptum which appears as a cluster of vesicles resembling frog spawn. If treatment is needed, excision has to be wide and deep as dilated lymphatic channels and cisterns extend to the subcutaneous tissue.

*Glomus tumours* These are derived from the cells surrounding small arteriovenous shunts. Solitary lesions are painful and most common on the extremities and under the nails. Multiple lesions are seldom painful and may affect other parts of the body. Painful lesions can be removed; others may be left.

*Pyogenic granulomas* These badly named lesions are in fact common benign acquired haemangiomas, often seen in children and young adults. They develop at sites of trauma, over the course of a few weeks, as bright red raised, sometimes pedunculated and raspberry-like lesions which bleed easily (Fig. 20.55).

The important differential diagnosis is from an amelanotic malignant melanoma and, for this reason, the histology should always be checked. A pyogenic granuloma shows leashes of vessels of varying calibre covered by a thin, often ulcerated, epidermis.

Lesions should be removed by curettage under local anaesthetic with cautery to the base. Rarely, this is followed by recurrence or an eruption of satellite lesions around the original site.

## Other benign dermal tumours

### Dermatofibromas (histiocytomas)

These benign tumours are firm, discrete, usually solitary dermal nodules (Fig. 20.56), often on the

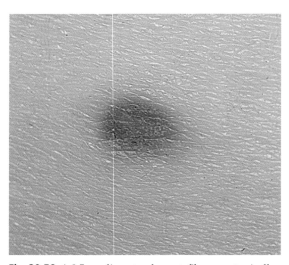

**Fig. 20.56** A 0.5 cm diameter dermatofibroma – typically these lesions feel larger than they look. Its depressed surface became more obvious when the surrounding skin was pinched.

extremities of young adults. The lesions have an 'iceberg' effect in that they feel larger than they look. The overlying epidermis is often lightly pigmented and dimples when the nodule is squeezed. Some lesions seem to follow minor trauma or an insect bite. Histologically, the proliferating fibroblasts merge into the sparsely cellular dermis at the margins. A straightforward lesion may be left alone but, if there is any diagnostic doubt, it should be excised.

### Neurofibromas

Although solitary tumours occur occasionally, multiple neurofibromas are most common and are usually seen as part of the inherited condition of neurofibromatosis. The clinical features of the tumour are described on p. 350.

### Neuroma

This rare benign tumour is usually solitary. It may appear spontaneously but is seen most often as a result of nerve injury at the site of trauma or a surgical wound. There is nothing specific about the appearance of the skin-coloured dermal nodule but the tumour is frequently painful, even with gentle pressure. ENGLAND is a useful acronym for painful tumours (eccrine spiradenoma, neuroma, glomus tumour, leiomyoma, angiolipoma, neurofibroma (rarely) and dermatofibroma (rarely)).

### Keloid (see also pp. 212–213)

This is an overgrowth of dense fibrous tissue in the skin, arising in response to trauma, however trivial. The tendency to develop keloids is genetically inherited. Keloids are common in Negroids and may be familial. Keloid formation is encouraged by infection, foreign material and by wounds (including surgical ones), especially those not lying along the lines of least tension or the skin creases. Even in Caucasoids, keloids and hypertrophic scars are seen often enough on the presternal area, the neck, upper back and deltoid region of young adults to make doctors think twice before removing benign lesions there. Silicone sheeting and intralesional steroid injections are helpful but treatment should be given early, preferably for developing lesions.

**Fig. 20.57** Multiple lipomas.

### Lipomas

Lipomas are common benign tumours of mature fat cells in the subcutaneous tissue. There may be one or many (Fig. 20.57) and lipomas are rarely a familial trait. They are most common on the proximal parts of the limbs but can occur at any site. They have an irregular lobular shape and a characteristic soft rubbery consistency. They are rarely painful. They need to be removed only if there is doubt about the diagnosis or if they are painful, unsightly or interfere with activities such as sitting back against a chair.

### Lymphocytoma cutis

This small dermal nodule is caused by reactive proliferation of B lymphocytes. The purplish lesions may be single or multiple or grouped and are found usually on the face. Some may follow insect bites, scabies nodules and tattoos. If spontaneous regression does not occur, intralesional corticosteroid injection may help.

### Mastocytosis (urticaria pigmentosa)

This term describes the various conditions in which the skin, and occasionally other tissues, contains an excess of mast cells. All types are characterized by a tendency for the skin to wheal after being rubbed (Darier's sign). The main types are as follows.
- *Mastocytoma* Usually presents as a solitary pink or brown itchy papule which wheals on rubbing. There are no systemic features.

**Fig. 20.58** Juvenile type of mastocytosis.

● *Juvenile mastocytosis*  This is the most common type. Numerous pink or brown papules develop over the trunk and limbs (Fig. 20.58). There is no systemic involvement, and the condition is often mistaken for multiple melanocytic naevi.

● *Diffuse cutaneous mastocytosis*  This is rare and seen mostly in infants, being characterized by persistent dermographic wheals that appear after minor friction. The skin is diffusely infiltrated with mast cells, producing a thickened appearance like pigskin. The bone marrow, liver and spleen may be involved. Flushing is common. Death from massive histamine release is a real risk. Spontaneous improvement usually occurs.

● *Adult type*  Pink or pink–brown telangiectatic macules appear in early adult life and can spread to cover the whole body. The liver, spleen and bone are involved in up to 20% of cases but systemic features such as headaches, flushing and palpitations are unusual. Serum tryptase levels correlate with systemic mast cell burden.

## Malignant dermal tumours

### Kaposi's sarcoma

This malignant tumour of proliferating capillaries and lymphatics may be multifocal. There are two types: the classic, and that associated with immunosuppression. Human herpes virus type 8 (HHV8) has been isolated from, and linked to, both types.

*Classic Kaposi's sarcoma* is seen most often in Africans and in elderly Jews of European origin. The tumours are usually on the feet and ankles but may be seen on the hands and on cold parts of the skin (e.g. the ears and nose). Initially, they are dark blue–purple macules progressing to tumours and plaques which ulcerate and fungate. The rate of spread is variable but often slow. Tumours may metastasize to lymph nodes and spread to internal organs; oedema of the legs may be severe.

These tumours are very sensitive to radiotherapy which is the treatment of choice during the early stages; chemotherapy, with chlorambucil or vinblastine, helps when there is systemic involvement. Life expectancy is 5–9 years.

*Kaposi's sarcoma and immunosuppression* (see Figs 16.32–16.34) Smaller and more subtle (e.g. bruise-like) lesions may occur in an immunodeficient host. This tumour has become well known because of its association with AIDS (p. 244) caused by the human immunodeficiency virus (HIV-1). Lesions of AIDS-related Kaposi's sarcoma can appear anywhere but are most common on the upper trunk and head and neck. The initial bruise-like lesions tend to follow tension lines; they become raised, increasingly pigmented and evolve into nodules and plaques. Lesions frequently arise on the oral mucous membranes. The observation in the early years of the AIDS pandemic that HIV-positive intravenous drug abusers did not develop Kaposi's sarcoma as often as did HIV-positive homosexuals is now explained by the discovery that an infectious agent (HHV8) is an important cause. The prognosis of AIDS patients with Kaposi's sarcoma used to be poor, with most developing opportunistic infections and having a life expectancy of around 1 year. The advent of highly active antiretroviral therapy (HAART) has changed this and even multiple lesions of HIV-associated Kaposi's sarcoma usually resolve with this treatment.

> **Learning points**
>
> ● Early Kaposi's sarcomas often look trivial but odd in those with immunosuppression. Keep HIV in mind
> ● Turn back to page 317 if you can't remember which benign nodules are painful

## Lymphomas and leukaemias

The latest (2005) WHO-EORTC classification (see Further reading) is too detailed for most non-specialists. These conditions are rare and it is convenient to group skin involvement in them into two broad categories.

1 Disorders that arise in the skin or preferentially involve it:

- cutaneous T-cell lymphoma (mycosis fungoides) and its variants: subcutaneous panniculitis-like T-cell lymphoma, anaplastic large cell CD30[+] lymphoma, granulomatous slack skin, pagetoid reticulosis and folliculotrophic mycosis fungoides;
- Sézary syndrome;
- lymphoma associated with HIV infection.

2 Those arising extracutaneously, but that sometimes involve the skin:

- Hodgkin's disease;
- B-cell lymphoma;
- leukaemia.

### *Cutaneous T-cell lymphoma (CTCL; sometimes called mycosis fungoides)*

This lymphoma of skin-associated helper T lymphocytes usually evolves slowly. There are three clinical phases: the patch, plaque and tumour stages, with involvement of lymph nodes and other tissues occurring late in the disease.

The *patch stage* (formerly termed 'premycotic' to denote an early phase of mycosis fungoides) may last for years (see Fig. 6.9). Most commonly it consists of scattered, barely palpable, erythematous, slightly pigmented, sharply marginated, scaly patches rather like psoriasis or seborrhoeic dermatitis (p. 97). Often they have a bizarre outline (e.g. arciform or horseshoe-shaped) and, on close inspection, atrophy with surface wrinkling is usually evident. Their distribution is usually asymmetrical. Less commonly, the patch stage can be a widespread poikiloderma, with atrophy, pigmentation and telangiectasia (Fig. 20.59). As the lymphoma develops, some patches become indurated and palpable: *the plaque stage*. Some then turn into frank tumours which may become large (occasionally like mushrooms, hence the term 'mycosis fungoides') and ulcerate (Fig. 20.60). The patch stage of CTCL may be difficult to diagnose clinically, but the plaque and

**Fig. 20.59** Poikiloderma vasculare atrophicans may be a precursor of the tumour stage of cutaneous T-cell lymphoma (CTCL).

**Fig. 20.60** An ulcerated tumour of mycosis fungoides against a background of plaques.

tumour stages are usually characteristic. The first two phases of the disease may occupy 20 years or more, but the tumour stage is often short, with spread and death usually within 3 years.

### *Variants*

- Subcutaneous panniculitis-like T-cell lymphomas resemble an ulcerating panniculitis, especially lupus panniculitis profundus (p. 143).

● Anaplastic large cell CD30⁺ lymphomas present as rapidly growing tumours which sometimes regress spontaneously.

● Granulomatous slack skin affects young patients. Indurated plaques become atrophic and the skin then becomes pendulous in the affected areas.

● Pagetoid reticulosis is seen most often on the acral parts and again affects the young. It appears as a slow-growing psoriasiform or verrucous plaque.

● Folliculotrophic mycosis fungoides usually appears as itchy pink scaly plaques with follicular prominence. This is followed by alopecia although this may be subtle.

● The Sézary syndrome is also a CTCL caused by a proliferation of helper T lymphocytes. Generalized skin erythema and oedema are associated with pruritus and lymphadenopathy. Abnormal T lymphocytes, with large convoluted nuclei, are found circulating in the blood (Sézary cells).

### Histology

The histological hallmarks of plaque stage CTCL are:
● intra-epidermal lymphocytic micro-abscesses (Pautrier micro-abscesses);
● a band of lymphoid cells in the upper dermis, infiltrating the epidermis; and
● atypical lymphocytes.

The histology of the patch stage poses more problems and may differ little from dermatitis. In lymphomas, T cells are clonal with most of the cells in the lesion having the same T-cell receptor. Immunophenotyping and T-cell receptor gene rearrangement studies (p. 23) may sometimes, but not always, be helpful in reaching a definitive diagnosis. Many biopsies, over several years, may be needed to prove that a suspicious rash is indeed an early stage of CTCL. Clinico-pathological correlation is essential.

### Differential diagnosis

The patch and plaque stages may be mistaken for psoriasis or parapsoriasis (Chapter 5), seborrhoeic dermatitis (p. 97) or tinea corporis (p. 249). However, they respond poorly to treatment for these disorders; the bizarre shapes of the patches and their asymmetrical distribution often raise suspicion. In the early stages, skin scrapings may be needed to exclude tinea. Patients with lymphomatoid papulosis develop papules or small cutaneous nodules of clonal T cells with a worrying malignant histology but a benign clinical course.

### Treatment

Moderately potent or potent local steroids, and UVB treatment, may provide prolonged palliation in the patch stage. In the plaque stage, psoralen with ultraviolet A (PUVA), oral retinoids and α-interferon are helpful. If lesions become more indurated, electron beam therapy may be used. Topical nitrogen mustard paint has also been used with success in both patch and plaque stages. Individual tumours respond well to low-dose radiotherapy. Systemic chemotherapy is disappointing, except for patients with the Sézary syndrome. For these patients, treatment with extracorporeal photopheresis (irradiating psoralenized blood with UVA in a machine) or with a targeting monoclonal antibody carrying diphtheria toxin may help destroy circualting malignant cells.

## Extracutaneous lymphomas

### Hodgkin's disease

This is of interest to dermatologists because it may present with severe generalized pruritus (p. 332). Patients with unexplained pruritus must be examined for lymphadenopathy and hepatosplenomegaly. Only rarely does Hodgkin's disease affect the skin directly, as small nodules and ulcers.

### Leukaemia

Rarely, the first sign of leukaemia is a leukaemic infiltrate in the skin. Clinically, this shows as plum-coloured plaques or nodules or, less often, a thickening and rugosity of the scalp (cutis verticis gyratum). More often, the rashes associated with leukaemia are non-specific red papules ('leukaemids'). Other non-specific manifestations include pruritus, herpes zoster, acquired ichthyosis and purpura.

**Fig. 20.61** Immunopathology showed that these nodules were caused by a B-cell lymphoma.

**Fig. 20.62** Several scalp metastases arising from a breast carcinoma.

## B-cell lymphomas

B-lymphocytic lymphomas presenting with skin lesions are rare. They appear as scattered plum-coloured nodules (Fig. 20.61). Histologically, a B-cell lymphoma infiltrates the lower dermis in a nodular or diffuse manner. Immunophenotyping shows a monoclonal expansion of B lymphocytes, all with either lambda or kappa light chains. Treatment is with radiotherapy and systemic chemotherapy.

## Other malignant tumours

### Dermatofibrosarcoma protuberans

Dermatofibrosarcoma protuberans is a slowly growing malignant tumour of fibroblasts, arising usually on the upper trunk. At first it seems like a dermatofibroma or keloid but, as it slowly expands, it turns into a plaque of red or bluish nodules with an irregular protuberant surface. It seldom metastasizes. It should be removed with extra wide margins, and even then will sometimes recur.

### Cutaneous metastases

About 3% of patients with internal cancers have cutaneous metastases. They usually arise late and indicate a grave prognosis, but occasionally a solitary cutaneous metastasis is the first sign of the occurrence of a tumour.

The most common cutaneous metastases come from breast cancer. The skin of the breast is also most often involved by the direct extension of a tumour. This may show up as a sharply demarcated and firm area of erythema (carcinoma erysipeloides), firm telangiectatic plaques and papules (carcinoma telangiectoides) or as skin like orange peel (*peau d'orange*) caused by blocked and dilated lymphatics. Carcinoma of the breast may also send metastases to the scalp, causing patches of alopecia (Fig. 20.62), or to other areas as firm and discrete dermal nodules.

Other common primaries metastasizing to the skin are tumours of the lung, gastrointestinal tract, uterus, prostate and kidney. The most frequent sites for secondary deposits are the umbilicus and the scalp.

## Further reading

Australian Cancer Network (1997) *Guidelines for the Management of Cutaneous Melanoma*. Stone Press, Epping.

Cox NH, Eedy DJ & Morton CA. (1999) Guidelines for the management of Bowen's disease. *British Journal of Dermatology* **141**, 633–641.

Kim EJ, Hess S, Richardson SK, *et al.* (2005) Immunopathogenesis and therapy of cutaneous T cell lymphoma. *Journal of Clinical Investigation* **115**, 798–812.

Motley R, Kersey P & Lawrence C. (2002) Multiprofessional guidelines for the management of the patient with primary cutaneous squamous cell carcinoma. *British Journal of Dermatology* **146**, 18–25.

Rigel DS, Friedman R, Dzubow MD, Reintgen MD, Bystryn J-C & Marks R. (2005) *Cancer of the Skin*. Elsevier-Saunders, Philadelphia.

Roberts DLL, Anstey AV, Barlow RJ, *et al.* (2002) UK guidelines for the management of cutaneous melanoma. *British Journal of Dermatology* **146**, 7–17. (Also at www.bad.org.uk)

Telfer NR, Colver GB & Bowers PW. (1999) Guidelines for the management of basal cell carcinoma. *British Journal of Dermatology* **141**, 415–423.

Thompson JF, Scolyer RA & Kefford RF. (2005) Cutaneous melanoma. *Lancet* **365**, 687–701.

Willemze R, Jaffe ES, Burg G, *et al.* (2005) WHO-EORTC classification for cutaneous lymphomas. *Blood* **105**, 3768–3785.

# 21 The skin in systemic disease

Only selected aspects of this huge subject can be covered here. In the first part of this chapter, the skin changes seen in particular diseases (e.g. sarcoidosis) or groups of diseases (e.g. internal malignancies) are described. The second part covers some individual skin conditions that can be associated with a wide range of internal disorders (e.g. pyoderma gangrenosum).

## The skin and internal malignancy

Obvious skin signs can be seen if a tumour invades the skin, or sends metastases to it, but there are other more subtle ways in which tumours can affect the skin. Sometimes they act physiologically, causing, for example, the acne seen with some adrenal tumours, flushing in the carcinoid syndrome and jaundice with a bile duct carcinoma. These cast-iron associations need no further discussion here. However, the presence of some rare but important conditions should alert the clinician to the possibility of an underlying neoplasm.

**1** *Acanthosis nigricans* is a velvety thickening and pigmentation of the major flexures. Setting aside those cases caused by obesity (Fig. 21.1), the metabolic syndrome (including type 2 diabetes with insulin resistance) or by drugs such as nicotinic acid used to treat hyperlipidaemia, the chances are high that a malignant tumour is present, usually within the abdominal cavity.

**2** *Erythema gyratum repens* is a shifting pattern of waves of erythema covering the skin surface and looks like the grain on wood.

**3** *Acquired hypertrichosis lanuginosa* ('malignant down') is an excessive and widespread growth of fine lanugo hair.

**4** *Necrolytic migratory erythema* is a figurate erythema with a moving crusted edge. When present, usually with anaemia, stomatitis, weight loss and diabetes, it signals the presence of a glucagon-secreting tumour of the pancreas.

**5** *Bazex syndrome* is a papulosquamous eruption of the fingers and toes, ears and nose, seen with some tumours of the upper respiratory tract.

**6** *Dermatomyositis*, other than in childhood (p. 136). About 30% of adult patients have an underlying malignancy. Pay special attention to the ovaries where ovarian cancer may lurk undetected.

**7** *Generalized pruritus.* One of its many causes is an internal malignancy, usually a lymphoma (p. 332).

**8** *Superficial thrombophlebitis.* The migratory type has traditionally been associated with carcinomas of the pancreas.

**9** *Acquired ichthyosis.* This may result from a number of underlying diseases (p. 50) but it is always important to exclude malignancy, especially lymphomas, as the cause.

**Fig. 21.1** Acanthosis nigricans – in this case caused by obesity.

**Fig. 21.2** Acute febrile neutrophilic dermatosis (Sweet's syndrome).

**10** *Genetic conditions.* One example is the Muir–Torre syndrome in which sebaceous adenomas are accompanied by surprisingly unaggressive visceral malignancies.

**11** *Acute febrile neutrophilic dermatosis* (Sweet's syndrome; Fig. 21.2 and p. 113). The classic triad found in association with the red oedematous plaques consists of fever, a raised erythrocyte sedimentation rate (ESR) and a raised blood neutrophil count. The most important internal association is with myeloproliferative disorders.

**12** *Paraneoplastic pemphigus* (Chapter 9). This is similar to pemphigus vulgaris but with extensive and persistent mucosal ulceration. The blisters on the palms and soles can look like erythema multiforme. It is associated with myeloproliferative malignancies as well as underlying carcinomas.

**13** *Others.* Pachydermoperiostosis is a coarsening and thickening of the skin seen in association with severe clubbing. It can be inherited as an autosomal dominant trait, or be a result of the standard causes of clubbing which include conditions such as bronchial carcinoma.

## The skin and diabetes mellitus

The following are more common in those with diabetes than in others.

**1** *Necrobiosis lipoidica.* Less than 3% of diabetics have necrobiosis, but 11–62% of patients with necrobiosis will have diabetes. Non-diabetic necrobiosis patients should be screened for diabetes as some will have impaired glucose tolerance or diabetes, and some will become diabetic later. The association is with both type 1 (previously termed 'insulin dependent') and type 2 (previously termed 'non-insulin dependent') diabetes. The lesions appear as one or more discoloured areas on the fronts of the shins (Fig. 21.3). Early plaques are violaceous but atrophy as the inflammation goes on and are then shiny, atrophic and brown–red or slightly yellow. The underlying blood vessels are easily seen through the atrophic skin and the margin may be erythematous or violet. Minor knocks can lead to slow-healing ulcers; biopsy can do the same.

No treatment is reliably helpful The atrophy is permanent; the best one can expect from medical treatments is halting of disease progression. The disease is caused by inflammation, yet treatment

**Fig. 21.3** Necrobiosis lipoidica: shiny yellowish patch with marked telangiectasia.

with topical steroids may add to the atrophy. A strong topical corticosteroid applied to the edge of an enlarging lesion may halt its expansion. There is little evidence that good control of the diabetes will help the necrobiosis. A padded dressing should help those whose legs are subjected to trauma.

**2** *Granuloma annulare*. The cause of granuloma annulare is not known; it now seems that there is no association between the common type and diabetes. An association applies to a few adults with extensive superficial granuloma annulare, characterized by dull red or purple macules. Clinically, the lesions of the common type of granuloma annulare often lie over the knuckles and are composed of dermal nodules fused into a rough ring shape (Fig. 21.4). On the hands the lesions are skin-coloured or slightly pink; elsewhere a purple colour may be seen. Although a biopsy is seldom necessary, the histology shows a diagnostic palisading granuloma, like that of necrobiosis lipoidica. Lesions tend to go away over the course of a year or two. Stubborn ones respond to intralesional triamcinolone injections. Cosmetically disfiguring cases may warrant treatment with psoralen and ultraviolet A (PUVA).

**3** *Diabetic dermopathy*. In about 50% of type 1 diabetics, multiple small (0.5–1 cm in diameter) slightly sunken brownish scars can be found on the limbs, most obviously over the shins.

**4** *Candidal infections* (p. 252).

**5** *Staphylococcal infections* (p. 225).

**Fig. 21.4** Granuloma annulare.

**6** *Vitiligo* (p. 281).

**7** *Eruptive xanthomas* (p. 330).

**8** *Stiff thick skin* (diabetic sclerodactyly or cheiroarthropathy) on the fingers and hands, demonstrated by the 'prayer sign' in which the fingers and palms cannot be opposed properly (Fig. 21.5).

**9** *Atherosclerosis* with ischaemia or gangrene of feet.

**10** *Neuropathic foot ulcers*.

## The skin in sarcoidosis

About one-third of patients with systemic sarcoidosis have skin lesions; it is also possible to have cutaneous sarcoidosis without systemic abnormalities (also

**Fig. 21.5** Diabetic cheiropathy – the prayer sign. Poor finger apposition in the diabetic hand (on the left) compared with the normal one (on the right).

**Fig. 21.6** Sarcoidosis: plum-coloured plaques on the cheek.

**Fig. 21.7** Solitary spider naevus showing the central feeding vessel. No underlying liver disease in this case.

known as sarcoid). The most important skin changes are as follows.

**1** *Erythema nodosum* (p. 112; see Fig. 8.10). This occurs in the early stages of sarcoidosis, especially in young women, and is almost always associated with hilar adenopathy.

**2** Sarcoidal granulomas in the skin. Histology reveals a 'naked' tubercle comprising foci of macrophages and giant cells without many surrounding lymphocytes. These are seen clinically as:

* *Scar sarcoidosis* Granulomatous lesions arising in long-standing scars should raise suspicions of sarcoidosis;
* *Lupus pernio* Dusky infiltrated plaques appear on the nose and fingers, often in association with sarcoidosis of the upper respiratory tract.
* *Papular, nodular and plaque forms* (Fig. 21.6) These brownish-red, violaceous or hypopigmented papules and plaques are indolent although often symptom free. Sometimes they are annular or psoriasis-like. Lesions vary in number, size and distribution. Sarcoid is a 'great imitator' of many diseases.

### Treatment

Intralesional and topical corticosteroids are sometimes helpful and hydroxychloroquine and chloroquine (Formulary 2, p. 405) have been used successfully. Chronic lesions respond poorly to any line of treatment short of systemic steroids, which are usually best avoided if involvement is confined to the skin.

## The skin in liver disease

Some of the associated abnormalities are the following.

**1** *Pruritus* This is related to obstructive jaundice and may precede it (p. 332).

**2** *Pigmentation* With bile pigments and sometimes melanin (Chapter 19).

**3** *Spider naevi* (Fig. 21.7) These are often multiple in chronic liver disease (p. 148).

**4** *Palmar erythema* (p. 147).

**5** *White nails* These associate with hypoalbuminaemia.

**6** *Lichen planus* (p. 72) and cryoglobulinaemia (p. 159) with hepatitis C infection.

**7** *Polyarteritis nodosa* (p. 159) with hepatitis B infection.

**8** *Porphyria cutanea tarda* (p. 115).

**9** *Xanthomas* With primary biliary cirrhosis (p. 328).

**10** *Hair loss and generalized asteatotic eczema* may occur in alcoholics with cirrhosis who have become zinc deficient.

## The skin in renal disease

The main changes associated with chronic renal failure are as follows.

**1** *Pruritus* and a generally dry skin.

**2** *Pigmentation* A yellowish sallow colour and pallor from anaemia.

**3** *Half-and-half nail* The proximal half is white and the distal half is pink or brownish.

**4** *Perforating disorders* Small papules in which collagen or elastic fibres are being extruded through the epidermis.

**5** *Pseudoporphyria* (p. 329).

Some skin changes may be caused by the conditions leading to renal disease (e.g. leucocytoclastic vasculitis, p. 113; connective tissue disorders, Chapter 10, and Fabry's disease, p. 331).

## Graft-vs.-host disease

Allogeneic haematopoietic stem cell transplantation is now a well-established treatment for several disorders including aplastic anaemia and leukaemia. Recently, bone marrow as a source for stem cells has been replaced by peripheral blood stem cells. Umbilical cord blood grafts are increasingly used. Immunologically competent donor lymphocytes, however, may still cause problems by reacting against host tissues, especially the skin, liver and gut.

Acute graft-vs.-host (GVH) disease appears within 4 weeks. Fever accompanies malaise and a worsening morbilliform rash, which often starts on the palms and soles and behind the ears. It may progress to a generalized desquamation or even toxic epidermal necrolysis. Histology in the early stage may help to confirm the diagnosis. Typical features include degeneration of basal keratinocytes and/or single cell necrosis of keratinocytes with a surrounding cluster of lymphocytes ('satellite cell necrosis').

Chronic GVH disease, occurring a minimum of 100 days after transplantation, affects about 50% of patients; its skin changes are variable but may be like those of lichen planus (p. 72) or a pigmented scleroderma (p. 138). The skin changes may be severe enough to need treatment with systemic prednisolone and azathioprine, PUVA or ciclosporin (Formulary 2, p. 399). Painful skin ulcers complicate severe cases.

## Malabsorption and malnutrition

Some of the most common skin changes are listed in Table 21.1.

**Table 21.1** Skin changes in malabsorption and malnutrition.

| Condition | Skin changes |
|---|---|
| Malnutrition | Itching |
| | Dryness |
| | Symmetrical pigmentation |
| | Brittle nails and hair |
| Protein malnutrition (kwashiorkor) | Dry red–brown hair |
| | Pigmented 'cracked skin' |
| Iron deficiency | Pallor |
| | Itching |
| | Diffuse hair loss |
| | Koilonychia |
| | Smooth tongue |
| Vitamin A (retinol) deficiency | Dry skin |
| | Follicular hyperkeratoses |
| | Xerophthalmia |
| Vitamin $B_1$ (aneurin) deficiency | Beri-beri oedema |
| Vitamin $B_2$ (riboflavine) deficiency | Angular stomatitis |
| | Smooth purple tongue |
| | Seborrhoeic dermatitis-like eruption |
| Vitamin $B_6$ (pyridoxine) deficiency | Ill-defined dermatitis |
| Vitamin $B_7$ (niacin) deficiency | Pellagra with dermatitis, dementia and diarrhoea |
| | Dermatitis on exposed areas, pigmented |
| Vitamin C deficiency (scurvy) | Skin haemorrhages especially around follicular keratoses containing coiled hairs |
| | Bleeding gums |
| | Oedematous 'woody' swellings of limbs in the elderly |

# The porphyrias

There are at least eight enzymes in the metabolic pathway that lead to the synthesis of haem. There are also eight different types of porphyria, each being caused by a deficiency of one of these enzymes, and each having its own characteristic pattern of accumulation of porphyrin and porphyrin precursors. Formed porphyrins, but not porphyrin precursors, cause the photosensitivity (to ultraviolet radiation of wavelength 400 nm, which is capable of penetrating through window glass) that is the cardinal feature of the cutaneous porphyrias.

The different types can be separated on clinical grounds, aided by the biochemical investigation of urine, faeces and blood. Only five varieties are mentioned here.

## Congenital erythropoietic porphyria

This is very rare, caused by mutations in the uroporphyrinogen III-cosynthase gene, and inherited as an autosomal recessive trait. Severe photosensitivity is noted soon after birth, and leads to blistering, scarring and mutilation of the exposed parts, which become increasingly hairy. The urine is pink and the teeth are brown, although fluorescing red under Wood's light. A haemolytic anaemia is present. Treatment is unsatisfactory but must include protection from and avoidance of sunlight. The hairy appearance, discoloured teeth and the tendency to avoid daylight may have given rise to legends about werewolves.

## Erythrohepatic protoporphyria (erythropoietic protoporphyria)

In this more common, autosomal dominant condition, caused by mutations in the ferrochelatase gene, a less severe photosensitivity develops during infancy. A burning sensation occurs within minutes of exposure to sunlight. Soon the skin becomes swollen and crusted vesicles sometimes appear, leading to pitted scars. Liver disease and gallstones occur. In addition to sun avoidance and the use of sunscreens (Formulary 1, p. 383), skin-yellowing doses of beta-carotene may be given orally.

## Cutaneous hepatic porphyria (porphyria cutanea tarda)

There are two types: a sporadic type (accounting for 80% of cases) and a type inherited as an autosomal dominant trait (20%). Both are characterized by low hepatic uroporphyrinogen decarboxylase activity. The sporadic type is usually seen in men, but rarely in women, who have damaged their livers by drinking too much alcohol but may also occur in women taking oestrogens. It has also been shown that a few cases are caused by haemochromatosis or previous hepatitis C virus infection. Blisters, erosions and milia form on the exposed parts of the face, and on the backs of the hands (Figs 21.8 and 21.9), in response to sunlight or to minor trauma. These areas become scarred and hairy. The urine is pink and fluoresces a bright coral-pink under Wood's light (p. 38) as a result of excessive uroporphyrins (Fig. 21.10). Treatment is based on avoiding alcohol

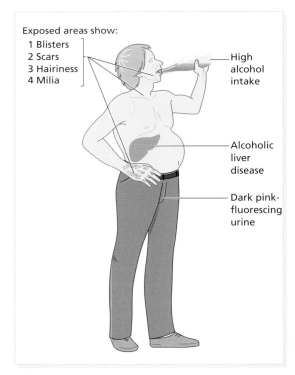

**Fig. 21.8** Cutaneous hepatic porphyria (porphyria cutanea tarda).

**Fig. 21.9** Blisters, milia and erosions on the side of a finger.

**Fig. 21.10** Cutaneous hepatic porphyria. Coral-red fluorescence of urine under Wood's light denoting excessive uroporphyrins (chloroform extraction).

and oestrogens, but other measures are usually needed too, including iron depletion by regular venesection or very low-dose hydroxychloroquine therapy (e.g. 100 mg twice weekly) under specialist supervision. Higher doses cause toxic hepatitis in these patients.

## Acute intermittent porphyria

This condition, inherited as an autosomal dominant trait as the result of mutations of the porphobilinogen deaminase gene, is most common in Scandinavia. Skin lesions do not occur. Attacks of abdominal pain, accompanied by neuropsychiatric symptoms and the passage of dark urine, are sometimes triggered by drugs (especially barbiturates, griseofulvin, oestrogens and sulphonamides).

## Variegate porphyria

This disorder, inherited as an autosomal dominant trait and the result of mutations of the protoporphyrinogen oxidase gene, is particularly common in South Africa. It shares the skin features of porphyria cutanea tarda and the systemic symptoms and drug provocation of acute intermittent porphyria.

## 'Pseudoporphyria'

This term is used when skin and histological changes like those of cutaneous hepatic porphyria occur without an underlying abnormality of porphyrin metabolism. It has been linked with chronic renal failure and haemodialysis, ultraviolet radiation and sun beds and can be induced by many drugs, notably furosemide, non-steroidal anti-inflammatory drugs, beta-lactam antibiotics and azole antifungals. In the differential diagnosis, be sure to rule out epidermolysis bullosa acquisita (p. 125).

## Some metabolic disorders

### Amyloidosis

Amyloid is a protein that can be derived from several sources, including immunoglobulin light chains and keratins. It is deposited in the tissues in combination with a P component derived from the plasma. Skin changes are prominent in primary systemic amyloidosis, and also in the amyloid associated with multiple myeloma. In contrast, systemic amyloidosis of the type that is secondary to chronic inflammatory disease, such as rheumatoid arthritis or tuberculosis, tends not to affect the skin. Skin blood vessels infiltrated with amyloid rupture easily, causing 'pinch purpura' to occur after minor trauma. The waxy deposits of amyloid, often most obvious around the eyes, may also be purpuric. More diffuse deposits suggest scleroderma. Distinct from the systemic amyloidoses are localized deposits of amyloid. These are uncommon and usually take the form of macular areas of rippled pigmentation, or of plaques made up of coalescing papules. Both types are itchy.

**Table 21.2** Xanthomas: clinical appearance and associations.

|  | Clinical appearance | Types of hyperlipidaemia (Frederickson classification) and associated metabolic abnormalities |
| --- | --- | --- |
| Xanthelasma palpebrarum (Fig. 21.11) | Soft yellowish plaques on the eyelids | None or type II, III or IV |
| Tuberous xanthomas (Fig. 21.12) | Firm yellow papules and nodules, most often on points of knees and elbows | Types II, III and secondary |
| Tendinous xanthomas | Subcutaneous swellings on fingers or by Achilles tendon | Types II, III and secondary |
| Eruptive xanthomas | Sudden onset, multiple small yellow papules<br>Buttocks and shoulders | Types I, IV, V and secondary (usually in diabetes) |
| Plane xanthomas (Fig. 21.13) | Yellow macular areas at any site<br>Yellow palmar creases | Type III and secondary |
| Generalized plane xanthomas | Yellow macules over wide areas | Myeloma |

## Mucinoses

The dermis becomes infiltrated with mucin in certain disorders. Skin biopsy specimens readily show the mucin, especially when stained with Giemsa.

**1** *Myxoedema* In the puffy hands and face of patients with hypothyroidism.

**2** *Pretibial myxoedema* Pink or flesh-coloured mucinous plaques are seen on the lower shins, together with marked exophthalmos, in some patients with hyperthyroidism. They may also occur after the thyroid abnormality has been treated.

**3** *Scleromyxoedema* A diffuse thickening and papulation of the skin may occur in connection with an immunoglobulin G (IgG) monoclonal paraproteinaemia. In lichen myxoedematosis deposits are more discrete and nodular.

**4** *Follicular mucinosis* In this condition, the infiltrated plaques show a loss of hair. Some cases are associated with a lymphoma.

## Xanthomas

Deposits of fatty material in the skin and subcutaneous tissues (xanthomas) may provide the first clue to important disorders of lipid metabolism.

*Primary hyperlipidaemias* are usually genetic. They fall into six groups, classified on the basis of an analysis of fasting blood lipids and electrophoresis of plasma lipoproteins. All, save type 1, carry an increased risk of atherosclerosis – in this lies their importance and the need for treatment.

*Secondary hyperlipidaemia* can be found in a variety of diseases including diabetes, primary biliary cirrhosis, the nephrotic syndrome and hypothyroidism.

The clinical patterns of xanthoma correlate well with the underlying cause. The main patterns and their most common associations are shown in Table 21.2 (Figs 21.11–21.13). Lipid-regulating drugs (e.g. statins and fibrates) not only stop xanthomas from appearing, but they also allow them to resolve. More importantly, they help reduce the risk of vascular occlusions such as coronary artery disease.

**Fig. 21.11** Xanthelasma: flat yellow lesions on the eyelids, often with normal blood lipids.

**Fig. 21.12** Tuberous xanthoma on the points of the elbows – a mixture of nodules and papules.

**Fig. 21.13** Plane xanthoma with yellow palmar creases.

**Learning point**

Check the blood lipids in all types of xanthoma, including xanthelasma of the eyelids. Abnormalities are remediable with statins and fibrates

## Phenylketonuria

Phenylketonuria is a rare metabolic cause of hypopigmentation. Its prevalence is about 1 in 25 000. It is inherited as an autosomal recessive trait caused by a deficiency of the liver enzyme phenylalanine hydroxylase, which catalyses the hydroxylation of phenylalanine to tyrosine. This leads to the accumulation of phenylalanine, phenylpyruvic acid and their metabolites.

Affected individuals have fair skin and hair. They often develop eczema, usually suggesting the atopic type, and they may be photosensitive. The accumulation of phenylalanine and its metabolites damages the brain during its phase of rapid development just before and just after birth. Mental retardation, epilepsy and extrapyramidal manifestations such as athetosis may then occur.

Oculocutaneous albinism (p. 280) can usually be distinguished by its eye signs. The Guthrie test, which detects raised blood phenylalanine levels, is carried out routinely at birth in most developed countries.

A low-phenylalanine diet should be started as soon as possible to prevent further neurological damage.

## Alkaptonuria

In this rare, recessively inherited disorder, based on a homogentisic acid oxidase deficiency, dark urine may be seen in childhood, and in adult life pigment, ranging from grey–blue to brown–black, may be deposited in various places including the ears and sclera (ochronosis). Arthropathy may occur.

## Fabry's disease (angiokeratoma corporis diffusum)

A deficiency of the enzyme α-galactosidase A is found in this sex-linked disorder (chromosome region Xq21.3-22); abnormal amounts of glycolipid are deposited in many tissues as a result. Treatment with intravenous enzyme replacement therapy is now available. The skin lesions are grouped, almost black, small telangiectatic papules especially around the umbilicus and pelvis. Progressive renal failure occurs in adult life. Most patients have attacks of excruciating unexplained pain in their hands. Some female carriers have skin changes, although these are usually less obvious than those of affected males. Similar skin lesions may be seen in lysosomal storage disorders such as fucosidosis.

## Generalized pruritus

Pruritus is a symptom with many causes, but not a disease in its own right. Itchy patients fall into two groups: those whose pruritus is caused simply by surface causes (e.g. eczema, lichen planus and scabies), which seldom need much investigation; and those who may or may not have an internal cause for their itching. These patients require a detailed physical examination, including a careful search for lymphadenopathy, and investigations including a full blood count, iron status, urea and electrolytes, liver function tests, thyroid function tests and a chest X-ray. The underlying cause for the pruritus may turn out to be one of the following.

**1** *Liver disease* Itching signals biliary obstruction. It is an early symptom of primary biliary cirrhosis. Colestyramine may help cholestatic pruritus, possibly by promoting the elimination of bile salts. Other treatments include naltrexone, rifampicin and ultraviolet B.

**2** *Chronic renal failure* Urea itself seems not to be responsible for this symptom, which plagues about one-third of patients undergoing renal dialysis. Ultraviolet B phototherapy, naltrexone or administration of oral activated charcoal may help.

**3** *Iron deficiency* Treatment with iron may help the itching.

**4** *Polycythaemia* The itching here is usually triggered by a hot bath; it has a curious pricking quality and lasts about an hour.

**5** *Thyroid disease* Itching and urticaria may occur in hyperthyroidism. The dry skin of hypothyroidism may also be itchy.

**6** *Diabetes* Generalized itching may be a rare presentation of diabetes.

**7** *Internal malignancy* The prevalence of itching in Hodgkin's disease may be as high as 30%. It may be unbearable, yet the skin often looks normal. Pruritus may occur long before other manifestations of the disease. Itching is uncommon in carcinomatosis.

**8** *Neurological disease* Paroxysmal pruritus has been recorded in multiple sclerosis and in neurofibromatosis. Brain tumours infiltrating the floor of the

**Fig. 21.14** An example of the butterfly sign. This lady could not reach her upper back but could scratch her skin everywhere else. In other patients, the spared area is shaped more like a butterfly.

fourth ventricle may cause a fierce persistent itching of the nostrils.

**9** *Diffuse scleroderma* may start as itching associated with increasing pigmentation and early signs of sclerosis. Itching is usually severe throughout the course of this debilitating disease.

**10** The skin of the elderly may itch because it is too dry, or because it is being irritated.

**11** *Pregnancy* (Chapter 15).

**12** *Drugs* The history is the most useful indicator of this diagnosis.

The search for a cause has to be tailored to the individual patient, and must start with a thorough history and physical examination. The presence of a 'butterfly sign' (Fig. 21.14) sometimes suggests an internal cause for the itching. Unless a treatable cause is found, therapy is symptomatic and consists of sedative antihistamines (Formulary 2, p. 398), skin moisturizers, and the avoidance of rough clothing, overheating and vasodilatation, including that brought on by alcohol. Ultraviolet B often helps all kinds of itching, including the itching associated with chronic renal and liver disease. Local applications include calamine and mixtures containing small amounts of menthol or phenol (Formulary 1, p. 384).

> **Learning points**
>
> - Learn how to spell pruritus (not pruritis) but do not accept it as a diagnosis in its own right
> - Ponder underlying causes in those with no primary skin disease

**Fig. 21.15** Pyoderma gangrenosum: a plum-coloured lesion with a typical cribriform appearance.

**Fig. 21.16** Another manifestation of Crohn's disease: grossly oedematous vulva with interconnecting sinuses. Biopsy at the site arrowed showed a granulomatous histology.

## Pyoderma gangrenosum

An inflamed nodule or pustule breaks down centrally to form an expanding ulcer with a polycyclic or serpiginous outline, and a characteristic undermined bluish edge (Fig. 21.15). The condition is not bacterial in origin but its pathogenesis, presumably immunological, is not fully understood. It may arise in the absence of any underlying disease, but tends to associate with the following conditions.

1 Inflammatory bowel disease (ulcerative colitis and Crohn's disease; Fig. 21.16). Of these patients, 2% develop pyoderma, with peristomal pyoderma being a particular complication in those with abdominal stomas.

2 Conditions causing polyarthritis, including rheumatoid arthritis (Fig. 21.17).

3 Haematological malignancies – particularly of myeloid origin (with a bullous form of pyoderma).

Lesions may be single or multiple, and pustular and bullous variants occur. Pyoderma severity does not appear to be related to the activity of inflammatory bowel disease or rheumatoid arthritis when these are the cause. It responds to systemic – and

**Fig. 21.17** This long-standing ulcer was pyoderma gangrenosum secondary to the patient's rheumatoid arthritis.

in mild cases highly potent topical – corticosteroids, sometimes with adjunctive minocycline. Lesions heal leaving papery scars. Alternative treatments include ciclosporin and the anti TNF-α agent infliximab.

## Further reading

Braverman IM. (1998) *Skin Signs of Systemic Disease*, 3rd edn. W.B. Saunders, Philadelphia, PA.

Brooklyn T, Dunnill G & Probert C. (2006) Diagnosis and treatment of pyoderma gangrenosum. *British Medical Journal* **333**, 181–184.

Lebwohl M. (2004) *The Skin and Systemic Disease: A Color Atlas and Text*, 2nd edn. Churchill Livingstone, Edinburgh.

Provost TT & Flynn JA. (2001) *Cutaneous Medicine: Cutaneous Manifestations of Systemic Disease*. B.C. Decker, Ontario.

Savin JA, Hunter JAA & Hepburn NC. (1997) *Skin Signs in Clinical Medicine: Diagnosis in Colour*. Mosby-Wolfe, London.

# 22 Cosmetic dermatology

As our population ages, its desire for cosmetic dermatology increases as the aim of cosmetic dermatology is not to alleviate disease, but to try and make the skin look young again. Perhaps the desire to look young and beautiful seems frivolous, but success has measurable benefits. Studies consistently show that good-looking men and women earn more, are more successful at interviews and have a higher sense of self-worth. In contrast, well-constructed trials and impartial data on the results of cosmetic dermatological procedures are scanty.

In the UK, with its relatively few dermatologists, hardly any deal only with cosmetic skin problems, but in the USA the proportion is much higher. Nevertheless, all dermatologists should know which cosmetic procedures can be performed, and their risks and benefits. This chapter gives an overview of the most common techniques in current use.

The over-the-counter cosmetics industry is worth $160 billion/year worldwide, and in the USA more is spent on beauty products than on education. However, the definition of what is a cosmetic, as opposed to a medicine, is still confusing. In 1938, the American Food and Drug Administration (FDA) defined a cosmetic as anything that can be 'poured, sprinkled or sprayed on, introduced into, or otherwise applied to the human body . . . for cleansing, beautifying, promoting attractiveness, or altering the appearance *without affecting the body's structure or functions'*. This has led to confusion when the cosmetic industry wants to claim rejuvenating properties for its products, but not such dramatic ones that they become classified as medicines, and so available only with a medical prescription. This discourages the open publication of research carried out by the industry, as the absence of effect of their products will not help sales, and the finding of true alterations in the structure of the skin carries the risk of having the product classified as a medicine. European regulations are

less conservative, and state 'almost every product usually perceived as a cosmetic . . . does, in some way or another, modify physiological function . . . *the modification has to be more than significant'* for the Medicinal Product Directive to apply.

## Ageing of the skin (see also p. 275)

Ageing of skin is a mixture of chronological ageing and environmental influences, chief among which are ultraviolet radiation (p. 275) and smoking. Chronological (intrinsic) ageing is characterized by a finely wrinkled, smooth skin, with few histological changes. In contrast, environmentally aged skin is more deeply wrinkled, with reduced elasticity and an epidermis showing solar lentigines and keratoses, and scattered pigmentation. Photoaged skin has reduced levels of the fibrillar collagens, a major structural element in healthy dermis, and a disrupted elastic fibre network. The loss of collagen correlates with the depth and number of wrinkles, and is the result of a combination of reduced procollagen synthesis and increased breakdown by matrix metalloproteinase (MMP) enzymes. Ultraviolet radiation generates free radicals in the dermis and epidermis that alter protein structure directly, as well as initiating signal transduction cascades that activate MMPs. Histologically, the epidermis is thinned, with reduced proliferation and a flattened rete ridge pattern.

The Glogau scoring system can be used as a clinical indicator of degree of photoageing (Table 22.1).

## Cosmetic treatments

In medical dermatology, several different treatments may be needed over time to treat, for example, a psoriatic patient. Similarly, in cosmetic dermatology no one technique can reverse all the changes of photoageing, and treatments must be tailored

**Table 22.1** Glogau photoageing grade.

| | |
|---|---|
| I | No wrinkles |
| | Mild pigmentary changes |
| II | Wrinkles in motion |
| | Early senile lentigines |
| | Palpable but invisible keratoses |
| III | Wrinkles at rest |
| | Dyschromia and telangiectases |
| | Visible keratoses |
| IV | Yellow–grey skin colour |
| | Prior skin malignancies |
| | Wrinkled throughout |

to the individual. The techniques used most commonly are the application of emollients and retinoid creams, facial peels, injection of botulinum toxin and dermal fillers, and laser and light sources. As a general rule, the choice of treatment depends on the depth of the pathological changes. Superficial changes, such as pigmentary ones and early keratoses (Glogau I and II), are best treated with agents acting on the epidermis, such as topical retinoids and shallow facial peels. In contrast, wrinkles caused by dermal changes need treatment that reaches the deeper layers of the skin – such as ablative laser therapy or the injection of fillers.

## Emollients and retinoids

Even mildly aged skin looks better after the application of moisturizers. The scaliness of aged skin is caused by corneocytes (p. 14) clumping together into lamellae, instead of being shed separately. Emollients help to 'unstick' the corneocytes, and contain two main types of ingredient: occlusives and humefactants. Over-the-counter preparations are usually mixtures of these, prepared either as oil-in-water emulsions (creams and lotions) or water-in-oil emulsions (hand creams). Occlusives (such as soft white paraffin or lanolin) are poorly permeable to water, and so reduce transepidermal water loss when applied to the skin. Humefactants absorb water, generally from the environment, but also from the epidermis. They draw water into the stratum corneum, and the resulting swelling of corneocytes gives an impression of wrinkle reduction, although this is only temporary. Over-the-counter moisturizers advertised as 'antiwrinkle creams'

usually rely on this mechanism. Urea, glycerine and hydroxy acids are all humefactants.

Trial data confirm that topical tretinoin improves the appearance of mild to moderate photodamage. Fine and coarse wrinkles, pigmentary changes and keratoses all improve as new collagen is formed in the dermis. Skin irritation is common, and both this and the improvement in appearance correlate with the concentration of tretinoin used.

## Botulinum toxin

*Clostridium botulinum* was identified at the end of the 19th century as the organism responsible for the potentially fatal disease botulism, in which paralysis of the cranial and autonomic nerves follows the ingestion of its toxin. There are seven serotypes of botulinum toxin, of which A, B and E account for the majority of human disease. The toxins work at the neuromuscular junction, where they produce a chemical denervation by binding irreversibly at the presynaptic junction and blocking the release of acetylcholine. Despite the permanent binding of the toxin, paralysis wears off after several months as collateral axonal sprouts develop and are able to release acetylcholine.

Botulinum toxin was first used clinically in the 1980s to correct squints and cervical dystonia, but moved rapidly into cosmetic use when it was found to be effective at reducing wrinkles. Its use is one of the most popular cosmetic procedures because it is easy to administer and starts to work after only a few days.

### Types of botulinum toxin

Four types of botulinum toxin are available in the UK (Table 22.2). Vistabel® (Botox cosmetic® in the USA) is a type A botulinum toxin, and licensed to

**Table 22.2** Types of botulinum toxin.

| Toxin type | Trade name | UK licence for cosmetic use? |
|---|---|---|
| Type A toxin | Vistabel (Botox cosmetic) | Yes |
| | Botox | No |
| | Dysport | No |
| Type B toxin | Neurobloc (Myobloc) | No |

treat glabellar lines, for which it should now be used in place of the identical Botox®. Dysport® is also a type A botulinum toxin, while Neurobloc® is a type B toxin. None of the latter three is licensed for cosmetic use, and this must be explained to patients for whom they may be considered. Type A botulinum toxins do not take effect for several days after injection, and their actions last for 3–4 months. Neurobloc® (Myobloc in the USA) has a shorter action of around 6 weeks. The potencies of Vistabel®/ Botox® and Dysport® are calculated differently, with 1 unit of Vistabel® being roughly equivalent to 4 units of Dysport®.

## Uses of botulinum toxin

Botulinum toxin is primarily used to treat 'dynamic wrinkles' (i.e. wrinkles produced by muscle contraction). The upper part of the face is most amenable to treatment, as wrinkles here are caused by the contraction of specific muscles, such as the frontalis (leading to horizontal wrinkles on the forehead), procerus and corrugator (causing vertical glabellar frown lines).

A glabellar frown typically needs injection into each corrugator and the procerus muscle. To treat horizontal wrinkles, botulinum toxin is injected roughly every 2 cm across the forehead (Fig. 22.1). A more feminine arched brow appearance can be created by injecting the toxin in a V, rather than a horizontal pattern (Fig. 22.2). The area 1 cm above the medial end of the orbital rim should be avoided to lessen the risk of ptosis. 'Crow's feet' (periocular rhytides) are treated with injections lateral to the lateral canthus.

Botulinum toxin is not suitable for the 'static wrinkles' associated with dermal collagen loss, for which dermal fillers are more effective. It is therefore most commonly used in younger patients. Potential side-effects include bruising, ptosis and an asymmetrical or unwanted appearance, but fortunately these go away as the effects of the toxin wear off.

Botulinum toxin is also used to treat hyperhidrosis (p. 175).

## Dermal fillers

'Wrinkles at rest' respond poorly to botulinum toxin. The underlying cause here is a loss of dermal volume and elasticity, and the aim of using dermal fillers

(a)

(b)

**Fig. 22.1** Before (a) and after (b) photographs of the effect of botulinum toxin injections on horizontal frown lines.

**Fig. 22.2** Typical sites for injection of botulinum toxin to reduce glabellar rhytids.

(a)

(b)

**Fig. 22.3** Before and after photographs showing reduction in nasolabial fold wrinkles following injection of a hyaluronic acid filler.

is to replace that volume. An ideal filler would be non-inflammatory, non-allergenic, non-carcinogenic, long-lasting and providing a natural appearance. However, no such product exists and there are few trials comparing the different agents.

Fillers are based on naturally derived or synthetic polymers – usually of collagen or hyaluronic acid. Most are injected into the upper or mid-dermis and are useful for wrinkles at rest, acne scars and wrinkles in the lower two-thirds of the face where botulinum toxin is less effective. They are commonly used for the nasolabial folds (Fig. 22.3), 'marionette lines' (which radiate from the lateral border of the mouth to the chin), crow's feet and for augmenting the lips.

## Collagen fillers

Bovine collagen and its derivatives have been used for 20 years to augment soft tissue, and, with over 1 million subjects treated, have a long safety record. Various products are available (e.g. Zyderm, Zyplast). They differ in their concentration of collagen – with lower concentrations being used for the more superficial, finer wrinkles. Products such as Zyplast contain collagen cross-linked with glutaraldehyde; this slows the breakdown of the collagen by host collagenases and lengthens its action to around 4 months. Unmodified collagen begins to lose its effect after 2–4 months. The major drawback of bovine collagen is the 3% incidence of delayed hypersensitivity reactions. For this reason, an intradermal test injection is given into the volar forearm first, and read 4 weeks later. A positive test is shown by erythema, itching and induration, and precludes the use of bovine collagen.

Bovine collagen has been used less in recent years, largely because of the need for preliminary skin testing. Human collagen, either taken from cadavers or more commonly produced by human dermal fibroblasts cultured in the laboratory (e.g. CosmoDerm™/CosmoPlast™), is now frequently being used as an alternative. It has the advantage that there is no need for preliminary skin testing. Its effects last for around 3 months.

## Hyaluronic acid fillers

Hyaluronic acid-based products can be used instead of collagens. Hyaluronic acid is a glycosaminoglycan found naturally in the ground substance of the dermis (p. 20). It is strongly hydrophilic and so 'plumps up' the dermis by attracting water. In its unmodified state, hyaluronic acid would rapidly be broken down, but chemical modification prevents this. There are a growing number of hyaluronic acid-based products used worldwide, but two main forms are used in Europe: Hylaform® comes from rooster combs; Restylane® is synthesized by genetically engineered streptococci. Both have a longer action than collagen – usually around 4 months – and as delayed hypersensitivity reactions are unusual, preliminary skin testing is not needed.

## Longer lasting fillers

A number of permanent and semi-permanent fillers are becoming available, intended to provide longer lasting effects. These generally contain synthetic polymers. The benefits of a more permanent effect must be balanced against the higher risk of developing granulomatous reactions and nodules. Poly-l-lactic acid is one of the recently introduced synthetic polymers. It acts differently from hyaluronic acid and collagen, in that it stimulates fibroblasts to produce collagen. As a result its action starts more slowly, but lasts for 1–2 years. It was initially licensed for the treatment of HIV-related lipoatrophy, but is now more widely used as a cosmetic agent in non-HIV patients to treat lines deeper than those that respond to volumetric fillers.

Dermal fillers do have side-effects, but there are no comparative trial data on these. Bovine collagens probably create the most problems with hypersensitivity reactions, but prior skin testing should lessen this risk. Foreign body reactions, granulomas, lumps resulting from maldistribution, local tissue necrosis and infection have been reported for all types of filler.

Autologous fat transfer is used in some centres and has the advantage that it obviates the risk of a foreign body reaction. The patient's own fat is harvested from donor sites such as the buttocks or thighs by gentle aspiration, under local anaesthetic. The aspirate is gently centrifuged down, and fat injected into the area of lipoatrophy. This technique is particularly useful for the peri-orbital and malar areas, and fat can also be frozen and stored for incremental 'touch ups' over time.

## Chemical peels

Variations in pigmentation, and the epidermal lesions of ageing, are best treated with chemical peels or with lasers.

Chemical peels are categorized by their depth of action. All rely on the application of a chemical exfoliant, which induces removal or necrosis and inflammation of the epidermis, and sometimes of the dermis too. Superficial peels induce necrosis of part or all of the epidermis; medium-depth peels produce destruction of the epidermis and inflammation of the papillary dermis; deep chemical peels create inflammation down to the deep reticular dermis.

The mainstay of chemical peels are hydroxy acids, classified as α and β hydroxy acids (AHAs and BHAs), depending on the position of the hydroxyl group. Typical AHAs include lactic, glycolic and citric acids, while salicylic acid is the only BHA in clinical use. In the short term, AHAs affect corneocyte cohesiveness in the lower stratum corneum, and in the longer term they thicken the epidermis and papillary dermis, with increased acid mucopolysaccharides and collagen in the dermis. Salicylic acid has been used as a keratolytic for decades, and enhances the shedding of corneocytes by reducing intercellular stickiness. Resorcinol is a phenol derivative which has keratolytic properties, but is also useful in treating hyperpigmentation.

Most chemical peels rely on a combination of agents. The depth of the peel depends on the agents used, the vehicle in which they are delivered and the length of time for which they are applied. Typical of the combination peels is Jessner's solution – a mixture of resorcinol, salicylic acid and lactic acid in ethanol. 'Frosting' resulting from the precipitation of salicylic acid occurs on treated skin, and can be used as a guide when applying the solution. Single applications of a superficial chemical peel produce only subtle changes, and treatments repeated every few weeks are needed to improve actinic damage, lentigines and melasma.

Trichloracetic acid (TCA) at concentrations of 35–40% is the standard solution for medium-depth facial peels. It produces epidermal and dermal necrosis, without serious systemic toxicity, although it may induce post-inflammatory hyperpigmentation in dark-skinned subjects, in whom it should not be used. TCA can be used alone (Fig. 22.4), or after preliminary treatment with a superficial peeling agent to achieve a deeper effect. 'Frosting' of the skin occurs shortly after TCA is applied, but here is caused by the precipitation of denatured proteins in the epidermis.

Superficial peels are generally safe, but can cause allergic or irritant contact dermatitis. Salicylate poisoning has been reported, but only after large areas were treated. Post-inflammatory pigmentation may occur, subjects with darker skins being at greater risk. Medium-depth TCA peels inevitably lead to erythema and desquamation of the epidermis, at its worst about a week after treatment. While re-epithelialization is occurring, patients should avoid sun exposure. Prophylactic antiviral

(a)          (b)          (c)

**Fig. 22.4** Before (a), seven days (b)and six months (c) after a 25% TCA peel. Once the post-treatment crusting has settled, there is a reduction in peri-oral wrinkles and signs of epidermal photoaging.

medication is often used to prevent the recurrence of a herpes simplex infection in subjects with a history of this.

## Laser resurfacing (p. 378)

This is the most effective treatment for deeper changes in the skin such as rhytides and scarring, and also improves epidermal photodamage. Its disadvantage is the greater morbidity inevitable in a procedure that induces a partial-thickness burn. Carbon dioxide ($CO_2$) and erbium yttrium aluminium garnett (Er:YAG) lasers selectively vaporize the epidermis and papillary dermis, allowing the epidermis to re-epithelialize and new collagen and elastic tissue to be laid down in the upper dermis. The wavelengths of these lasers ($CO_2$ $\lambda = 10\ 600$ nm and Er:YAG $\lambda = 2094$ nm) are predominantly absorbed by water in the skin, generating heat and thermal destruction. The millisecond pulse widths of modern $CO_2$ lasers ensure efficient tissue vaporization, and minimize non-selective thermal damage. The $CO_2$ laser (Fig. 22.5) penetrates deeper than the Er:YAG laser, removing 25–50 µm of tissue with each pass and producing thermal wounding of the dermis. A degree of immediate skin tightening follows, because of denaturation and shrinkage of

type I dermal collagen, and dermal remodelling continues for several months afterwards. The shorter wavelength of the Er:YAG laser is absorbed more efficiently by water and penetrates less deeply – usually 15–20 µm each pass – with more rapid healing but less clinical improvement.

Laser resurfacing hurts and patients need systemic analgesics and topical or even general anaesthesia. Oral antiviral prophylaxis is given before and after the procedure. Postoperatively, emollients and wet dressings must be applied to the treated area for at least the first week, and patients must be warned to expect oedema and exudation. Careful patient selection should ensure that only those with realistic expectations, who can tolerate the discomfort of the procedure and will follow the instructions for post-treatment care, are chosen. Possible side-effects include a dissemination of concurrent bacterial or viral infections, pain and pruritus. Longer term complications include hyper- and hypopigmentation, prolonged erythema, scarring and ectropion. The concurrent use of oral isotretinoin is an absolute contraindication because of an increased risk of hypertrophic scarring.

Techniques devised to avoid the morbidity of laser resurfacing include fractional resurfacing and non-ablative treatments. In fractional resurfacing, small non-contiguous areas of skin are treated. This allows faster healing to occur from adjacent non-treated tissue. Its drawbacks are that several treatments are required, and the early reports suggest that resurfacing is not as effective as that achieved by conventional laser treatment. Non-ablative treatment has been described, with a number of other laser sources intended to cause the beneficial changes seen after conventional laser resurfacing, but without epidermal coagulation necrosis. In the absence of convincing clinical trial data, the place of this technique remains uncertain.

---

**Learning points**

1 Dynamic wrinkles respond to treatment with botulinum toxin. Wrinkles at rest are better treated with a dermal filler.
2 Match the treatment to the depth of the skin changes. More superficial ageing signs such as lentigines and keratoses will respond to superficial or mid-depth peels. Deeper changes – rhytides or scarring – will need deep peels, or CO2 laser.

---

Aside from resurfacing, lasers can be used to treat pigmentary lesions of the skin, whether resulting from melanin or unwanted tattoos. The type of laser must be matched to the target chromophore, but as a general rule the best results are obtained when there is a large colour difference between the normal skin and the lesion treated.

## Further reading

Baumann L. (2002) *Cosmetic Dermatology: Principles and Practice*. McGraw-Hill, New York.

Coleman-Moriarty K. (2004) *Botulinum Toxin in Facial Rejuvenation*. Mosby, Edinburgh.

Ratner D, Tse Y, Marchell N, *et al.* (1999) Cutaneous laser resurfacing. *Journal of the American Academy of Dermatology* **41**, 365–389.

Samuel M, Brooke RCC, Hollis S & Griffiths CEM. (2005) Interventions for photodamaged skin. *Cochrane Database of Systematic Reviews* **1**, CD001782. DOI: 10.1002/14651858.

The beauty business. *The Economist* 22 May 2003.

# 23 The skin and the psyche

Most people accept that there are strong links between the skin and the emotions. Embarassment causes blushing. Anxiety causes cold, sweaty palms. Anger causes the face to redden. However, only a few skin disorders, such as dermatitis artefacta, have emotional factors as their direct cause. The relationships between the mind and the skin are usually subtle and complex. Nevertheless, patients with skin disorders do have a higher prevalence of psychiatric abnormalities than the general population, although specific personality profiles and disorders can seldom be tied to specific skin diseases. Similarly, it is still not clear how, or even how often, psychological factors trigger, worsen or perpetuate such everyday problems as atopic eczema or psoriasis.

Each school of psychiatry has its own theories on the subject, but their explanations do not satisfy everyone. Do people really damage their skin to satisfy guilt feelings? Does their skin 'weep' because they have themselves suppressed weeping? Until more is known, it may be wise to adopt a simpler and more pragmatic approach, in which interactions between the skin and psyche are divided into two broad groups:

- emotional reactions to the presence of skin disease, real or imagined; and
- the effects of emotions on skin disease (Fig. 23.1).

## Reactions to skin disease

The presence of disfiguring skin lesions can distort the emotional development of a child: some become withdrawn, others become aggressive, but many adjust well. The range of reactions to skin disease is therefore wide. At one end lies indifference to grossly disfiguring lesions and, at the other, lies an obsession with skin that is quite normal. Between these extremes are reactions ranging from natural anxiety over ugly skin lesions to disproportionate worry over minor blemishes.

A chronic skin disease such as psoriasis can undoubtedly spoil the lives of those who suffer from it. It can interfere with work, and with social activities of all sorts including sexual relationships, causing patients to feel like outcasts. The heavy drinking of so many men with severe psoriasis is one result of these pressures. An experienced dermatologist will be on the lookout for depression and the risk of suicide, as up to 10% of patients with psoriasis have had suicidal thoughts. However, these reactions do not necessarily correlate with the extent and severity of the eruption as judged by an outside observer. Who has the more disabling problem: someone with 50% of their body surface covered in psoriasis, but who largely ignores this and has a happy family life and a productive job, or one with 5% involvement whose social life is ruined by it? The concept of 'body image' is useful here.

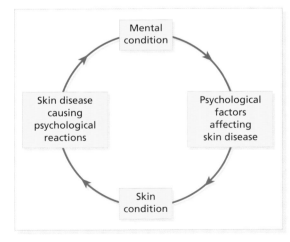

**Fig. 23.1** Mind–skin interactions.

## Body image

All of us think we know how we look, but our ideas may not tally with those of others. The nose, face, hair and genitals tend to rank high in a person's 'corporeal awareness', and trivial lesions in those areas can generate much anxiety. The facial lesions of acne, for example, can lead to a huge loss of self-esteem, and, for some reason, feelings of shame.

## Dermatological delusional disease

### Dysmorphophobia

This is the term applied to distortions of the body image. Minor and inconspicuous lesions are magnified in the mind to grotesque proportions.

#### Dermatological 'non-disease'

This is a form of dysmorphophobia. The clinician can find no skin abnormality, but the distress felt by the patient leads to anxiety, depression or even suicide. Such patients are not uncommon. They expect dermatological solutions for complaints such as hair loss, or burning, itching and redness of the face or genitals. The dermatologist, who can see nothing wrong, cannot solve matters and no treatment seems to help. Such patients are reluctant to see a psychiatrist although some may have a monosymptomatic hypochondriacal psychosis.

### Other delusions

These patients sustain single hypochondriacal delusions for long periods, in the absence of other recognizable psychiatric disease. They may become eccentric and live in social isolation. Some believe that they have syphilis, AIDS or skin cancer. Others hide in shame from an inapparent body odour. Still other patients have the delusion that their skin is infested with parasites.

### Delusions of parasitosis (Fig. 23.2)

This term is better than 'parasitophobia', which implies a fear of becoming infested. Patients with delusions of parasitosis are unshakably convinced that they are already infested. No rational argument can convince them that they are not. Many see parasites move on their skin, or feel them crawl or need to dig them out. The pest control agencies that they have called in, and their medical advisers, therefore must both be wrong. Patients often bring to the clinic a box of specimens of the 'parasite' at different stages of its supposed life cycle. These must be examined microscopically but usually turn out to be fragments of skin, hair, clothing, haemorrhagic crusts or unclassifiable debris. The skin changes may include gouge marks and scratches, but it is correct to consider these patients separately from those with dermatitis artefacta.

These patients become angry if doubts are cast on their ideas, or if they are referred to a psychiatrist. How could treatment for mental illness possibly be expected to kill parasites? Family members may share their delusions and much tact is needed to secure any co-operation with treatment. Direct confrontations are best avoided; sometimes it may be best simply to treat with psychotropic drugs, explaining that these may be able to help some of the symptoms.

The delusions of a few of these patients are based on an underlying depression or schizophrenia, and of a further few on organic problems such as vitamin deficiency or cerebrovascular disease. Other patients are addicted to metamphetamine or narcotics. These disorders must be treated on their own merits. However, most patients have monosymptomatic hypochondriacal delusions, which can often be suppressed by treatment with drugs, accepting that these will be needed long term. Otherwise, the outlook for resolution is poor.

Pimozide is probably the best treatment for this condition, but high doses carry cardiac risks. If pimozide is used, an electrocardiogram (ECG) should be performed before starting treatment and the drug should not be given to those with a prolonged Q-T interval or with a history of cardiac dysrhythmia. Fortunately, most patients respond to low doses of 2–4 mg/day. Patients on high doses need periodic ECG checks. Tardive dyskinesia may develop and persist despite withdrawal of the drug. Risperidone, olanzapine and sulpiride are reasonable,

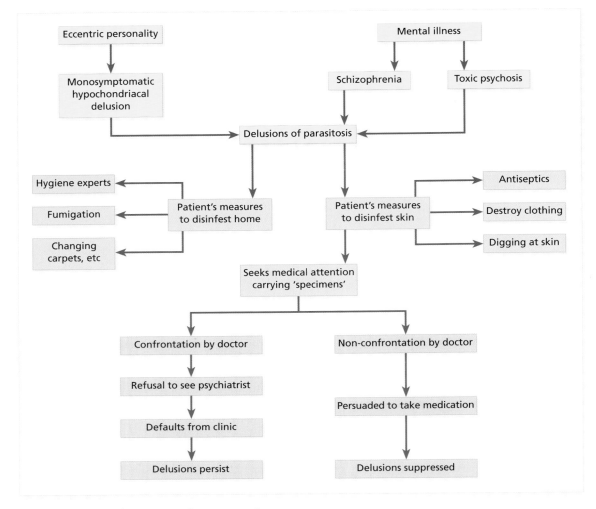

**Fig. 23.2** Delusions of parasitosis – the sequence of events.

and perhaps safer, alternatives. Some patients gain insight and relief. Others hint that their parasites still persist although this no longer disables them. Many fail to keep their follow-up appointments.

## Dermatitis artefacta

Here the skin lesions are caused and kept going by the patient's own actions, but parasites are not held to be to blame. Patients with dermatitis artefacta deny self-trauma but, naturally, if treatment is left to them to carry out, their problems do not improve. Lesions will heal under occlusive dressings, but this does not alter the underlying psychiatric prob-

lems, and lesions may recur or crop up outside the bandaged areas or the bandages get removed. Different types of dermatitis artefacta are listed in Table 23.1.

The lesions favour accessible areas, and do not fit with known pathological processes. The diagnosis is often difficult to make, but an experienced clinician will suspect it because there are no primary lesions and because of the bizarre shape or grouping of the lesions, which may be rectilinear or oddly grouped (Fig. 23.3). Areas damaged by burning (Fig. 23.4), corrosive chemicals (Fig. 23.5) or by digging have their own special appearance. Histology varies depending on cause, but many show epidermal necrosis.

**Table 23.1** Types of dermatitis artefacta.

| Type | Personality |
|------|-------------|
| Minor habits (e.g. excoriated acne) | Relatively normal or obsessive |
| More obvious lesions | Hysterical or neurotic (secondary gain) |
| Bizarre | Psychotic |
| Malingering | Criminal |

**Fig. 23.5** Dermatitis artefacta: denials of self-trauma did not convince us that this was caused by any other skin disease.

**Fig. 23.3** Obvious dermatitis artefacta: back your own judgement against the patient's here.

**Fig. 23.4** A lighted cigarette was responsible for this appearance.

More subtle changes are seen in 'dermatological pathomimicry', in which patients reproduce or aggravate their skin disease by deliberate contact with materials to which they know they will react.

Apart from frank malingerers, the patients are often young women with some medical knowledge, perhaps a nurse. Some form of 'secondary gain' from having skin lesions may be obvious. The psychological problems may be superficial and easily resolved, but usually psychiatric help is needed and the artefacts are part of a prolonged psychiatric illness. A few patients respond to banal treatments if given the chance to save face. Direct confrontation and accusations are usually best avoided, but the physician must make efforts to help by working to get the patient to see a psychiatrist and to convince those caring for them that the wounds are self-inflicted.

**Learning points**

- Do not reward a delusion with a treatment for scabies
- Direct confrontations with patients with dermatitis artefacta or delusions of parasitosis may make you feel better, but do little for them

**Fig. 23.6** Unusually extensive neurotic excoriations.

**Fig. 23.7** The excoriated nodules of prurigo nodularis.

## Neurotic excoriations

Patients with neurotic excoriations differ from those with other types of dermatitis artefacta in that they admit to picking and digging at their skin. This habit affects women more often than men and is most active at times of stress. The clinical picture is mixed, with crusted excoriations, peripherally healing irregular ulcers and pale scars, often with a hyperpigmented border, lying mainly on the face, neck, shoulders and arms (Fig. 23.6). The condition may last for years and psychotherapy is seldom successful. Selective serotonin uptake inhibitors such as fluoxetine help some patients, especially those with compulsive needs to pick and squeeze skin.

## Acne excoriée

Here the self-inflicted damage is based to some extent on the lesions of acne vulgaris, which may in themselves be mild, but become disfiguring when dug and squeezed to excess. The patients are usually young girls who may leave themselves with ugly scars. A psychiatric approach is often unhelpful; many patients have insight and recognize their compulsive need to pick at every blemish. A daily ritual of attacking the lesions, helped by a magnify-

ing mirror, may persist for years. Again, selective serotonin uptake inhibitors may help.

## Localized neurodermatitis (lichen simplex)

This term refers to areas of itchy eczematization and lichenification, perpetuated by bouts of scratching in response to itching and stress. The condition is not uncommon and can occur on any area of skin. In men, lesions are often on the posterior calves; in women, they favour the nape of the neck where the redness and scaling look rather like psoriasis. Some examples of persistent itching in the anogenital area are caused by lichen simplex there.

Patients with localized neurodermatitis develop scratch responses to minor itch stimuli more readily than controls. Local therapy does not alter the underlying cause, but topical steroids, sometimes only the most potent ones, ameliorate the symptoms. Occlusive bandaging of suitable areas clears only those lesions that are covered.

Nodular prurigo (Fig. 23.7) may be a variant on this theme as manifested in atopic subjects, who scratch and rub remorselessly at their extremely itchy nodules. These patients readily agree that they prefer the pain of excoriations to the itch of the nodules.

## Hair-pulling habit

Trichotillomania is too dramatic a word for what is usually only a minor comfort habit in children, ranking alongside nail-biting and lip-licking. Perhaps the term should be dropped in favour of 'hair-pulling habit'. It is usually of little consequence, and children who twist and pull their hair, often as they are going to sleep, seldom have major psychiatric disorders. The habit often goes away most quickly if it is ignored. However, more severe degrees of hair-pulling are sometimes seen in disturbed adolescents and in those with learning difficulties; then the outlook for full regrowth is less good, even with formal psychiatric help.

The diagnosis can usually be made on the history, but some parents do not know what is going on. The bald areas do not show the exclamation-mark hairs of alopecia areata, or the scaling and inflammation of scalp ringworm. The patches are irregular in outline and hair loss is never complete. Those hairs that remain are bent or broken, and of variable short lengths.

## Dermatoses precipitated or perpetuated by emotional factors

Popular candidates for inclusion in this group of diseases are psoriasis, urticaria, atopic eczema, pompholyx, discoid eczema, alopecia areata, lichen simplex and lichen planus. Fancy rather than fact still rules here, but a scientific basis for these effects is gradually being established. For example, in psoriasis, stress increases the neuropeptide content of lesions, with a concomitant drop in the activity of enzymes that degrade neuropeptides, especially mast-cell chymase. In addition, the blood concentrations of certain neuromediators, especially β-endorphin, change during exacerbations and the hypothalamic–pituitary axis response to social stress appears to differ in psoriatics who feel that stress worsens their disease, compared with those in whom it does not. Yet an aura of doubt lingers on – for a variety of reasons. The concept of stress is not a simple one, and the terms in which it is discussed are sometimes used rather vaguely. Each type of stress may well provoke its own pattern of response. For this reason many investigators have preferred to record damaging life events rather than to speculate about the presence of stress itself. However, there are problems with this approach too, as a barrage of minor daily annoyances may well be more important than major life events. Every dermatologist will have seen apparent examples of associations between external stress and exacerbations of most of these conditions, but proof that stress causes them is hard to find. No one questions that stress can cause sweating of the palms, but some studies suggest that chronic hyperhidrosis of the palms and soles, once thought to be simply an accentuated response to stress, has no relationship to chronic anxiety at all.

## Further reading

Arck PC, Slominski A, Theoharides TC, Peters EMJ & Paus R. (2006) Neuroimmunology and stress: skin takes center stage. *Journal of Investigative Dermatology* **126**, 1697–1704.

Elmer KB, George RM & Peterson K. (2000) Therapeutic update: use of risperidone for the treatment of monosymptomatic hypochondriacal psychosis. *Journal of the American Academy of Dermatology* **43**, 683–686.

Gupta MA & Gupta K. (1996) Psychodermatology: an update. *Journal of the American Academy of Dermatology* **34**, 1030–1046.

Koblenzer CS. (2000) Dermatitis artefacta: clinical features and approaches to treatment. *American Journal of Clinical Dermatology* **1**, 47–55.

Koblenzer CS. (2005) The emotional impact of chronic and disabling skin disease: a psychoanalytic perspective. *Dermatologic Clinics* **23**, 619–627.

Koo JY, Do JH & Lee CS. (2000) Psychodermatology. *Journal of the American Academy of Dermatology* **43**, 848–853.

Picardi A, Abeni D, Melchi CF, Puddu P & Pasquini P. (2000) Psychiatric morbidity in dermatological outpatients: an issue to be recognized. *British Journal of Dermatology* **143**, 983–991.

Steinhoff M, Bienenstock J, Schemltz M, Maurer M, Wei E & Biro T. (2006) Neurophysiological, neuroimmunological, and neuroendocrine basis for pruritus. *Journal of Investigative Dermatology* **126**, 1705–1718.

# 24 Other genetic disorders

The human genome consists of 23 pairs of chromosomes carrying an estimated 30 000 genes. The pairs of matching chromosomes as seen at colchicine-arrested metaphase are numbered in accordance with their size. A centromere divides each chromosome into a shorter (p) and a longer (q) arm.

Any individual's chromosomal makeup (karyotype) can be expressed as their total number of chromosomes with their sex chromosome constitution. A normal male therefore is 46XY. A shorthand notation exists for recording other abnormalities such as chromosome translocations and deletions.

The precise location of any gene can be given by naming the chromosome, the arm of the chromosome (p or q) and the numbers of the band and subband of the chromosome, as seen with Giemsa staining, on which it lies. Filaggrin, one of the genes important for atopic eczema, for instance, lies on chromosome 1q21.3 (i.e. on the long arm of chromosome 1 at band 21, subband 3).

Several techniques can be used to identify the position of a gene.

1 A clue may emerge by finding that some affected individuals have chromosomal deletions or unbalanced translocations, suggesting that the gene in question lies on the abnormal segments.

2 *Linkage analysis* Genes are linked if they lie close together on the same chromosome; they will then be inherited together. The closer together they are, the less is the chance of their being separated by crossovers, one to six of which, depending on length, occur on each chromosome at meiosis. Each member of an affected family has to be examined both for the presence of the trait to be mapped, and also for a marker, usually a DNA probe, which has already been mapped. If linkage is established then the two loci will be close on the same chromosome. The probability of the results of such a study representing true linkage can be expressed as a logarithm of the odds (Lod) score. A score of three or more suggests that the linkage is likely to be genuine.

3 *Somatic cell hybridization* A hybrid made by fusing a human cell with a mouse cell will at first have two sets of chromosomes. Later, human chromosomes are lost randomly until a stable state is reached. Those cells that produce a particular human protein must contain the relevant chromosome. A panel of such hybrid cells can be created which differ in their content of human chromosomes. By comparing these, the chromosomal site of the relevant gene can be deduced.

4 *In situ hybridization* A cloned sequence of DNA, if made single-stranded by heat, will stick to its complementary sequence on a chromosome. Radioactive or fluorescent labelling can be used to indicate its position there.

## Non-Mendelian genetics

Traditional genetics has also been extended by the introduction of several new non-Mendelian concepts of importance in dermatology. These include the following.

1 *Mosaicism* A mosaic is a single individual made up of two or more genetically distinct cell lines. The concept is important in several skin disorders including incontinentia pigmenti (p. 353) and segmental neurofibromatosis (p. 349). The mutation of a single cell in a foetus (a post-zygotic mutation) may form a clone of abnormal cells. In the epidermis these often adopt a bizarre pattern of lines and whorls – Blaschko's lines, named after the dermatologist who recorded them in linear epidermal naevi in 1901.

2 *Contiguous gene deletions* Complex phenotypes occur when several adjacent genes are lost. In this way, for example, X-linked ichthyosis may associate with hypogonadism or anosmia.

**3** *Genomic imprinting* means that genes may differ in their effect depending on the parent from which they are inherited. Genes from the father seem especially important in psoriasis, and from the mother in atopy (p. 91).

**4** *Uniparental disomy* occurs when both of a pair of genes are derived from the same parent so that an individual lacks either a maternal or a paternal copy. In this way, a disorder usually inherited as a recessive trait can arise even though only one parent is a carrier.

**5** *Mitochondrial mutations* can cause genodermatoses (e.g. one type of palmoplantar keratoderma). The condition is passed from the mother to both male and female offspring, but affected males do not pass it on to their offspring.

Two other important genetic concepts are 'clinical heterogeneity' (when clinically distinct phenotypes are produced by different mutations within the same gene, such as red hair variants caused by different polymorphisms of the *MC1R* gene) and 'genetic heterogeneity' (when the same clinical picture can be produced by mutations in different genes as in tuberous sclerosis).

Inheritance is important in many of the conditions discussed in other chapters and this has been highlighted in the sections on aetiology. This chapter includes some genetic disorders not covered elsewhere.

## Red hair

Red hair is not, of course, a disease but it is the first normal variation in human appearance for which a causative genetic polymorphism has been found. The melanocortin-1 receptor (*MC1R*) gene is found at 16q24.3. While at least 30 genetic variants have been described, three in particular are associated with an increased phaeo- (red) to eu- (black) melanin ratio (p. 277). Individuals homozygous or heterozygous for one or two of these 'red hair alleles' are likely to have pale skin, red hair and poor tanning ability.

## Neurofibromatoses

These relatively common disorders affect about 1 in 3000 people and are inherited as an autosomal dominant trait. There are two main types: von Recklinghausen's neurofibromatosis (*NF1*; which accounts for 85% of all cases) and bilateral acoustic neurofibromatosis (*NF2*); these are phenotypically and genetically distinct.

### NF1

#### Cause

The *NF1* gene has been localized to chromosome 17q11.1. It is unusually large (300 kb) and many different mutations within it have now been identified. The *NF1* gene is a tumour suppressor gene, the product of which, neurofibromin, interacts with the product of the *RAS* proto-oncogene. This may explain the susceptibility of *NF1* patients to a variety of tumours. The inheritance of *NF1* is as an autosomal dominant trait but about half of index cases have no preceding family history.

#### Clinical features

The physical signs include the following.
● Six or more *café au lait* patches (light brown oval macules; Fig. 24.1), usually developing in the first year of life.

**Fig. 24.1** Neurofibromatosis: one large but benign neurofibroma has ulcerated over the sacrum. Several *café au lait* patches are visible.

**Fig. 24.3** Lisch nodules: best seen with a slit-lamp.

**Fig. 24.2** Freckling of the axilla and a *café au lait* patch – both markers of neurofibromatosis.

- Axillary freckling (Fig. 24.2) in two-thirds of affected individuals (Crowe's sign).
- Variable numbers of skin neurofibromas, some small and superficial, others larger and deeper, ranging from flesh-coloured to pink, purple or brown (Fig. 24.1). Most are dome-like nodules, but others are irregular raised plaques. Some are firm, some soft and compressible through a deficient dermis ('button-hole' sign); others feel 'knotty' or 'wormy'. Neurofibromas may not appear until puberty and become larger and more numerous with age.
- Small circular pigmented hamartomas of the iris (Lisch nodules; Fig. 24.3), appear in early childhood.

Nearly all *NF1* patients meet the criteria for diagnosis by the age of 8 years, and all do so by 20 years. The usual order of appearance of the clinical features is *café au lait* macules, axillary freckling, Lisch nodules and neurofibromas.

### Diagnosis

The *café au lait* marks, axillary freckling and Lisch nodules should be looked for, as they appear before the skin neurofibromas. A segmental form of *NF1* is caused by a post-zygotic mutation. Isolated neuro-

fibromas are not uncommon in individuals without neurofibromatosis and are of little consequence unless they are painful.

### Complications

A neurofibroma will occasionally change into a neurofibrosarcoma. Other associated features may include kyphoscoliosis, learning impairment, epilepsy, renal artery stenosis and an association with phaeochromocytoma. Forme fruste variants occur (e.g. segmental neurofibromatosis).

### Management

Ugly or painful lesions, and any suspected of undergoing malignant change, should be removed. The chance of a child of an affected adult developing the disorder is 1 in 2 – parents should be advised about this. Those who are affected should be kept under review and have their blood pressure checked regularly.

### NF2

### Cause

The inheritance of *NF2* is also autosomal dominant. Mapping to chromosome 22q12.21 followed the observation of changes in chromosome 22 in meningiomas as these tumours may be seen in *NF2*. This gene also normally functions as a tumour suppressor gene, the product of which is known as Merlin.

## Clinical features

- Bilateral acoustic neuromas;
- Few, if any, cutaneous manifestations;
- No Lisch nodules;
- Other tumours of the central nervous system may occur, especially meningiomas and gliomas.

## Management

All *NF2* patients and their families should have access to genetic testing as presymptomatic diagnosis improves clinical management. Clinical screening for at-risk family members can start at birth.

## Tuberous sclerosis

This uncommon condition, with a prevalence of about 1 in 12 000 in children under 10 years, is inherited as an autosomal dominant trait, with variable expressivity even within the same family. Fertility is reduced, so transmission through more than two generations is rare.

## Cause

Inactivating mutations at two different loci can, independently, cause clinically identical tuberous sclerosis. Both genes are tumour suppressors. The product of one (*TSC1* on chromosome 9q34) is hamartin; that encoded by the other (*TSC2* on 16p13.3) is tuberin. Hamartin and tuberin form a complex, and this may explain why changes in the production of either causes a similar disease phenotype. In fact, *TSC2* gene mutations are responsible for 80–90% of cases.

## Clinical features

The skin changes include the following.
- *Small oval white patches* ('ash leaf macules') occur in 80% of those affected. These are important as they may be the only manifestation at birth.
- *Angiofibromas* (known as adenoma sebaceum) occur in 85% of those affected. They develop at puberty as pink or yellowish acne-like papules on the face, often around the nose (Fig. 24.4). These
- *Periungual fibromas* occur in 50% of patients. These

**Fig. 24.4** Tuberous sclerosis. The patient with adenoma sebaceum, understandably, was referred to the acne clinic.

develop in adult life as small pink sausage-like lesions emerging from the nail folds (Fig. 24.5).
- *Connective tissue naevi* ('shagreen patches') are seen in 40% of patients. Cobblestone, somewhat yellow plaques often arise in the skin over the base of the spine.

Other features may include:
- epilepsy (in 75% of patients);
- mental retardation (in 50% of patients);

**Fig. 24.5** The periungual fibromas of tuberous sclerosis are found in adult patients.

**Fig. 24.6** Computed tomography scan of a patient with tuberous sclerosis. Modern imaging techniques can sometimes show cortical tubers (white) even when the skin changes are minimal.

● ocular signs, including retinal phakomas and pigmentary abnormalities (in 50% of patients);
● hyperplastic gums;
● gliomas along the lateral walls of the lateral ventricles (80% of cases) and calcification of the basal ganglia; and
● renal and heart tumours.

### Diagnosis and differential diagnosis

Any baby with unexplained epilepsy should be examined with a Wood's light (p. 38) to look for ash leaf macules. Skull X-rays and computed tomography scans (Fig. 24.6) help to exclude involvement of the central nervous system and kidneys. The lesions of adenoma sebaceum (a misnomer, as histologically they are angiofibromas) may be mistaken for acne.

### Management

Affected families need genetic counselling. Apparently unaffected parents with an affected child will wish to know the chances of further children being affected. Before concluding that an affected child is the result of a new mutation, the parents should be examined with a Wood's light and by an ophthalmologist to help exclude the possibility of genetic

transmission from a subtly affected parent. As the gene defects become established, prenatal screening of DNA should indicate those at risk.

Facial angiofibromas may improve cosmetically after electrodessication, dermabrasion or destruction by laser but tend to recur.

## Xeroderma pigmentosum

Xeroderma pigmentosum is a heterogeneous group of autosomal recessive disorders, characterized by the defective repair of DNA after its damage by ultraviolet radiation. The condition is rare, affecting about 5 per million in Europe.

### Cause

Ultraviolet light damages DNA by producing covalent linkages between adjacent pyrimidines. These distort the double helix and inhibit gene expression. Cells from xeroderma pigmentosum patients lack the ability of normal cells to repair this damage.

DNA repair is a complex process using a large number of genes that encode a variety of interacting products that locate and prepare damaged sites for excision and replacement. It is not surprising therefore that several genetic defects have been shown to lead to a similar clinical picture.

### Clinical features

There are many variants but all follow the same pattern.
● The skin is normal at birth.
● Multiple freckles, roughness and keratoses on exposed skin appear between the ages of 6 months and 2 years (Fig. 24.7). Photosensitivity increases thereafter.
● The atrophic facial skin shows telangiectases and small angiomas.
● Many tumours develop on light-damaged skin: these include basal cell carcinomas, squamous cell carcinomas and malignant melanomas. Many patients die before the age of 20 years.
● Eye problems are common and include photophobia, conjunctivitis and ectropion.
● The condition may be associated with microcephaly, mental deficiency, dwarfism, deafness and ataxia (De Sanctis–Cacchione syndrome).

**Fig. 24.7** Xeroderma pigmentosum: obvious freckling on neck. Scars on nose mark the spots where tumours have been removed.

## Diagnosis

This becomes evident on clinical grounds, although variants with minor signs may cause difficulty. The DNA repair defect can be detected in a few laboratories after the ultraviolet irradiation of cultured fibroblasts or lymphocytes from the patient.

## Treatment

Skin cancers can be prevented by strict avoidance of sunlight, the use of protective clothing, wide-brimmed hats and of reflectant sunscreens and dark glasses. If possible, patients should not go out by day. Early and complete removal of all tumours is essential. Radiotherapy should be avoided. Cutaneous gene therapy may be a possibility in the future.

## Incontinentia pigmenti

This rare condition is inherited as an X-linked dominant disorder. It is usually lethal before birth in males whereas affected females, mosaic as a result of X-inactivation, can survive. The bizarre patterning of the skin is caused by this random X-inactivation (Lyonization). The lines of affected and normal skin represent clones of cells in which either the abnormal or normal X chromosome is active. The gene for one type of incontinentia pigmenti has been mapped to Xq28: it is a component of a signalling pathway (the NF-κB pathway) that controls the expression of several genes responsible for cytokines.

## Clinical features

Skin changes are usually present at birth but may sometimes come up over the first few days of life. There are three stages in their evolution.
1 *Vesicular* Linear groups of blisters occur more on the limbs than trunk.
2 *Warty* After a few weeks the blisters dry up and the predominant lesions are papules with a verrucous hyperkeratotic surface.
3 *Pigmented* A whorled or 'splashed' macular pigmentation, ranging from slate-grey to brown, replaces the warty lesions. Its bizarre patterning is a strong diagnostic pointer.

Occasionally, the vesicular and warty stages occur *in utero*; warty or pigmented lesions may therefore be the first signs of the condition. There is also a variant in which pale rather than dark whorls and streaks are seen.

Associated abnormalities are common. One-quarter of patients have defects of their central nervous system, most commonly mental retardation, epilepsy or microcephaly. Skull and palatal abnormalities may also be found. Delayed dentition, and even a total absence of teeth, are recognized features. The incisors may be cone- or peg-shaped. Ocular defects occur in one-third of patients, the most common being strabismus, cataract and optic atrophy.

## Differential diagnosis

Diagnosis is usually made in infancy when bullous lesions predominate so the differential diagnosis includes bullous impetigo (p. 222), candidiasis (p. 252), and the rarer linear immunoglobulin A (IgA) bullous disease of childhood (p. 125) and epidermolysis bullosa (p. 128).

## Investigations

There is frequently an eosinophilia in the blood. Biopsy of an intact blister reveals an intra-epidermal vesicle filled with eosinophils.

## Management

This is symptomatic and includes measures to combat bacterial and candidal infection during the vesicular phase. Family counselling should be available.

## Ehlers–Danlos syndrome

Many subtypes have now been recognized and this complicated subject has earned its own scientific group, which continuously updates classification and molecular biology.

### Cause

All varieties of the Ehlers–Danlos syndrome are based on abnormalities in the formation or modification of collagen and the extracellular matrix, but are not necessarily a result of mutations in the collagen genes themselves. Established defects include lysyl hydroxylase deficiency, abnormalities in pro-alpha-1 (V) collagen chains, mutations in type III collagen genes, a deficiency of procollagen protease, and a fibronectin defect.

### Clinical features

- Soft hyperelastic skin;
- Hyperextensibility of the joints;
- Fragility of skin and blood vessels;
- Easy bruising; and
- Curious ('cigarette paper') scars.

Sometimes these changes are so mild that the condition is not recognized.

### Complications

These depend on the type. They include subluxation of joints, varicose veins in early life, an increased liability to develop hernias, kyphoscoliosis, aortic aneurysms and ruptured large arteries, and intraocular haemorrhage. Affected individuals may be born prematurely as a result of the early rupture of fragile fetal membranes.

### Diagnosis and treatment

The diagnosis is made on the clinical features and family history. The frequent skin lacerations and prominent scars may suggest child abuse. The diagnosis and type can sometimes be confirmed by enzyme studies on isolated fibroblasts. There is no effective treatment but genetic counselling is needed.

## Pseudoxanthoma elasticum

This is the classic inherited connective tissue disorder affecting the elastic structures in the body – most obviously in the skin, blood vessels and eyes.

### Cause

It is inherited as an autosomal recessive condition, the result of mutations in a gene (the *ABCC6* gene on chromosome 16p13.1) encoding for a transmembrane transporter protein, which is a member of the ABC transporters superfamily. It is still not clear how this causes the disease.

### Pathology

The elastic fibres in the mid-dermis become swollen and fragmented; their calcification is probably a secondary feature. The elastic tissue of blood vessels and of the retina may also be affected.

### Clinical features

The skin of the neck and axillae, and occasionally of other body folds, is loose and wrinkled. Groups of small yellow papules give these areas a 'plucked chicken' appearance (Fig. 24.8). Breaks in the retina show as angioid streaks, which are grey, poorly defined areas radiating from the optic nerve head. Arterial involvement may lead to peripheral, coronary or cerebral arterial insufficiency.

**Fig. 24.8** The 'plucked chicken' appearance of pseudoxanthoma in the antecubital fossa.

## Complications

The most important are hypertension, recurrent gut haemorrhages, ischaemic heart disease and cerebral haemorrhage. Pregnancy is always accompanied by striae and there is an increased risk of miscarriage.

## Diagnosis and treatment

The diagnosis is made clinically and confirmed by the histology. There is no effective treatment. Blood pressure should be carefully monitored and controlled.

> **Learning point**
>
> In all genodermatoses, the decision to have children, or not, must lie with the family concerned. Make sure they have all of the facts before them

## Further reading

Harper J. (1996) *Inherited Skin Disorders: the genodermatoses*. Butterworth-Heinemann, Oxford.

Huson SM. (2006) The neurofibromatoses: more than just a medical curiosity. *Journal of the Royal College of Physicians Edinburgh* **36**, 44–50.

Irvine MD & McLean WHI. (2003) The molecular genetics of the genodermatoses: progress to date and future directions. *British Journal of Dermatology* **148**, 1–13.

Matthew C. (2001) Postgenomic technologies: hunting the genes for common disorders. *British Medical Journal* **122**, 1031–1034.

Moss C & Savin JA. (1995) *Dermatology and the New Genetics*. Blackwell Science, Oxford.

Online Mendelian Inheritance in Man (OMIM) website: http://www.ncbi.nlm.nih.gov/omim/

Rees JL. (2000) Genetics, past and present, and the rise of systems dermatology. *British Journal of Dermatology* **143**, 41–46.

# 25 Drug eruptions

Almost any drug can cause a cutaneous reaction, and many inflammatory skin conditions can be caused or exacerbated by drugs. A drug reaction can reasonably be included in the differential diagnosis of most skin diseases.

## Mechanisms

These are many and various (Table 25.1), being related both to the properties of the drug in question and to a variety of host factors. Indeed, pharmaceutical companies study genes to predict responders and non-responders, and to detect patients who may be unable to metabolize a drug normally. For example, drug-induced lupus erythematosus occurs more commonly among 'slow acetylators' who take hydralazine. However, not all adverse drug reactions have a genetic basis; the excess of drug eruptions seen in the elderly may reflect drug interactions associated with their high medication intake.

### Non-allergic drug reactions

Not all drug reactions are based on allergy. Some are a result of overdosage, others are due to to the accumulation of drugs or to unwanted pharmaco-logical effects (e.g. stretch marks from systemic steroids; Fig. 25.1). Other reactions are idiosyncratic (an odd reaction peculiar to one individual) or a result of alterations of ecological balance (see below).

Cutaneous reactions can be expected from the very nature of some drugs. These are normal but unwanted responses that patients show when a drug is given in a high dose, or even in a therapeutic dose. For example, mouth ulcers may occur as a result of the cytotoxicity of methotrexate. Silver-based preparations, given for prolonged periods, can lead to a slate-grey colour of the skin (argyria). Acute vaginal candidiasis occurs when antibiotics remove the normal resident bacteria from the female genital tract and so foster colonization by yeasts. Dapsone or rifampicin, given to patients with lepromatous leprosy, may cause erythema nodosum leprosum as the immune response to the bacillus is re-established.

Non-allergic reactions are often predictable. They affect many, or even all, patients taking the drug at a sufficient dosage for a sufficient time. Careful studies before marketing should indicate the types of reaction that can be anticipated.

**Table 25.1** Some mechanisms involved in drug reactions.

Pharmacological
Caused by overdosage or failure to excrete or metabolize
Cumulative effects
Altered skin ecology
Allergic
   IgE-mediated
   Cytotoxic
   Immune complex-mediated
   Cell-mediated
Idiosyncratic
Exacerbation of pre-existing skin conditions

**Fig. 25.1** Gross striae caused by systemic steroids.

## Allergic drug reactions

Allergic drug reactions are less predictable. They occur in only a minority of patients receiving a drug and can do so even with low doses. Allergic reactions are not a normal biological effect of the drug and usually appear after the latent period required for induction of an immune response. Chemically related drugs may cross-react.

The majority of allergic drug reactions are caused by cell-mediated immune reaction (p. 30), which can present in a number of forms, most commonly a maculopapular eruption or morbilliform erythema. Rarer allergic reactions include bullae, erythroderma, pruritus, toxic epidermal necrolysis (TEN), acute generalized exanthematous pustulosis, and the drug rash with eosinophilia and systemic signs (DRESS) syndrome. Helper CD4+ T cells occur more frequently in the more common morbilliform eruptions, while cytotoxic CD8+ T cells predominate in blistering eruptions (TEN, Stevens–Johnson syndrome) and fixed drug eruptions. Other types of drug reaction include urticaria and angio-oedema, generally brought about by immunoglobulin E (IgE) mediated type I hypersensitivity reactions, and vasculitis generally caused by type III immune complex-mediated reactions (p. 9). The factors that lead to particular clinical patterns of cutaneous adverse drug reactions remain largely unexplained.

## Presentation

### Some drugs and the reactions they can cause

Experience helps here, together with a knowledge of the reactions most likely to be caused by individual drugs, and also of the most common causes of the various reaction patterns. Any unusual rash should be suspected of being a drug reaction, and approached along the lines listed in Table 25.2.

### Antibiotics

Penicillins and sulphonamides are among the drugs most commonly causing allergic reactions. These are often morbilliform (Fig. 25.2), but urticaria, erythema multiforme and fixed eruptions are

**Table 25.2** The six vital questions to be asked when a drug eruption is suspected.

**1** Can you exclude a simple dermatosis (e.g. scabies or psoriasis) and the known skin manifestations of an underlying disorder (e.g. systemic lupus erythematosus)?
**2** Does the rash itself suggest a drug eruption (e.g. urticaria, erythema multiforme)?
**3** Does a past history of drug reactions correlate with current prescriptions?
**4** Was any drug introduced a few days or weeks before the eruption appeared?
**5** Which of the current drugs most commonly cause drug eruptions (e.g. penicillins, sulphonamides, thiazides, allopurinol, phenylbutazone)?
**6** Does the eruption fit with a well-recognized pattern caused by one of the current drugs (e.g. an acneiform rash from lithium)?

**Fig. 25.2** Symmetrical erythematous maculopapular rash as a result of ampicillin.

common too. Viral infections are often associated with exanthems, and many rashes are incorrectly blamed on an antibiotic when, in fact, the virus was responsible. Most patients with infectious mononucleosis develop a morbilliform rash if ampicillin is administered. Penicillin is a common cause of severe anaphylactic reactions, which can be life-threatening. Minocycline can accumulate in the tissues and produce a brown or grey colour in the mucosa, sun-exposed areas or at sites of inflammation, as in the lesions of acne. Minocycline can rarely cause the hypersensitivity syndrome reaction, hepatitis, worsen lupus erythematosus or elicit a transient lupus-like syndrome.

### Penicillamine

Like penicillin itself, this can cause morbilliform eruptions or urticaria, but the drug has also been incriminated as a cause of haemorrhagic bullae at sites of trauma, of the extrusion of elastic tissue through the skin, and of pemphigus.

### Oral contraceptives

Reactions to these are less common now that their hormonal content is small. The hair fall that may follow stopping the drug is like that seen after pregnancy (telogen effluvium; p. 184). Melasma, hirsutism, erythema nodosum, acne and photo-sensitivity are other reactions.

### Gold

This frequently causes rashes. Its side-effects range from pruritus to morbilliform eruptions, to curious papulosquamous eruptions such as pityriasis rosea or lichen planus. Erythroderma, erythema nodosum, hair fall and stomatitis may also be provoked by gold.

### Steroids

Cutaneous side-effects from systemic steroids include a ruddy face, cutaneous atrophy, striae (Fig. 25.1), hirsutism, an acneiform eruption and a susceptibility to cutaneous infections, which may be atypical.

### Anticonvulsants

Skin reactions to phenytoin, carbamazepine, lamotrigine and phenobarbital are common and include erythematous, morbilliform, urticarial and purpuric rashes. TEN, erythema multiforme, exfoliative dermatitis, DRESS syndrome and a lupus erythematosus-like syndrome are fortunately rarer. About 1% of patients taking lamotrigine develop Stevens–Johnson syndrome or TEN. A phenytoin-induced pseudolymphoma syndrome has also been described in which fever and arthralgia are accompanied by generalized lymphadenopathy and hepatosplenomegaly and, sometimes, some of the above skin signs. Long-term treatment with phenytoin may cause gingival

**Fig. 25.3** Gingival hyperplasia caused by long-term phenytoin treatment.

hyperplasia (Fig. 25.3) and coarsening of the features as a result of fibroblast proliferation.

### Highly active antiretroviral drugs

Long-term highly active antiretroviral treatment (HAART) has been commonly associated with lipodystrophy, producing a gaunt facies with sunken cheeks. Interactions between HAART and anti-tuberculous drugs are common.

### Biological agents

Cetuximab and ertlotinib both target epidermal growth factor receptors (EGFR) and are used to treat bowel and lung cancers. These antineoplastic antibodies and their cousins commonly cause a distinctive widespread eruption with follicular pustules which resembles acne. This is because sweat and hair follicle cells express EGFR and the drug causes changes in these structures leading to follicular eruptions. Other side-effects are xerosis, fissures of the palms and soles, altered hair growth and paronychia. Many experts feel this is dose-related and not allergic; they may be able to reinstitute the drug at lower dosage, after 1–2 weeks, without recurrence.

## Some common reaction patterns and drugs that can cause them

### Toxic (reactive) erythema

This vague term describes the most common type

**Fig. 25.4** Toxic erythema with urticarial features.

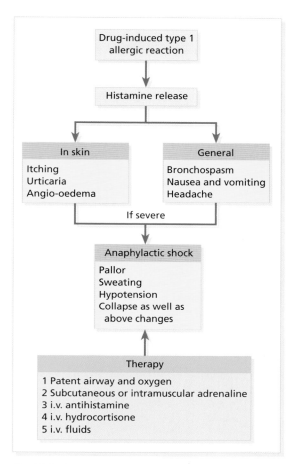

**Fig. 25.5** The cause, clinical features and treatment of anaphylaxis.

of drug eruption, looking sometimes like measles or scarlet fever, and sometimes showing prominent urticarial (Fig. 25.4) or erythema multiforme-like elements. Itching and fever may accompany the rash. Culprits include antibiotics (especially ampicillin), sulphonamides and related compounds (diuretics and hypoglycaemics), barbiturates, phenylbutazone and para-aminosalicylate (PAS).

## *Urticaria* (Chapter 8)

Many drugs may cause this but salicylates are the most common, often working non-immunologically as histamine releasers. Antibiotics are also often to blame. Insect repellents and nitrogen mustards can cause urticaria on contact. Urticaria may be part of a severe and generalized reaction (anaphylaxis) that includes bronchospasm and collapse (Fig. 25.5).

## *Allergic vasculitis* (Chapter 8)

The clinical changes range from urticarial papules, through palpable purpura, to necrotic ulcers. Erythema nodosum may occur. Sulphonamides, beta-lactam antibiotics, diuretics, non-steroidal anti-inflammatory drugs (NSAIDs), phenytoin and oral contraceptives are among the possible causes.

These disorders are caused by circulating immune complexes of drug and antibody (Type III reaction; p. 29). Fever, gut and joint inflammations may be present (serum sickness). Nephropathy is usually mild here, if present at all.

## *Erythema multiforme* (Chapter 8)

Target-like lesions appear mainly on the extensor aspects of the limbs, and bullae may form. In the Stevens–Johnson syndrome, the patients are often ill and the mucous membranes are severely affected. Sulphonamides, barbiturates, lamotrigine and phenylbutazone are known offenders.

## Purpura

The clinical features are seldom distinctive apart from the itchy brown petechial rash on dependent areas that is characteristic of carbromal reactions. Thrombocytopenia and coagulation defects should be excluded (Chapter 11). Thiazides, sulphonamides, phenylbutazone, sulphonylureas, barbiturates, quinine and anticoagulants are among the drugs causing purpura.

## Bullous eruptions

Some of the reactions noted above can become bullous (e.g. Stevens–Johnson syndrome). Bullae may also develop at pressure sites in drug-induced coma. Vancomycin, lithium, diclofenac, captopril, furosemide and amiodarone are associated with development of linear IgA bullous disease (p. 125). Granulocyte–macrophage colony-stimulating factor can induce an eosinophilia and unmask a dormant bullous pemphigoid or epidermolysis bullosa acquisita. Like porphyria cutanea tarda, pseudoporphyria makes photoexposed skin fragile, prone to blisters, and causes scarring, but porphyrin studies are normal. Suspect NSAIDs, furosemide, retinoids or tetracyclines.

## Eczema

This is not a common pattern and occurs mainly when patients sensitized by topical applications are given the drug systemically. Penicillin, sulphonamides, neomycin, phenothiazines and local anaesthetics should be considered.

## Exfoliative erythroderma

The entire skin surface becomes red and scaly. This can be caused by drugs (particularly phenylbutazone, PAS, isoniazid and gold), but can also be caused by widespread psoriasis, lymphomas and eczema.

## Fixed drug eruptions

Round erythematous or purple, and sometimes bullous plaques recur at the same site each time

**Fig. 25.6** Fixed drug eruption – an unusually severe bullous reaction.

the drug is taken (Fig. 25.6). Pigmentation persists between acute episodes. The glans penis seems to be a favoured site. The causes of fixed drug eruptions in any country follow the local patterns of drug usage there but these change as old drugs drop out of use and are replaced by new ones with an unknown potential for causing this type of reaction. For example, in the UK, three of the four most common causes of fixed drug eruptions in 1970 (barbiturates, phenolphthalein and oxyphenbutazone) are no longer common causes. Paracetamol is currently the most common offender in the UK; trimethoprim-sulfa leads the list in the USA. NSAIDs (including aspirin), antibiotics, systemic antifungal agents and psychotropic drugs lie high on the list of other possible offenders.

## Acneiform eruptions

Lithium, iodides, bromides, oral contraceptives, androgens or glucocorticosteroids, antituberculosis and anticonvulsant therapy may cause an acneiform rash (Chapter 12) as may the monoclonal antibody drugs targeting EGFR.

## Lichenoid eruptions

These resemble lichen planus (Chapter 6, p. 72), but not always very closely as mouth lesions are uncommon and scaling and eczematous elements may be seen. Consider antimalarials, NSAIDs, gold, phenothiazines and PAS.

**Fig. 25.7** Acute generalized exanthematous pustulosis precipitated by amoxicillin.

## Toxic epidermal necrolysis (p. 127)

In adults, this 'scalded skin' appearance is often drug-induced (e.g. sulphonamides, cephalosporins, quinolones, barbiturates, phenylbutazone, oxyphenbutazone, phenytoin, oxicams, carbamazepine, lamotrigine and penicillin).

## Acute generalized exanthematous pustulosis (Fig. 25.7)

Acute generalized exanthematous pustulosis (AGEP) suggests acute pustular psoriasis, with a dramatic generalized eruption of red plaques studded with tiny non-follicular pustules. Patients have fever and leucocytosis. Antibiotics and diltiazem are the most common drugs to induce AGEP, which usually develops after only a few days.

## Drug rash with eosinophilia and systemic signs syndrome

Drug rash with eosinophilia and systemic signs (DRESS) syndrome includes the triad of fever, rash (from morbilliform to exfoliative dermatitis) and internal organ involvement (hepatitis, pneumonitis, nephritis and haematological abnormalities). An eosinophilia and lymphadenopathy also commonly occur. It characteristically develops 3–8 weeks after starting the causative drug. The most common culprits are anticonvulsants (particularly phenytoin, phenobarbital and carbamazepine), minocycline, allopurinol and sulphonamides.

## Hair loss

This is a predictable side-effect of acitretin and cytotoxic agents, an unpredictable response to some anticoagulants and sometimes seen with antithyroid drugs. Diffuse hair loss may occur during, or just after, the use of an oral contraceptive.

## Hypertrichosis

This is a dose-dependent effect of diazoxide, minoxidil and ciclosporin.

## Pigmentation (see also p. 287)

Melosma (p. 286) may follow an oral contraceptive plus sun exposure. Large doses of phenothiazines impart a blue–grey colour to exposed areas (Fig. 25.8); heavy metals can cause a generalized browning; clofazimine makes the skin red; mepacrine turns the skin yellow; and minocycline turns areas of leg skin a curious greenish grey colour that suggests a bruise.

## Photosensitivity

This is dealt with in Chapter 18. Always exclude the common drug causes (thiazides, tetracyclines, phenothiazines, sulphonamides and psoralens).

## Xerosis

The skin can become rough and scaly in patients receiving oral retinoids, nicotinic acid or lithium.

## Exacerbation of pre-existing skin conditions

Psoriasis and acne are good examples of this. Psoriasis may be made worse by giving beta-blockers,

**Fig. 25.8** Note sparing of skin creases and area shielded by spectacle frames in this patient with photorelated hyperpigmentation from a phenothiazine drug.

antimalarials, terbinafine or lithium. Glucocorticoids, progesterone, androgens, anticonvulsants, bromides, iodidies and lithium may exacerbate acne.

## Course

The different types of reaction vary so much that a brief summary is not possible. If an allergic reaction occurs during the first course of treatment, it characteristically begins late, often about the ninth day, or even after the drug has been stopped. In such cases, it has taken that lag time to induce an immune reaction. In previously exposed patients the common morbilliform allergic reaction starts 2–3 days after the administration of the drug. The speed with which a drug eruption clears depends on the type of reaction and the rapidity with which the drug is eliminated.

## Differential diagnosis

The differential diagnosis ranges over the whole subject of dermatology depending on which disease is mimicked. For instance, toxic erythema reactions can look very like measles. The general rule is never to forget the possibility of a drug eruption when an atypical rash is seen. Six vital questions should be asked (Table 25.2).

## Treatment

The first approach is to withdraw the suspected drug, accepting that several drugs may need to be stopped at the same time. This is not always easy as sometimes a drug is necessary and there is no alternative available. At other times the patient may be taking many drugs and it is difficult to know which one to stop. The decision to stop or continue a drug depends upon the nature of the drug, the necessity of using the drug for treatment, the availability of chemically unrelated alternatives, the severity of the reaction, its potential reversibility and the probability that the drug is actually causing the reaction.

Assessment depends upon clinical detective work (Table 25.2). Judgements must be based on probabilities and common sense. Every effort must be made to correlate the onset of the rash with prescription records. Often, but not always, the latest drug to be introduced is the most likely culprit. Prick tests and *in vitro* tests for allergy are still too unreliable to be of value. Re-administration, as a diagnostic test, is usually unwise except when no suitable alternative drug exists.

Non-specific therapy depends upon the type of eruption. In urticaria, antihistamines are helpful. In some reactions, topical or systemic corticosteroids can be used, and applications of calamine lotion may be soothing. Plasmapheresis and dialysis can be considered in certain life-threatening situations.

Anaphylactic reactions require special treatment (Fig. 25.5) to ensure that the airway is not compromised (e.g. oxygen, assisted respiration or even emergency tracheostomy). One or more injections of adrenaline (epinephrine) (1 : 1000) 0.3–0.5 mL should be given subcutaneously or intramuscularly in adults before the slow (over 1 min) intravenous injection of chlorphenamine maleate (10–20 mg diluted in syringe with 5–10 mL blood). Although the action of intravenous hydrocortisone (100 mg) is delayed for several hours, it should be given to prevent further deterioration in severely affected patients. Patients should be observed for 6 h after their condition is stable, as late deterioration may occur. If an anaphylactic reaction is anticipated, patients should be taught how to self-inject adrenaline, and may be given a salbutamol inhaler to use at the first sign of the reaction.

To re-emphasize, the most important treatment is to stop the responsible drug. Desensitization, seldom advisable or practical, may rarely be carried out when therapy with the incriminated drug is essential and when there is no suitable alternative (e.g. with some anticonvulsants, antituberculous and antileprotic drugs). An expert, usually a physician with considerable experience of the drug concerned, should supervise desensitization.

---

**Learning points**

- This whole chapter is a warning against polypharmacy. Do your patients really need all the drugs they are taking?
- Consider the possiblity of a drug reaction when a rash appears suddenly
- Watch out for eruptions from new drugs
- Avoid provocation tests unless there are very strong indications for them
- Fever, lymphadenopathy, internal organ involvement suggest a potentially severe drug reaction, especially if the skin is red, swollen, blistered, purpuric or shedding

---

# Further reading

Bachot N & Roujeau JC. (2003) Differential diagnosis of severe cutaneous drug reactions. *American Journal of Clinical Dermatology* **4**, 561–572.

Chave TA, Mortimer MJ, Hall AP & Hutchinson PE. (2005) Toxic epidermal necrolysis: current evidence, practical management and future directions. *British Journal of Dermatology* **153**, 241–253.

Greenberger PA. (2006) Drug allergy. *Journal of Allergy and Clinical Immunology* **117** (2 Supplement Mini-Primer), S464–470.

Katz HI. (1998) *Guide to Adverse Treatment Interactions for Skin, Hair, and Nail Disorders.* Lippincott-Raven, Philadelphia.

Knowles S, Shapiro L & Shear NH. (1999) Drug eruptions in children. *Advances in Dermatology* **14**, 399–415.

Lieberman P. (2006) Anaphylaxis. *Medical Clinics of North America* **90**, 77–95.

Litt JZ. (2006) *Drug Eruption Reference Manual* (with CD ROM), 12th edn. Parthenon, London.

Roujeau JC. (2005) Clinical heterogeneity of drug hypersensitivity. *Toxicology* **209**, 123–129.

Wolverton SE. (2001) *Comprehensive Dermatologic Drug Therapy.* W.B. Saunders, Philadelphia.

# 26 Medical treatment of skin disease

An accurate diagnosis, based on a proper history and examination (Chapter 3), must come before a rational line of treatment can be chosen; and even when a firm diagnosis has been reached, each patient must be treated as an individual. For some, no treatment may even be the best treatment, especially when the disorder is cosmetic or if the treatment would be worse than the condition itself. A patient with minimal vitiligo, for example, may be helped more by careful explanation, reassurance and camouflage than by an extended course of enthusiastic treatment producing only marginal improvement.

If a diagnosis cannot be reached, the doctor has to decide whether a specialist opinion is needed or whether it is best to observe the rash, perhaps treating it for a while with a bland application. In either case, the indiscriminate use of topical corticosteroids or other medications, in the absence of a working diagnosis, often confuses the picture and may render the future diagnosis more difficult.

However, provided the steps described in Chapter 3 are followed, a firm diagnosis can usually be made, and a sensible course of treatment can be planned. Even then the results are often better when patients understand their disease and the reasons behind their treatment. The cause and nature of their disease should be explained to them carefully, in language they are familiar with, and they must be told what can realistically be expected of their treatment. False optimism or undue pessimism, by patients or doctors, leads only to an unsound relationship. Too often patients become discontented, not because they do not know the correct diagnosis but because they have not been told enough about its cause or prognosis. Even worse, they may have little idea of how to use their treatment and what to expect of it; poor compliance often follows poor instruction. If the treatment is complex, instruction

sheets are helpful; they reinforce the spoken word and answer unasked questions.

The principal steps in diagnosis and management therefore are as follows:
- history;
- examination;
- investigations;
- diagnosis;
- explanation of the condition, its cause and prognosis;
- choice of treatment and instructions about it;
- discussion of expectations; and
- follow-up, if necessary.

> **Learning points**
> - One correct diagnosis is worth a hundred therapeutic trials
> - The doctor who fails to have a placebo effect on his patients should become a pathologist or anaesthetist (J.N. Blau)
> - Disease thrives on pessimism (W.B. and E.D. Shelley)

## Therapeutic options

Some of the treatments used in dermatology are listed in Table 26.1.

**Table 26.1** Therapeutic options in dermatology.

| Drugs | Topical |
| | Systemic |
| Physical | Surgical |
| |   excision |
| |   curettage |
| | Intralesional injection |
| | Electrodessication |
| | Cryotherapy |
| | Radiotherapy |
| | Phototherapy |
| | Laser therapy |

## Topical vs. systemic therapy

The great advantage of topical therapy is that the drugs are delivered straight to where they are needed, at an optimum concentration for the target organ. Systemic side-effects from absorption are less than those expected from the same drug given systemically: with topical treatment, vital organs such as the marrow, liver and kidneys are exposed to lower drug concentrations than is the skin. However, topical treatment is often messy, time-consuming and incomplete, whereas systemic treatment is clean and quick and its effect is uniform over the entire skin surface. Cost must also be considered.

Some drugs can only be used topically (e.g. permethrin for scabies and mupirocin for bacterial infections), while others only work systemically (e.g. azathioprine for pemphigus and methotrexate for psoriasis).

When a choice exists and both possibilities are equally effective, then local treatment is usually to be preferred. Most cases of mild pityriasis versicolor, for example, respond to topical antifungals alone so systemic itraconazole is not the treatment of first choice.

## Topical treatment

### Percutaneous absorption

A drug (the 'active ingredient') used on the skin must be dissolved or suspended in a vehicle (base). The choice of the drug and of the vehicle are both important and depend on the diagnosis and the state of the skin. For a drug to be effective topically, it must pass the barrier to diffusion presented by the horny layer (Chapter 2). This requires the drug to be transferred from its vehicle to the horny layer, from which it will diffuse through the epidermis into the papillary dermis. Passage through the horny layer is the rate-limiting step.

The transfer of a drug from its vehicle to the horny layer depends on its relative solubility in each (measured as the 'partition coefficient'). Movement across the horny layer depends both upon the concentration gradient and on restricting forces (its 'diffusion constant'). In general, non-polar substances penetrate more rapidly than polar ones. Low

molecular weight drugs penetrate the epidermis better than high molecular weight ones. A rise in skin temperature and in hydration, both achieved by covering a treated area with polyethylene occlusion, encourages penetration.

Some areas of skin present less of a barrier than do others. Two extreme examples are palmar skin, with its impermeable thick horny layer, and scrotal skin, which is thin and highly permeable. The skin of the face is more permeable than the skin of the body. Body fold skin is more permeable than nearby unoccluded skin. In humans, absorption through the hair follicles and sweat ducts is of little significance and the amount of hair on the treated site is no guide to its permeability.

In many skin diseases, the horny layer becomes abnormal and loses some of its barrier function For example, the abnormal nucleated (parakeratotic) horny layers of psoriasis and chronic eczema, although thicker than normal, have lost much of their protective qualities. Water loss is increased and therapeutic agents penetrate more readily. Similarly, breakdown of the horny layer by chemicals (e.g. soaps and detergents) and by physical injury will allow drugs to penetrate more easily. Conversely, as the skin heals, the barrier function of the horny layer returns and drug absorption diminishes.

In summary, the penetration of a drug through the skin depends on the following factors:

- its molecular weight;
- its polarity;
- its concentration;
- the base;
- its partition coefficient;
- its diffusion constant;
- the thickness of the horny layer;
- the state, including hydration, of the horny layer;
- temperature.

### Active ingredients

These include corticosteroids, tar, dithranol, antibiotics, antifungal and antiviral agents, benzoyl peroxide, retinoic acid and many others (Formulary 1, p. 381). The choice depends on the action required, and prescribers should know how each works. As topical corticosteroids are the mainstay of much local dermatological therapy, their

**Table 26.2** The pharmacology of topical corticosteroid applications.

| | |
|---|---|
| Active constituents | Include hydrocortisone and synthetic halogenated derivatives<br>Halogenation increases activity |
| Bases | Available as solutions, lotions, creams, ointments, sprays, mousses, foams, masks and tapes |
| Penetration | Readily penetrate via the horny layer and appendages<br>Form a reservoir in the horny layer<br>Polyethylene occlusion and high concentrations increase penetration |
| Metabolism | Some minor metabolism in epidermis and dermis (e.g. hydrocortisone converts to cortisone and other metabolites)<br>Leave skin via dermal vascular plexus and enter general metabolic pool of steroids<br>Further metabolism in liver |
| Excretion | As sulphate esters and glucuronides |
| Actions | Anti-inflammatory<br>1 Vasoconstrict<br>2 Decrease permeability of dermal vessels<br>3 Decrease phagocytic migration and activity<br>4 Decrease fibrin formation<br>5 Decrease kinin formation<br>6 Inhibit phospholipase $A_2$ activity and decrease products of arachidonic acid metabolism<br>7 Depress fibroblastic activity<br>8 Stabilize lysosomal membranes<br>Immunosuppressive<br>Antigen – antibody interaction unaffected but inflammatory consequences lessened by above mechanisms and by inhibiting cytokines (e.g. IFN-$\gamma$, GM-CSF, IL-1, IL-2, IL-3 and TNF-$\alpha$)<br>Lympholytic<br>Decrease epidermal proliferation |
| Side-effects | 1 Thinning of epidermis<br>2 Thinning of dermis<br>3 Telangiectasia and striae (caused by 1 and 2; Figs 26.1 and 26.2)<br>4 Bruising (caused by 2 and vessel wall fragility)<br>5 Hirsutism<br>6 Folliculitis and acneiform eruptions<br>7 May worsen or disguise infections (bacterial, viral and fungal)<br>8 Systemic absorption (rare but may be important in infants, when applied in large quantities under polyethylene pants)<br>9 Tachyphylaxis – lessening of clinical effect with the same preparation<br>10 Rebound – worsening, sometimes dramatic on withdrawing treatment |
| Uses | Eczema, psoriasis in some instances (facial, flexural, and palms/soles)<br>Many non-infective, inflammatory dermatoses |

IL, interleukin; INF-$\gamma$, $\gamma$-interferon; GM-CSF, granulocyte–macrophage colony-stimulating factor; TNF, tumour necrosis factor.

pharmacology is summarized in Table 26.2 (Figs 26.1 and 26.2).

## Vehicles (bases)

Most vehicles are a mixture of powders, water and greases (usually obtained from petroleum), to which emulsifiers, stabilizers and preservatives are often added. Figure 26.3 shows that blending these bases together produces preparations that retain the characteristics of each of their components.

A vehicle should maximize the delivery of topical drugs but may also have useful properties in its own right. A base of petrolatum decreases water loss. Used carelessly, vehicles may do harm. A tincture (containing alcohol) may dry out the skin and injure

**Fig. 26.1** Stretch marks behind the knee caused by the topical corticosteroid treatment of atopic eczema.

**Fig. 26.2** Often attributed to Cushing's disease, or to local corticosteroid therapy – but stretch marks across the back are common in normal fast-growing teenagers.

it. Suggested indications are shown in Table 26.3. The choice of vehicle depends upon the action desired, availability, messiness, ease of application and cost.

**Fig. 26.3** The derivation of vehicles.

### Individual vehicles

Dusting powders are used in the folds to lessen friction between opposing surfaces. They may repel water (e.g. talc) or absorb it (e.g. starch); zinc oxide powder has an absorptive power midway between these extremes. Powders ought not to be used in moist areas where they tend to cake and abrade.

Watery lotions evaporate and cool inflamed areas. This effect is hastened by adding an alcohol. Both glycerol and arachis oil slow evaporation and retain skin moisture. Substances that precipitate protein (astringents, e.g. silver nitrate) lessen exudation.

Shake lotions are watery lotions to which powder has been added so that the area for evaporation is increased. These lotions dry wet weeping skin. When water has evaporated from the skin, the powder particles clump together and may become abrasive. This is less likely if an oil such as glycerol has been added.

Creams are used for their cooling, moisturizing and emollient effects. They are either oil-in-water emulsions (e.g. aqueous cream, UK; acid mantle cream, USA) or water-in-oil emulsions (e.g. oily cream, UK; cold cream, USA). Emulsifying agents are added to increase the surface area of the dispersed phase and that of any therapeutic agent in it.

Ointments are used for their occlusive and emollient properties. They allow the skin to remain supple by preventing the evaporation of water from the horny layer. There are three main types:
1 those that are water-soluble (macrogols, polyethylene glycols);
2 those that emulsify with water (e.g. hydrophilic petrolatum);

**Table 26.3** Vehicles and their properties.

| Base | Used on | Effect | Points of note |
| --- | --- | --- | --- |
| Dusting powders | Flexures (may be slightly moist) | Lessen friction | If too wet, clump and irritate |
| Alcohol-based application (tinctures) | Scalp hair | Clean vehicle for corticosteroid application | Cosmetically elegant, do not matt hair<br>May sting raw areas |
| Watery and shake lotions | Acutely inflamed skin (wet and oozing) | Drying, soothing and cooling | Tedious to apply<br>Frequent changes (lessened by polyethylene occlusion)<br>Powder in shake lotions may clump |
| Creams | Both moist and dry skin | Cooling, emollient and moisturizing | Short shelf life<br>Fungal and bacterial growth in base<br>Sensitivities to preservatives and emulsifying agents |
| Ointments | Dry and scaly skin | Occlusive and emollient | Messy to apply, soil clothing<br>Removed with an oil |
| Pastes | Dry, lichenified and scaly skin | Protective and emollient | Messy and tedious to apply (linen or calico needed)<br>Most protective if applied properly |
| Sprays | Weeping acutely inflamed skin<br>Scalp | Drying, non-occlusive | Vehicle evaporates rapidly<br>No need to touch skin to treat it |
| Gels | Face and scalp | Vehicle for corticosteroids, salicylic acid and tretinoin | May sting when applied to inflamed skin can be covered by makeup |
| Mousse | Scalp | Clean vehicle for corticosteroid application | Does not matt the hair |

**3** those that repel water (mineral oils, and animal and vegetable fats).

Gels may be hydrophilic or hydrophobic. They are especially suitable for scalp applications (because they are less greasy than ointments), treating individual lesions such as insect bites (because they dry on the skin quickly and do not need to be rubbed in) and for use in patients who dislike greasy preparations.

Pastes are used for their protective and emollient properties and usually are made of powder added to a mineral oil or grease, such as petrolatum. The powder lessens the oil's occlusive effect.

Variations on these themes have led to the numerous topical preparations available today. Rather than use them all and risk confusion, doctors should limit their choice to one or two from each category. Table 26.3 summarizes the properties and uses of some common preparations.

## Preservatives

Water-in-oil emulsions, such as ointments, require no preservatives. However, many creams are oil-in-water emulsions that permit contaminating organisms to spread in a continuous watery phase. These preparations therefore, as well as lotions and gels, incorporate preservatives. Those in common use include the parahydroxybenzoic acid esters (parabens), chlorocresol, sorbic acid and imidazolidinyl urea. Some puzzling reactions to topical preparations are based on allergy to the preservatives they contain.

## Methods of application

Ointments and creams are usually applied sparingly twice daily, but the frequency of their application will depend on many factors including the nature, severity and duration of the rash, the sites involved, convenience, the preparation (some local corticosteroids need only be applied once daily; Formulary 1, p. 385) and, most important, on common sense. In extensive eruptions, a tubular gauze cover keeps clothes clean and hampers scratching (see Fig. 7.19).

Three techniques of application are more specialized: immersion therapy by bathing, wet dressings (compresses) and occlusive therapy.

## Bathing

Once-daily bathing helps to remove crusts, scales and medications. After soaking for about 10 min, the skin should be rubbed gently with a sponge, flannel or soft cloth; cleaning may be made easier by soaps, oils or colloidal oatmeal.

Medicated baths are occasionally helpful, the most common ingredients added to the bath water being bath oils, antiseptics and solutions of coal tar.

Besides cleaning, the most important function of a bath is hydration. The skin absorbs water and this can be held in the skin for some time if an occlusive ointment is applied immediately after getting out of the bath. Older patients may need help to get into a bath and should be warned about falling if the bath contains an oil or another slippery substance.

## Wet dressings (compresses)

These are used to clean the skin or to deliver a topical medication. They are especially helpful for weeping, crusting and purulent conditions such as eczema, and are described more fully on p. 84. Five or six layers of soft cloth (e.g. cotton gauze) are soaked in the solution to be used; this may be tap water, saline, an astringent or an antiseptic solution, and the compress is then applied to the skin. Open dressings allow the water to evaporate and the skin to cool. They should be changed frequently (e.g. every 15 min for 1 h).

Closed dressings are covered with a plastic (usually polyethylene) sheet; they do not dry out so quickly and are usually changed twice daily. They are especially helpful for débriding adherent crusts and for draining exudative and purulent ulcers.

## Occlusive therapy

Sometimes steroid-sensitive dermatoses will respond to a steroid only when it is applied under a plastic sheet to encourage penetration. This technique is best reserved for the short-term treatment of stubborn localized rashes. The drawback of this treatment is that the side-effects of topical steroid treatment (Table 26.2) are highly likely to occur. The most important is systemic absorption if a large surface area of skin, relative to body weight, is treated (e.g. when steroids are applied under the polyethylene pants of infants).

## Monitoring local treatment

One common fault is to underestimate the amount required. The guidelines given in Table 26.4 and Fig. 26.4 are not precise and are based on twice-daily applications. Lotions go further than creams, which go further than ointments and pastes. Inevitably there will be differences in the quantity of topical preparations needed for the various diseases that affect different age groups. For example, an adult with widespread eczema will need at least 500 g of emollient per week, wheras an adolescent with acne might need only 30 g of a topical gel per month.

Pump dispensers for some topical corticosteroids allow measured amounts to be applied but have not proved popular. Alternatively, the use of 'fingertip units' (Fig. 26.5) can increase the accuracy of prescribing. As a guide, one fingertip unit in an adult male from a standard nozzle provides 0.5 g ointment.

## Systemic therapy

Systemic treatment is needed if a skin condition is associated with systemic disease, or if the medicament of choice is inactive topically (e.g. methotrexate

**Table 26.4** Minimum amount of cream (g) required for twice-daily application for 1 week.

| Age | Whole body | Trunk | Both arms and legs |
| --- | --- | --- | --- |
| 6 months | 60 | 25 | 35 |
| 4 years | 80 | 35 | 45 |
| 8 years | 130 | 55 | 75 |
| 12 years | 185 | 75 | 110 |
| Adult (70 kg male) | 250 | 100 | 150 |

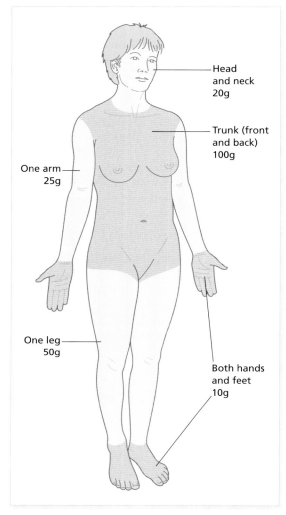

**Fig. 26.4** The minimum amount of a cream required in 1 week by an adult applying it twice daily.

**Fig. 26.5** A fingertip measures about 0.5 g ointment.

systemic upset. Examples of this are the depression that occurs in some patients affected with severe rashes, and high-output cardiac failure, which may occur in exfoliative dermatitis from the shunting of blood through the skin. A systemic upset caused by skin disease can be treated with drugs designed for such problems while the skin is being treated in other ways.

> **Learning points**
>
> - You know how much digoxin your patients are taking, but do you know how much of a topical corticosteroid they are applying? Keep a check on this
> - In some patients, drugs produce only side-effects (W.B. and E.D. Shelley)

## Further reading

Arndt KA. (1995) *Manual of Dermatologic Therapeutics*, 5th edn. Little, Brown, Boston, MA.

Greaves MW & Gatti S. (1999) The use of glucocorticoids in dermatology. *Journal of Dermatological Treatment* **10**, 83–91.

Lebwohl MG, Heymann WR, Berth-Jones J & Coulson I. (2006) *Treatment of Skin Disease*, 2nd edn. *Comprehensive Therapeutic Strategies*. Mosby, Edinburgh.

Shah VP, Behl CR, Flynn GL, Higuchi WI & Schaefer H. (1993) Principles and criteria in the development and optimization of topical therapeutic products. *Skin Pharmacology* **6**, 72–80.

Shelley WB & Shelley ED. (2001) *Advanced Dermatologic Therapy 11*. W.B. Saunders, Philadelphia.

Wakelin SH. (2002) *Handbook of Systemic Drug Treatment in Dermatology*. Manson, London.

and griseofulvin). The principles of systemic therapy in dermatology are no different from those in other branches of medicine: some drugs act specifically, others non-specifically. For example, antihistamines (H1 blockers) act specifically in urticaria, and non-specifically, by a sedative effect, on the most common skin symptom – itch.

Systemic disease coexists with skin disease in several ways (Chapter 21). Sometimes a systemic disease such as systemic lupus erythematosus may cause a rash; at other times, a skin disease causes a

# 27 Physical forms of treatment

The skin can be treated in many ways, including surgery, freezing, burning, ultraviolet radiation and lasers. Some broad principles are discussed here.

## Surgery

As our population ages and becomes more concerned about appearances, requests for skin surgery are becoming more common. The distinction between traditional dermatological surgery and cosmetic surgery is blurring. There are few over the age of 50 years who do not have a benign tumour (Chapter 20) that they consider unsightly and wish to have removed. There are also many who are unhappy with a skin damaged by cumulative sun exposure (p. 275), or concerned about medically trivial abnormalities on their face. To term the treatment of all these as 'cosmetic' seems harsh. Health care systems cannot cover the cost of treating all such problems but family doctors and dermatologists should be able to discuss with their patients any recent developments in phototherapy, laser treatment and specialized surgery that might help them. For example, doctors should be able to explain that diode lasers can remove unwanted hair permanently and without visible scarring, and the pros and cons of such treatment as well as supplying the names of specialists expert in it.

No surgery is minor. Always use an aseptic technique, if possible in a designated room with appropriate facilities. There are few exceptions but these include bedside biopsies on unconscious patients and those too ill to move. Prepacked sterile packs of instruments and swabs have made these procedures much easier.

## Skin biopsy

The indications for biopsy, and the techniques employed, are described in Chapter 3.

## Excision

Excision under local anaesthetic, using an aseptic technique, is a common way of removing small tumours (Figs 27.1 and 27.2). First, the lesion must be examined carefully and important underlying structures noted (e.g. the temporal artery). If possible, the incision should run along the line of a skin crease, especially on the face. If necessary, charts or

**Fig. 27.1** No surgery is minor. Always use an aseptic technique, in proper surroundings, with appropriate help.

**Fig. 27.2** Our standard pack is suitable for most skin surgery.

**Fig. 27.3** Skin wrinkle figures are helpful in deciding the direction of wounds following skin surgery. Those performing dermatological surgery should have ready access to them.

**Fig. 27.4** Suspicious pigmented lesions should be removed with a 2 mm margin marked out in advance.

**Fig. 27.5** A Gillies hook helps to remove an elliptical biopsy without damaging it.

pictures of standard skin creases should be consulted (Fig. 27.3). After injection of the local anaesthetic (usually 1 or 2% lidocaine [lignocaine] with or without 1 in 200 000 adrenaline [epinephrine]; p. 404), the lesion is excised as an ellipse with a margin of normal skin, the width of which varies with the nature of the lesion and the site (Fig. 27.4). The scalpel should be held perpendicular to the skin surface and the incision should reach the subcutaneous fat. The ellipse of skin is carefully removed with the help of a skin hook (Fig. 27.5) or fine-toothed forceps. Larger wounds, and those where the scar is likely to stretch (e.g. on the back), are closed in layers with absorbable sutures (e.g. Dexon) before apposing the skin edges without tension using non-absorbable interrupted or continuous subcuticular sutures such as nylon or Prolene (see Further reading at end of this chapter for precise techniques of suturing). Stitches are usually removed from the face in 4–5 days and from the trunk and limbs in 7–14 days. Artificial sutures (e.g. Steri-Strip) may be

used to take the tension off the wound edges after the stitches have been taken out.

## Shave excision

Many small lesions are removed by shaving them off at their bases with a scalpel tangential to the skin surface under local anaesthesia. This procedure is suitable only for exophytic tumours that are believed to be benign. Some cells at the base may be left and these, in the case of malignant tumours, would lead to recurrence.

## Saucerization excision

This modified shave excision extends into the subcutaneous fat. Instead of tangentially shaving off the growth, it is 'scooped' out, leaving a crater-like wound. The technique is used to remove certain small skin cancers and worrying melanocytic naevi. It leaves more scarring than a shave excision but the technique provides tissue that allows the dermatopathologist to determine if a tumour is invading and to measure tumour thickness if the lesion is a melanoma. Furthermore, the technique may ensure complete removal more adequately than shave excision.

## Curettage

Curettage under local anaesthetic is also used to treat benign exophytic lesions (e.g. seborrhoeic keratoses; Fig. 27.6) and, combined with electrodesiccation (Fig. 27.7), to treat some basal cell carcinomas. Its main advantage over purely destructive treatment is that histological examination can be carried out on the curettings. A sharp curette is used to scrape off the lesion and haemostasis is achieved by local haematinics, by electrocautery or electrodesiccation. The wound heals by secondary intention over 2–3 weeks, with good cosmetic results in most cases.

When a basal cell carcinoma is treated, the curette is scraped firmly and thoroughly along the sides and bottom of the tumour (the surrounding dermis is tougher and more resistant to curettage than the carcinoma) and the bleeding wound bed is then electrodesiccated aggressively. This stops bleeding and destroys a zone of tissue under and around the excised tumour to provide a tumour-free margin. The process is repeated once or twice at the same session to ensure that all of the tumour has been removed or destroyed. Only small basal cell carcinomas outside the skin folds should be treated in this way. The recurrence rates are relatively high for tumours in the nasolabial folds, over the inner canthi and on the nose, glabella and lips. The technique should not ordinarily be used for sclerosing basal cell carcinomas, invasive lesions larger than 1–2 cm, rapidly growing tumours or for those with micronodular features on histology.

## Microscopically controlled excision (Mohs' surgery)

This form of surgery for malignant skin tumours is time-consuming and expensive, but the probability of cure is greater than with excision or curettage. First, the tumour is removed with a narrow margin. The excised specimen is then marked at the edges, mapped and, after rapid histological processing, is immediately examined in horizontal section. If the tumour extends to any margin, further tissue is removed from the appropriate place, based on the markings and mappings, and again checked histologically. This process is repeated until clearance has been proved histologically at all margins. The resulting wound can then be closed directly, covered with a split skin graft or allowed to heal by secondary intention.

Mohs' surgery is useful to treat:
- basal cell carcinomas with a poorly defined edge;
- sclerosing basal cell carcinomas (can suggest an enlarging scar clinically);
- recurrent basal cell carcinomas;
- basal cell carcinomas lying where excessive margins of skin cannot be sacrificed to achieve complete removal of the tumour (e.g. near the eye);
- basal cell carcinomas in areas with a high incidence of recurrence such as the nose, glabella or nasolabial folds;
- some squamous cell carcinomas; and
- occasional malignant tumours other than basal and squamous cell carcinomas.

## Flaps and grafts

These can be used to reconstruct a defect left by the wide excision of a tumour or when a tumour

**Fig. 27.6** Curettage beats excision if a seborrhoeic wart has to be removed. Stretching the skin helps to hold the lesion steady.

is removed from a difficult site (e.g. the eyelid or tip of the nose; see Further reading at the end of this chapter as the techniques are beyond the scope of this book).

## Prevention of, and protection against, bloodborne infections after dermatological surgery

**1** *Bacterial* Antibiotic prophylaxis is effective in reducing bacteraemia during surgery, but it probably does not prevent endocarditis after simple skin surgery. British guidelines (see Further reading at the end of this chapter) suggest that antibiotic prophylaxis is not required for routine dermatological surgery even in the presence of a pre-existing heart lesion.

**2** *Viral* The risk of contracting a bloodborne virus infection from a patient by a needle stick or scalpel injury during a surgical procedure is low in the UK. It varies with the individual virus; it is higher with hepatitis B than with hepatitis C or HIV. The risk is especially high in those carrying the disease themselves (practising homosexuals, intravenous drug abusers who share needles and those coming from an endemic high-risk area). The risk of acquiring HIV through mucous membrane exposure is less than 1 in 1000 and there is no evidence of risk from blood in contact with intact skin.

These days, any patient can carry an undiagnosed infection, so gloves should be used for all surgical and other procedures where there is risk of contacting blood or body secretions. When operating on a high-risk patient the surgeon should wear not only gloves, but also a water-repellent gown, protective headwear and a mask with visor and protective footwear. Other good preventative measures include:
• good basic hygiene with regular hand washing;
• cover of existing wounds; and
• safe procedure for the handling and disposal of needles and blades.

Immunization is currently only effective against the hepatitis B virus. All medical staff who come into contact with blood or blood-related products should be immunized against this virus.

Immediate action after a needle or scalpel injury:
• wash off splashes on the skin with soap and running water;

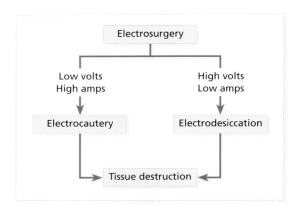

**Fig. 27.7** Types of electrosurgery.

• encourage bleeding if the skin is already broken;
• record the source and nature of the injury; and
• immediately consult the local medical adviser about risk assessment and prophylaxis with antiviral drug(s).

Further information can be found in the British Association of Dermatologists' guidelines (see Further reading at the end of this chapter).

## Electrosurgery

This is often combined with curettage, under local anaesthesia, to treat skin tumours. The main types are shown in Fig. 27.7.

## Cryotherapy

Freezing damages cells by intracellular ice formation. The ensuing thaw compounds this damage by osmotic changes across cell walls and by vascular stasis. The damage is semi-selective in that cellular components are more susceptible to cold injury than stromal ones. There is also some variation in susceptibility between different cells (e.g. melanocytes are more vulnerable to cold injury than keratinocytes).

Cryotherapy is a most convenient procedure for use in general outpatient and domiciliary practice. Further advantages include its cost-effectiveness, its speed and suitability for those who fear surgery, and its lessened chance of transmitting bloodborne infections. These have to be weighed up against its two main disadvantages: short-term pain and no histological confirmation of the lesion being treated.

**Fig. 27.8** Liquid nitrogen can be applied through a spray, or with a cotton wool bud direct from a vacuum flask (centre).

Several freezing agents are available. Liquid nitrogen (−196°C) is the most popular and is now used more than carbon dioxide snow ('dry ice', −79°C). It is effective and used often for viral warts, seborrhoeic keratoses, actinic cheilitis, actinic keratoses, simple lentigos and some superficial skin tumours (e.g. intra-epidermal carcinoma and lentigo maligna). It is applied either on a cotton bud or with a special spray gun (Fig. 27.8). The lesion is frozen until it turns white, with a 1–2 mm halo of freezing around. Two freeze–thaw cycles kill tissue more effectively than one but are usually unnecessary for warts and some keratoses (Fig. 27.9). Patients should be warned to expect pain and possible blistering after treatment. Care should be taken when treating warts on fingers as digital nerve damage can follow overenthusiastic freezing. Standard freeze–thaw times have been established for superficial tumours (see Further reading at end of this chapter) but temperature probes in and around deep tumours are needed to gauge the degree of freezing for their effective treatment. A crust, including the necrotic tumour, should slough off after about 2 weeks. As melanocytes (p. 277) are very sensitive to cold injury, hypopigmentation at a treated site is common and may be permanent.

(a)

(b)

**Fig. 27.9** Two freeze–thaw cycles with liquid nitrogen cleared this actinic keratosis.

## Radiotherapy

Superficial radiation therapy (50–100 kV) can be used to treat biopsy-proven skin cancers in those over 70 years old or who are too frail to tolerate surgery (Fig. 27.10). The usual dose is 3000 cGy, given in fractions over 5–10 days. The scars from radiotherapy worsen with time (Fig. 27.11) in contrast to surgical scars which improve. Nowadays, radiotherapy is seldom used for inflammatory conditions.

## Phototherapy

Chapter 18 deals mainly with adverse skin reactions to light. On the other side of the coin, the healing power of light has attracted much attention recently, as a result of technical advances in the manufacture of light sources for phototherapy. Knowledge of a

(a)

(b)

**Fig. 27.10** (a) A 90-year-old, unfit for surgery, did well with radiotherapy for this massive basal carcinoma. (b) The reaction was healing well after a few weeks.

**Fig. 27.11** Radiodermatitis with scarring, telangiectasia and hyperkeratosis.

few basic biophysical principles is required in order to understand tissue optics and photobiological reactions.

Visible light is a form of electromagnetic radiation with wavelengths lying between those of the warming infrared and high-energy ultraviolet radiation. The ultraviolet spectrum is divided into the UVC spectrum (wavelengths less than 290 nm), the UVB spectrum (wavelengths 290–320 nm) and UVA spectrum (from 320 nm to the most purple colour the eye can discern as light, roughly 420 nm).

The interaction of light with the skin depends on the amount of photons *reflected, scattered and absorbed*. *Reflected light* is perceived by the visual system as objects, including the appearances of skin disorders. Penetration of radiation is inversely proportional to its wavelength, so that visible light and infrared radiation penetrate the skin more deeply than ultraviolet radiation.

*Absorption* involves the transfer of energy from light to tissue. Photons are absorbed selectively by different chromophores (Chapter 18), depending on their absorption profile or 'spectrum'. These chromophores in turn determine the extent to which light penetrates the skin, as any photon that is absorbed is no longer capable of passing through the skin. With the possible exception of UVB phototherapy (p. 65 and p. 377), the specific chromophores for most light-based therapies are known and include haemoglobin, water, tattoo pigments and photosensitizing drugs (e.g. psoralens and photosensitizers used in photodynamic therapy). Energy from the photon is transferred to the chromophore to either generate heat (as with most lasers and intense pulsed lights) or drive photochemical reactions (as with ultraviolet phototherapy, excimer lasers and photodynamic therapy).

## Ultraviolet radiation therapy

Controlled trials have confirmed long-held beliefs that UVB helps some conditions (e.g. chronic plaque psoriasis, Chapter 5; atopic dermatitis; pityriasis rosea; the pruritus of renal failure; cutaneous T-cell lymphoma; and even pressure sores, see Table 18.4). Open trials show that UVB can improve acne, nummular eczema, neurodermatitis, pityriasis lichenoides chronica, some types of vitiligo, cholinergic urticaria, dermographism and eosinophilic pustular folliculitis.

Paradoxically, UVB is effective in 'desensitizing' patients with some photodermatoses, including polymorphic light eruption and solar urticaria. Not surprisingly, these conditions are usually provoked at the beginning of a course, but settle with continuing treatment. It is ironic that the chromophores, and the subsequent biological reactions involved in the most widely used and oldest form of phototherapy, UVB, remain debatable. Candidate chromophores include DNA, RNA, urocanic acid and melanin and the final reaction appears to result in cutaneous immunosuppression.

Although broadband UVB is still used for selected situations, most ultraviolet radiation treatment nowadays falls into two main categories: narrowband (311 nm) UVB therapy, and photochemotherapy with PUVA using wavelengths of UVA (p. 66).

**The advantages of narrowband UVB therapy over PUVA are that:**

- there is no need for pre- and post-treatment eye protection;
- it avoids systemic medication; and
- it may be less carcinogenic than PUVA treatment.

The advantages of oral PUVA therapy are that:

- treatment is less frequent than with narrowband UVB (twice versus three times weekly);
- it is probably the most effective of all ultraviolet radiation treatments;
- its carcinogenic risk is known; and
- the rays of UVA penetrate deeper into the skin, and so can affect disorders involving the deeper dermis.

After phototests on the skin or calculations based on the patient's skin type (p. 268) to establish a starting dose, irradiance is increased by small increments, aiming to produce no or minimal erythema after 24 h (UVB) or 48 h (PUVA). Close supervision by experienced staff is needed because extreme phototoxicity from an overdose, from sunlight or concomitant use of tanning booths, has produced severe burns and even death. A careful record should also be kept of the cumulative ultraviolet radiation dose as the risk of developing skin cancers, including malignant melanoma, may be increased when a patient has received a large cumulative dose. Patients who have had prolonged or repeated ultraviolet radiation should be screened for skin cancer at regular intervals (e.g. yearly) after courses.

## *Sunbeds*

Sunbeds, delivering UVA, are used widely throughout the world by those with skin types I–IV (p. 268) to obtain a tan. Some patients assume, often wrongly, that sunbeds also help their skin condition, usually one of those mentioned under Phototherapy above. Many sunbed users also believe, again mistakenly, that skin damage is avoided provided their skin does not burn. The potential short-term harmful effects (e.g. sunburn, itch, rashes) of sunbeds are known by many users but long-term damage to the skin is either too often understated or overlooked. It includes:

- premature ageing of the skin;
- skin cancer, including melanoma; and
- increased risk of cataracts.

Based on this evidence most dermatologists strongly discourage the use of sunbeds for cosmetic tanning.

## Photodynamic therapy

Photodynamic therapy (PDT) is used for superficial skin cancers such as superficial basal cell carcinoma less than 2 mm thick (p. 300) and precancers including intra-epidermal carcinoma (p. 305), the erythroplasia of Queyrat (p. 203) and actinic keratoses (p. 299). PDT has been increasingly used for benign conditions including sebaceous gland hyperplasia, acne vulgaris and the rejuvenation of photodamaged skin. Selective tissue destruction is achieved by incorporating the photosensitizer in the target tissue and then activating it with either a laser or non-laser light source. The most common combinations are the naturally occurring porphyrin precursor, aminolaevulinic acid (ALA) or its methyl derivative, and irradiation with a red light. In one regimen, water-soluble ALA (now commercially available in the USA and Europe) is applied topically, under occlusion, to the target tissue. After 4 h or so, when the ALA has been selectively absorbed by the tumour (Fig. 27.12), the area is exposed to the light for 15–60 min. The activated ALA converts molecular oxygen to cytotoxic singlet oxygen and free radicals, which in turn cause ischaemic necrosis of the target tissue by damaging cell membranes, especially those in the walls of blood vessels. PDT is carried out in an outpatient setting and its potential advantages over standard treatments include:

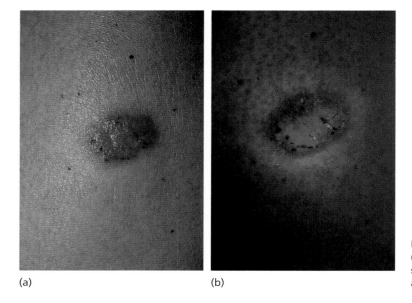

(a)                                        (b)

**Fig. 27.12** A basal cell carcinoma (a) showing, by fluorescence (b), selective uptake of aminolaevulinic acid (ALA)

(a)                                        (b)

**Fig. 27.13** (a) Hyperkeratotic Bowen's disease on a finger. (b) Treated successfully with photodynamic therapy. This would have been an awkward site for surgery.

- non-invasiveness;
- ability to treat many lesions at once;
- rarely causes ulceration and leads to a good cosmetic result;
- good patient acceptability (although the treatments do hurt);
- usefulness for treating tumours on sites that present surgical difficulty (e.g. the taut skin of the finger; Fig. 27.13).

A recent European trial suggests PDT may prevent new premalignant skin lesions in organ transplant recipients.

## Laser therapy

Lasers (acronym for **l**ight **a**mplification by the **s**timulated **e**mission of **r**adiation) are high-intensity coherent light sources of a specific wavelength.

The photons are absorbed by a target chromophore (e.g. a tattoo pigment, melanin in hair, oxyhaemoglobin in blood vessels) and, depending on the energy, the duration of the pulse of emission and the thermal relaxation time, cause local, sometimes microscopic, tissue destruction. The mechanisms of action of different lasers are deceptively simple and rely on one of the following tissue reactions.

• *Photothermal* The laser light is absorbed by the chromophore and converted to heat, resulting in coagulation or vaporization. Continuous wave lasers cause non-selective damage, and pulsed lasers selective damage.

• *Photomechanical* Laser energy, delivered fast for a few nanoseconds, causes mechanical damage to subcellular organelles containing melanin or exogenous pigment.

• *Photochemical* The laser light from, for example, excimer and photodynamic therapy lasers triggers a chemical reaction.

Cooling the skin surface with chilled probes, cryogen sprays or cold air fans helps to lessen collateral heat damage and to relieve pain. Lasers are now being used to treat many skin lesions including port-wine stains, tattoos, epidermal naevi, pigmented lesions, seborrhoeic keratoses, warts and tumours.

Technology has advanced rapidly and many types of laser are now available for clinical use. Most treatments can be carried out under local anaesthetic and as an outpatient. Port-wine stains can be treated successfully in children as well as in adults, using the flashlamp pulsed dye laser emitting light at 585 nm. Most tattoos can be removed by treatment with a Q-switched laser, causing selective photothermolysis; four wavelengths are available (ruby 694 nm; alexandrite 755 nm; neodymium:yttrium aluminium garnet [Nd:YAG] 532 and 1064 nm). Benign but unsightly pigmented lesions such as senile lentigines and naevi of Ota can be greatly improved by treatment with the flashlamp pumped pulsed dye laser (510 nm) and Q-switched lasers. Other pigmented lesions such as *café au lait* marks, melasma and Becker's naevi are less responsive to treatment but may be improved. The long pulse 532 nm Nd:YAG laser is more suitable for those with dark skin. Unwanted hair can be removed permamently with a pulsed diode laser (800 nm), with a Q-switched Nd:YAG laser emitting light at 1064 nm

**Fig. 27.14** Leucoplakia caused by chronic actinic damage – most suitable for laser resurfacing treatment.

or an intense pulsed light system (p. 380). Recently, there have been promising studies on the use of excimer lasers to clear stubborn plaques of psoriasis.

Rhinophyma, sebaceous gland hyperplasia, seborrhoeic keratoses, syringomas and many of the signs of chronic photodamage (e.g. rhytids, actinic cheilitis, actinic keratoses) can be helped by cutaneous resurfacing using $CO_2$ lasers emitting a wavelength of 10 600 nm (infrared), with which tissue water is the chromatophore, or a Q-switched erbium (Er):YAG laser emitting pulsed waves of 2940 nm in the near-infrared, which is absorbed by water 10 times more efficiently than the pulsed $CO_2$ laser beam (Fig. 27.14). Good postoperative care is important, as the patient is left with what is essentially a partial-thickness burn which heals by re-epithelialization from the cutaneous appendages. After profuse exudation for 24–48 h the treated area heals, usually in 5–15 days, but during this time the skin is unsightly. This excessive 'down time' and risks of scarring and pigmentations have led many to favour other forms of treatment for less severe cases. Absolute contraindications for laser resurfacing include the use of isotretinoin within the previous year, concurrent bacterial or viral infection and any hint of ectropion. Dark skin (skin types V and V1; p. 268) should be treated with special care as pigmentary irregularities after treatments are common. Cutaneous laser resurfacing is more effective on the face than on the neck and extremities.

If all of the above seems too complicated to the uninitiated then it is clear that laser treatments should be carried out only by fully trained specialists.

## Intense pulsed light therapy

This has become popular recently, partly as a result of its versatility and effective marketing to the public as well as to dermatologists. Intense pulsed light (IPL) sources are not lasers but polychromatic broadband flashlamps, equipped with optical filters, emitting preselected visible to infrared rays (see Fig. 18.2). They produce a photothermal effect. Because multiple wavebands (500–1200 nm) are delivered, several chromophores, including haemoglobin and melanin, can be targeted with a single exposure. Rejuvenation of photodamaged skin (lentigines, other pigmented lesions, telangiectasia, fine wrinkles and elastosis) may therefore be achieved with one rather than several devices (as would be required with lasers). Time and trials will define the niche for this treatment.

## Further reading

British Association of Dermatologists. Clinical Guidelines: antibiotic prophylaxis for endocarditis in dermatological surgery. www.bad.org.uk/healthcare. Accessed May 2007.

British Association of Dermatologists. Clinical Guidelines: guidelines for safe practice in patients with AIDS and hepatitis B. www.bad.org.uk/healthcare. Accessed May 2007.

British Association of Dermatologists. British Photodermatology Group consensus view on sunbeds for cosmetic tanning. www.bad.org.uk/public/skin/sunbeds/. Accessed May 2007.

Dover JS, Arndt KA, Dinehart SM, Fitzpatrick RE, Gonzales E & the Guidelines/Outcomes Committee. (1999) Guidelines of care for laser surgery. *Journal of the American Academy of Dermatology* **41**, 484–495.

Gold MH & Goldman MP. (2004) 5-Aminolevulinic acid photodynamic therapy: where we have been and where we are going. *Dermatologic Surgery* **30**, 1077–1083.

Goldberg MD. (2005) *Lasers and Lights*, Vols 1 and 2, *Procedures in Cosmetic Dermatology Series* (Dover JS, series editor). Elsevier Saunders, Philadelphia.

Kuflik EG. (1994) Cryosurgery updated. *Journal of the American Academy of Dermatology* **31**, 925–944.

Lawrence C. (2002) *An Introduction to Dermatological Surgery*, 2nd edn. Elsevier Churchill Livingstone, Edinburgh.

Morison WL. (2005) *Phototherapy and Photochemotherapy of Skin Disease*, 3rd edn. Taylor and Francis Group, Baltimore.

# Formulary 1 Topical treatments

Our selection has been determined by personal preferences and we accept that we have left out many effective remedies. However, the preparations listed here are those that we use most often. As a result some appear only in the UK column but not in the USA one, and vice versa. To conform with current prescribing recommendations whenever possible we have listed these products under their active ingredients, with their proprietary names in brackets. Up-to-date information can be found at www.bnf.org.uk or www.fda.gov.

| Type of preparation and general comments | UK preparations | USA preparations |
| --- | --- | --- |
| **Emollients**<br>These are used to make dry scaly skin smoother. Most are best applied after a shower or bath. The opposite of dry is wet, not greasy. While greasy formulations make the skin look moister, those containing humectants such as glycerin, urea or lactic acid generally moisturize better.<br>On the face, use moisturizers designed for the face to minimize acne cosmetica | Soft white paraffin BP<br>Emulsifying ointment BP<br>Aqueous cream BP – can be used as a soap substitute<br>Diprobase cream and ointment<br>E45 range<br>Oilatum range<br>Unguentum M – a useful diluent: contains propylene glycol and sorbic acid, which may sensitize<br>Neutrogena dermatological cream<br>Aquadrate and Calmurid creams contains urea<br>Dermol range – contain antimicrobials | Petrolatum alba USP<br>Vanacream – devoid of fragrances and many sensitizers<br>Aquaphor – a hydrophilic petrolatum<br>Plastibase – a hydrophilic polyglycol<br>Eucerin – hydrophilic petrolatum containing water<br>Aveeno range<br>Neutrogena range<br>Lubraderm<br>Carmol range – contains urea humectant<br>Tricream – creamed-dominant barrier repair<br>Complex 15 facial – phospholipids<br>Lacticare lotion – contains alphahydroxy acid |
| **Bath additives/shower gels**<br>These are a useful way of ensuring application to the whole skin. Most contain emollients that help with dry itchy skin. Others contain tar (Chapter 5) or antibacterials. Caution: makes bathtubs slippery | Balneum range<br>Emulsiderm – contains benzalkonium chloride<br>Oilatum range<br>Aveeno range<br>Hydromol bath emollient | Mineral oil bath emulsion (Keri Moisture Rich Shower and Bath Oil)<br>Colloidal oatmeal (Aveeno Moisturizing Formula Bath) |

| Type of preparation and general comments | UK preparations | USA preparations |
|---|---|---|
| **Shampoos**<br>All contain detergents which help to remove debris and scales; some have added ingredients to combat psoriasis, seborrhoeic eczema and bacterial infections. Most work best if their lather is left on the scalp for 5 min before being rinsed off | *Containing tar*<br>Alphosyl 2 in 1<br>Polytar range<br>T-Gel<br>Capasal – also contains salicylic acid<br><br>*Others*<br>Betadine – contains antibacterial povidone iodine<br>Ceanel concentrate – contains cetrimide, undecenoic acid<br>Selsun – contains selenium sulphide and can be used to treat pityriasis versicolor (p. 256)<br>Nizoral – contains ketoconazole and is useful for seborrhoeic dermatitis and pityriasis versicolor<br>Meted – contains salicylic acid and sulphur | *Containing tar*<br>Pentrax shampoo<br>Sebutone shampoo<br>Denorex shampoo – tingles on scalp<br>T-Gel<br>Polytar range<br><br>*Others*<br>Selsun contains selenium sulphide and can be used to treat pityriasis versicolor (p. 256)<br>Nizoral – contains ketoconazole and is useful for seborrhoeic dermatitis and pityriasis versicolor<br>Head and Shoulders, Zincon – contains zinc pyrethione<br>Sebulex, Scalpicin, T-sal, Salex – contain salicylic acid<br>Caprex – contains fluocinonide |
| **Cleansing agents**<br>These are used to remove debris and to combat infection. Some are astringents which precipitate protein and in doing so help to seal the moist surface of a weeping eczema or a stasis ulcer | Solution of sodium chloride 0.9% (Normasol) – used to clean wounds and ulcers<br>Potassium permanganate (Permitabs – one tablet in 4 L water makes a 0.01% solution) – will stain clothing and skin<br>Aluminium acetate lotion – use at 0.65% in water – is mildly astringent and used as wet dressing<br>Silver nitrate – use at 0.5% in water – is astringent, stains skin brown<br>Chlorhexidine/cetrimide (Hibicet Hospital Concentrate – dilute to 1 in 100) | Soaps<br>Syndets – neutral cleansers generally milder than soap (Dove)<br>Chlorhexidine 4% (Hibiclens) concentrate – use diluted to 1 in 100 (0.04% solution of chlorhexidine in water for skin disinfection)<br>Cetaphil gentle skin cleanser (lipid-free)<br>Benzalkonium chloride (Ionax line)<br>Triclosan (Dial, Lever 2000) – deodorant, antibacterial<br>Sulfacetamide/Sulphur (Plexion) – cleanser for rosacea<br>Alcohol gel (non-irritating disinfectant for hand washing – Purel) |
| **Barrier preparations**<br>These are used to protect the skin from irritants and are of value in the napkin (diaper) area and around stomas. Many contain the silicone, dimethicone. The choice of barrier creams for use at work depends upon individual circumstances: recommendations are not given here | Petrolatum<br>Zinc and castor oil ointment BP<br>Dimethicone and benzalkonium chloride (Conotrane)<br>Dimethicone and cetrimide (Siopel)<br>Dimethicone, calamine and zinc oxide (Vasogen) | Petrolatum<br>Zinc oxide ointment<br>Kerodex 51 (water-miscible)<br>Kerodex 71 cream (water-repellent)<br>Bentoquatum (Ivy Block Lotion) protective against toxicodendron (poison ivy allergy)<br>Dermaguard spray<br>Flexible collodion (film)<br>Zinc oxide, lanolin, talc and vitamins A and D (Desitin ointment)<br>Dimethicone (Diaper Guard Ointment)<br>Anusol (zinc oxide plus pramoxine)<br>Bag Balm (contains 8-hydroxyquinoline sulphate) |

| Type of preparation and general comments | UK preparations | USA preparations |
|---|---|---|
| **Depigmenting agents**<br>Most contain hydroquinone. The use of agents containing monobenzone causes permanent complete depigmentation | None in *BNF* but some preparations available over the counter | Hydroquinone 2–4% (Melanex topical solution – contains 3% hydroquinone; Solaquin forte – contains 4% hydroquinone and sunscreen; Glyquin – contains 10% glycolic acid and 4% hydroquinone), Lustra Ultra (contains 0.3% retinol and 4% hydroquinone)<br>Mequinol 2%, tretinoin 0.01% (Solagé)<br>Hydroquinone (4%), tretinoin (0.05%) and fluocinonide (0.01%) (Tri-Luma)<br>Monobenzene / monobenzyl ether of hydroquinone (Benaquin) (Caution: permanent depigmentation)<br>Azelaic Acid (Finacea gel 15%, Azalex cream 20%) |
| **Camouflaging preparations**<br>Blemishes that cannot be removed can often be made less obvious by covering them. Expert cosmetic advice may be needed to obtain the best colour match | Covermark range<br>Dermablend range<br>Keromask range | Covermark range of products<br>Dermablend<br>Powder Palette (Physician's Formula – Pierre Fabre) in green for correcting red blush of rosacea |
| **Sunscreens and sunblocks**<br>These help the light-sensitive but are not a substitute for sun avoidance and sensible protective clothing. The sun protection factor (SPF) is a measure of their effectiveness against UVB more than UVA, but those recommended here block UVA also. Allergic contact dermatitis from the sunscreen ingredients may be missed and the rash put down to a deterioration of the original photosensitivity | Titanium dioxide (E45 Sun range)<br>Cinnamate, oxybenzone and titanium dioxide (Sunsense Ultra, Roc Sante Soleil, Uvistat range, Delph range, Spectra Ban) | Cinnamates, benzophenones, and salicylates: Coppertone waterproof lines, Neutrogena sunblock lines, Presun active clear gel, Lubraderm daily UV lotion, SolBar Liquid)<br>Avobenzone 3%, Homosalate 12%, Octyl methoxycinnamate 7.5%, Octocrylene 1.5%, Oxybenzone 6% (Solbar PF)<br>Titanium dioxide (5% Ti-Screen Natural Moisturizing Titanium Dioxide Sunblock Lotion, 2.4% Neutrogena Natural Buff 50)<br>Zinc oxide (Zinc oxide ointment)<br>Octinoxate (Vanacream Sunscreen Sport with zinc oxide – fragrance free)<br>Zinc oxide 7.5%, titanium dioxide 7.5% (Vanicream 60 Sunscreen for sensitive skin)<br>Helioplex – stabilizes avobenzone and oxybenzone prolonging duration of protection (Neutrogena Ultra Sheer Dry Touch, Neutrogena Age Shield)<br>Mexoryl XL – contains a photostable UVA-absorbing chemical ecamsule (L'Oreal Anthelios SX) |

| Type of preparation and general comments | UK preparations | USA preparations |
| --- | --- | --- |
| **Antipruritics**<br>Remember that these are of limited value: try to make a firm diagnosis that will lead to an effective line of treatment | Calamine lotion BP<br>Oily Calamine lotion BP – contains arachis oil<br>Menthol (0.5%) or phenol (1.0%) in aqueous cream<br>Crotamiton cream and lotion (Eurax) – also used to treat scabies<br>Doxepin (Xepin cream) | Calamine lotion<br>Crotamiton (Eurax cream and lotion) also used to treat scabies<br>Menthol and camphor (Sarna lotion) contains menthol and camphor<br>Menthol, phenol and zinc oxide (Shamberg's lotion)<br>Doxepin (Zonalon cream)<br>Pramoxine (Prax, Pramegel, Itch-X)<br>Benzocaine (Boil ease ointment, solarcaine) – caution: may sensitize |
| **Antiperspirants**<br>Most antiperspirants are deodorants too, but many deodorants (e.g. triclosan) are not antiperspirants | Aluminium chloride hexahydrate 20% (Anhydrol Forte solution or Driclor solution). Botulinum toxin (Botox) injections – for local temporary anhidrosis of axillae or palms<br>Glycopyrronium bromide 0.05% solution by iontophoresis (Robinul) to palmar or plantar skin | Aluminum zirconium tetrachlorhydroxy gly (many drugstore products, e.g. Gillette and Speed stick lines,<br>Aluminum chlorate 20% (Drysol) 12.5% (CertainDri Roll-On), 6.25% (Xerac-AC)<br>Formaldehyde 10% solution (Lazerformaldehyde) – caution: may sensitize<br>Botulinum toxin (Botox) injections – for local temporary anhidrosis of axillae or palms<br>Glycopyrronium bromide 0.05% solution by iontophoresis (Robinul) to palmar or plantar skin |
| **Keratolytics**<br>These are used to counter an excessive production of keratin. Salicylic acid preparations should be used for limited areas only and not above 6%, as absorption and toxicity may follow their prolonged and extensive application, especially in infants | Salicylic acid, 2–4% in emulsifying ointment or soft white paraffin<br>Urea preparations (see Emollients above)<br>Propylene glycol, 20% in aqueous cream | Salicylic acid (6% Keralyt gel)<br>Salicylic acid, 2–4% in emulsifying ointment or soft white paraffin<br>Urea preparations at high concentrations (Carmol 20%, 40% Kerol 50%)<br>Propylene glycol (Epilyt) |
| **Depilatories**<br>Over-the-counter depilatories are used to remove unwanted facial hairs and are all irritating. Eflornithine inhibits ornithine decarboxylase in hair follicles | Eflornithine 11.5% (Vaniqa) retards hair regrowth | Sulfides (Magic Shaving Powder)<br>Thioglycollates (Nair line, Neet line)<br>Zip wax, Nair microwave wax – mechanical hair removal<br>Eflornithine 11.5% (Vaniqa) retards hair regrowth |

| Type of preparation and general comments | UK preparations | USA preparations |
|---|---|---|
| **Steroids**<br>Our selection here has had to be ruthless as so many brands and mixtures are now on the market. Conventionally, they are classified according to their potency. Your aim should be to use the least potent preparation that will cope with the skin disorder being treated. Side-effects and dangers are listed in Table 26.2 (p. 366)<br><br>Nothing stronger than 1% hydrocortisone should be used on the face (except in special circumstances, e.g. discoid lupus erythematosus) or in infancy. Be reluctant to prescribe more than 200 g/week of a mildly potent, 50 g/week of a moderately potent or 30 g/week of a potent preparation for any adult for more than a month<br><br>Most of the preparations listed are available as lotions, creams, oily creams and ointments; your choice of vehicle will depend upon the condition under treatment (p. 367). Use twice daily except for Cutivate and Elocon, which are just as effective if used once a day | *Mildly potent*<br>Hydrocortisone 0.5, 1.0, 2.5% preparations<br>Fluocinolone acetonide (Synalar cream 1 in 10)<br><br>*Moderately potent*<br>Alclometasone dipropionate (Modrasone cream and ointment)<br>Betamethasone valerate (Betnovate RD cream and ointment)<br>Clobetasone butyrate cream and ointment (Eumovate)<br><br>*Potent*<br>Betamethasone valerate (Betnovate range including scalp application, Betacap scalp application, Bettamousse scalp application)<br>Fluticasone propionate (Cutivate cream and ointment)<br>Mometasone furoate (Elocon range)<br>Hydrocortisone 17-butyrate (Locoid range)<br>Fluocinolone acetonide (Synalar range)<br><br>*Very potent*<br>Clobetasol propionate (Dermovate range)<br>Halcinonide (Halciderm cream)<br>Diflucortolone valerate (Nerisone Forte range) | *Mildly potent*<br>Hydrocortisone 0.5, 1.0, 2.5% (numerous manufacturers)<br>Desonide (Desowen, Tridesilon)<br>Alclometasone (Aclovate)<br><br>*Moderately potent*<br>Betamethasone valerate (Valisone)<br>Fluticasone (Cutivate)<br>Hydrocortisone valerate (Westcort)<br>Triamcinolone 0.025%, 0.1% (Kenalog, Aristocort, various manufacturers)<br><br>*Potent*<br>Betamethasone dipropionate (Diprosone)<br>Diflorasone (Elocon)<br>Fluocinonide .05% (Lidex)<br>Desoximetasone (Topicort 0.25%)<br>Fluocinonide 0.1% (Vanos)<br><br><br><br><br>*Very potent*<br>Clobetasol (Temovate)<br>Halobetasol (Ultravate)<br>Betamethasone dipropionate in enhanced vehicle (Diprolene)<br>Diflorasone (Psorcon)<br>Fluocinohide 0.1% (Vanos) |
| **Steroid combinations**<br>*With antiseptics* | *Mildly potent*<br>Hydrocortisone and clioquinol (Vioform-hydrocortisone cream and ointment)<br><br>*Potent*<br>Betamethasone valerate and clioquinol (Betnovate-C cream and ointment)<br>Hydrocortisone 17-butyrate with chlorquinaldol (Locoid-C cream and ointment)<br>Fluocinolone acetonide with clioquinol (Synalar-C cream and ointment) | *Mildly potent*<br>Clioquinol and hydrocortisone (1%)<br>Iodoquinol 1% and hydrocortisone 1% (Vytone cream) |

| Type of preparation and general comments | UK preparations | USA preparations |
|---|---|---|
| *With antibiotics* | *Mildly potent*<br>Hydrocortisone and fusidic acid (Fucidin H)<br><br>*Moderately potent and potent*<br>Betamethasone valerate and neomycin (Betnovate-N cream and ointment)<br>Fluocinolone acetonide and neomycin (Synalar-N cream and ointment) | *Mildly potent*<br>Neomycin, bacitracin, hydrocortisone 1% (Corticosporin) |
| *With antifungals* | *Mildly potent*<br>Hydrocortisone and clotrimazole (Canesten HC cream)<br>Hydrocortisone and miconazole (Daktacort cream and ointment)<br>Hydrocortisone and econazole (Econacort) | *Very potent*<br>Clotrimazole and betamethasone dipropionate (Lotrisone) |
| *With antibacterials and antifungals* | *Mildly potent*<br>Hydrocortisone, chlorhexidine and nystatin (Nystaform HC cream and ointment)<br>Hydrocortisone, benzalkonium, nystatin and dimeticone (a silicone) (Timodine cream)<br><br>*Moderately potent*<br>Clobetasone butyrate, oxytetracycline and nystatin (Trimovate cream)<br><br>*Very potent*<br>Clobetasol propionate, neomycin and nystatin (Dermovate NN cream and ointment) | *Moderately potent*<br>Neomycin, nystatin, triamcinolone 0.1% (Mycolog II) |
| *With tar* (for psoriasis) | *Mildly potent*<br>Hydrocortisone, allantoin and coal tar extract (Alphosyl HC cream) | |
| *With calcipotriol* (for psoriasis) | *Potent*<br>Betamethasone dipropionate (Dovobet ointment) | *Potent*<br>Betamethasone dipropionate (Taclonex ointment) |
| *With salicylic acid* | *Potent*<br>Betamethasone dipropionate and salicylic acid (Diprosalic ointment – and scalp application) | |

| Type of preparation and general comments | UK preparations | USA preparations |
| --- | --- | --- |
| **Preparations for use in the mouth** | | |
| *Useful mouth washes* | Benzydamine solution (Difflam oral rinse) – an analgesic for painful inflammation in the mouth<br>Chlorhexidine (Corsodyl mouth wash)<br>Hexetidine solution (Oraldene) – an antiseptic gargle | Cetylpyridinium (Cepacol antiseptic mouth wash)<br>Listerine antiseptic mouth rinse (contains thymol, eucalyptol, methylsalicylate, menthol)<br>'All-purpose mouth wash' – different formulations – e.g. compounded as nystatin suspension 100 000 U/mL, 120 mL; diphenhydramine elixir 12.5 mg/5 mL, 480 mL; hydrocortisone powder 240 mg; sodium carboxymethylcellulose 2%, 720 mL<br>'Magic mouth wash' – different formulations – e.g. compounded as equal parts Maalox (Magnesia and alumina oral suspension) and diphenhydramine elixir 12.5 mg/5 mL<br>Some also add dexamethasone |
| *Topical analgesics* | | Mucotrol – slow dissolving wafer<br>Diphenhydramine elixir 12.5 mg/5 mL |
| *Topical steroids* | Triamcinolone acetonide (Adcortyl in Orabase) – a paste that adheres to mucous membranes<br>Hydrocortisone pellets (Corlan pellets) to be dissolved slowly in mouth near the lesion – usually an aphthous ulcer | Triamcinolone acetonide (Kenalog in Orabase) – a paste that adheres to mucous membranes<br>Fluocinonide gel (Lidex gel)<br>Clobetasol gel (Temovate gel) |
| *For yeast infections* | Miconazole (Daktarin oral gel)<br>Amphotericin (Fungilin lozenges)<br>Nystatin (Nystan oral suspension) | Clotrimazole (Mycelex troches)<br>Nystatin oral suspension or pastilles (Nilstat, Mycostatin) |
| **Topical immunomodulators**<br>Long-term safety data not yet available, so should not generally be used as first-line agents | Pimecrolimus (Elidel cream 1%). For mild to moderate eczema<br>Tacrolimus (Protopic ointment 0.03%, 0.1%). For moderate to severe eczema | Pimecrolimus (Elidel cream 1%). For mild to moderate eczema<br>Tacrolimus (Protopic ointment 0.03%, 0.1%). For moderate to severe eczema |
| **Preparations for otitis externa**<br>Otitis externa, essentially an eczema, is often complicated by bacterial or yeast overgrowth – hence the combinations listed here | Aluminium acetate ear drops 8% – an effective astringent for the weeping phase: best applied on ribbon gauze<br>Hydrocortisone with neomycin and polymyxin (Otosporin drops)<br>Cotrimazole (Canesten solution) | Aluminium acetate ear drops 8% – an effective astringent for the weeping phase: best applied on ribbon gauze<br>Hydrocortisone, neomycin and polymyxin (Corticosporin drops)<br>Ciprofloxacin 0.2% and hydrocortisone 1% (Cipro HC Otic)<br>Acetic acid 2% with or without hydrocortisone (VoSol/VoSol-HC)<br>Tridesilon otic solution |

| Type of preparation and general comments | UK preparations | USA preparations |
| --- | --- | --- |
| **Antibacterial preparations**<br>The ideal preparation should have high antibacterial activity, low allergenicity, and the drug should not be available for systemic use; this combination is hard to find. Some compromises are given here | Mupirocin (Bactroban cream and ointment)<br>Fusidic acid (Fucidin ointment, cream or gel)<br>Neomycin and gramicidin (Graneodin ointment)<br>Polymyxin and bacitracin (Polyfax ointment)<br><br>*To eliminate nasal carriage of staphylococci*<br>Mupirocin (Bactroban Nasal cream)<br>Chlorhexidine and neomycin (Naseptin cream) | Retapamulin (Altabase ointment)<br>Mupirocin (Bactroban ointment)<br>Nitrofurazone (Furacin ointment, cream or solution)<br>Bacitracin (Baciguent ointment)<br>Gentamicin (Garamycin ointment)<br>Bacitracin and polymyxin (Polysporin ointment)<br>Silver sulfadiazine 1% cream – various manufacturers<br>Benzoyl peroxide 5–10% (antiseptic)<br><br>*To eliminate nasal carriage of staphylococci*<br>Mupirocin (Bactroban ointment) |
| **Antifungal preparations**<br>In our view imidazole, terbinafine, butenafine and amorolfine creams have now supplanted their messier, more irritant and less effective rivals (e.g. Whitfield's ointment). They are fungicidal and the fungistatic azoles such as ketoconazole and clotrimazole have the added advantage of combating yeasts as well as dermatophytes.<br>   Systemic therapy will be needed for tinea of the scalp, of the nails, and of widespread or chronic skin infections that prove resistant to topical treatment | Clotrimazole (Canesten cream)<br>Miconazole (Daktarin cream)<br>Terbinafine (Lamisil cream)<br>Amorolfine (Loceryl cream and nail lacquer)<br>Tioconazole (Troxyl nail solution) – applied locally it may increase the success rate of griseofulvin. Used by itself it may also cure or improve some nails<br>Ketoconazole (Nizoral cream) | Clotrimazole (Lotrimin cream, solution and powder)<br>Miconazole (Micatin cream)<br>Econazole (Spectazole cream)<br>Terbinafine (Lamisil cream)<br>Butenafine (Mentax cream)<br>Ciclopirox (Loprox cream and lotion, Penlac nail lacquer)<br>Naftifine (Naftin cream)<br>Oxiconazole (Oxistat cream and lotion)<br>Ketoconazole (Nizoral cream) |
| **Antiviral preparations**<br>Topical products have little part to play in the management of herpes zoster. However, if used early and frequently, they may help with recurrent herpes simplex infections | Aciclovir cream<br>Idoxuridine in dimethyl sulphoxide (Herpid application) – usually less effective than aciclovir | Penciclovir (Denavir cream)<br>Aciclovir (Zovirax cream) |
| **Wart treatments**<br>*Palmoplantar warts* | Salicylic acid and lactic acid (Salactol paint or Salatac and Cuplex gel)<br>Salicylic acid (at 26%, Occlusal solution: at 50%, Verrugon ointment)<br>Glutaraldehyde (Glutarol solution)<br>Formaldehyde (Veracur gel) | Salicylic acid (Duofilm, Occlusal-HP)<br>Salicylic acid plasters 40%<br>Salicylic acid, 15% in karaya (Transversal) |

| Type of preparation and general comments | UK preparations | USA preparations |
|---|---|---|
| *Anogenital warts*<br>Podophyllum should only be used for non-keratinized warts | Imiquimod (Aldara cream) — an immunomodulator (p. 238)<br>Podophyllin resin (Podophyllin paint compound) – irritant, use with care (p. 238)<br>Podophyllotoxin (Condyline solution) | Podophyllin resin, 15% (Podophyllin paint compound – use with care in (p. 238)<br>Podofilox (Condylox gel)<br>Imiquimod (Aldara cream) (p. 238) |
| **Preparations for treatment of scabies**<br>Poor results follow inefficient usage rather than ineffective preparations. We prefer permethrin or sulphur in young children, and pregnant and lactating women. Written instructions are helpful (p. 264) | Permethrin (Lyclear Dermal Cream)<br>Malathion (Quellada M liquid or Derbac-M liquid)<br>Benzyl benzoate application (BP). Irritant and less effective than malathion or permethrin<br>Crotamiton (Eurax cream) for use if itching persists after treatment with more effective scabicides | Permethrin (Elimite cream)<br>Lindane (Kwell lotion)<br>Crotamiton (Eurax cream) for use if itching persists after treatment with more effective scabicides<br>Precipitated sulphur 6% in soft white paraffin |
| **Preparations for treatment of pediculosis**<br>Resistance is a growing problem. Lotions left on for a minimum of 12 h are more effective, although less convenient than shampoos | Malathion (Prioderm alcohol-based lotion or Derbac-M aqueous lotion or Quellada lotion)<br>Permethrin (Lyclear Creme Rinse)<br>Phenothrin (Full Marks) | Malathione (Prioderm lotion and cream shampoo)<br>Permethrin (Nix)<br>Permethrin/piperonyl butoxide (Rid)<br>Benzyl benzoate solution 20–25%<br>Precipitated sulphur 6% in Nivea oil |
| **Preparations for acne**<br>*Active ingredient*<br>*Benzoyl peroxide* (an antibacterial agent) induces dryness during the first few weeks; this usually settles, even with continued use | Benzoyl peroxide (Panoxyl ranges)<br>Potassium hydroxyquinoline with benzoyl peroxide (Quinoderm range) | Benzoyl peroxide (Panoxyl, Benzac, Desquam-X, Oxy, Clearasil range 2.5, 5 and 10%)<br>With sulphur (Sulphoxyl) |
| *Retinoids*<br>Potent comedolytic agents, also used to reverse photoageing. May irritate. Must be avoided during pregnancy/lactation | Isotretinoin (Isotrex)<br>Tretinoin (Retin-A preparations)<br>Adapalene (Differin gel and cream) | Tretinoin (Retin-A preparations)<br>Tazarotene (Tazarac gel 0.05 and 0.1%)<br>Adapalene (Differin gel, lotion and cream) |
| *Antibiotics*<br>Bacterial resistance is increasing, but can be reduced by concomitant administration of benzoyl peroxide | Clindamycin (Dalacin-T solution or roll-on)<br>Erythromycin (Stiemycin solution)<br>Erythromycin and zinc acetate (Zineryt)<br>Erythromycin and benzoyl peroxide (Benzamycin) | Clindamycin (Cleocin-T solution and gel)<br>Erythromycin 2% solution – various manufacturers<br>Sulfacetamide (Klaron lotion)<br>Clindamycin and benzoyl peroxide (Clinderm, Benzaclin, Dual)<br>Erythromycin and benzoyl peroxide (Benzamycin)<br>Sulphur and sulfacetamide (Sulfacet-R) |
| *Azelaic acid and salicylic acid* | Azelaic acid (Skinoren cream)<br>Salicylic acid (Acnisal solution) | Azelaic acid (Azalex cream)<br>Salicylic acid (Neutrogena clear pore gel, Clearasil stick, Stridex gel) |

| Type of preparation and general comments | UK preparations | USA preparations |
|---|---|---|
| **Preparations for rosacea** | Metronidazole (Metrogel or Rozex gels) | Metronidazole gel, lotion, cream (Metrogel, Metrocream, Metrolotion, Noritate)<br>Sulphur and sulfacetamide (Sulfacet-R)<br>Sulfacetamide (Klaron) |
| **Preparations for psoriasis**<br>*Vitamin D derivatives*<br>Calcipotriol (calcipotriene, USA) and tacalcitol. Avoid using in patients with disorders of calcium metabolism | Calcipotriol (Dovonex cream, ointment and scalp solution). Maximum weekly doses: 6–12 years, 50 g; 12–16 years, 75 g; adults, 100 g. Can be irritant. Avoid on face<br>Calcitriol (Silkis ointment). Maximum daily dose for adults, 30 g. Less irritant than calcipotriol. Can be used on face/flexures<br>Tacalcitol (Curatoderm ointment). Maximum daily dose for adults, 10 g. Not recommended for children | Calcipotriene (Dovonex cream, lotion, and ointment)<br>Maximum doses same as UK<br>With betamethasone diproprionate (Taclonex ointment) |
| *Steroids*<br>Routine long-term treatment with potent or very potent steroids is not recommended. For indications see p. 63 | Calcipotriol with betamethasone diproprionate (Dovobet) | |
| Scalp applications | Betamethasone (Betnovate scalp application, Diprosalic scalp lotion – also contains salicylic acid)<br>Fluocinolone (Synalar gel) | Clobetasol (Temovate scalp application, Olux mousse)<br>Fluocinonide (Lidex solution)<br>Fluocinonide in peanut oil (Dermasmoothe FS)<br>Betamethasone valerate (Valisone lotion), Luxiq foam |
| For use elsewhere<br>Tar – steroid combinations are helpful | (See Topical steroids above) | |
| *Dithranol/anthralin*<br>Stains normal skin and clothing. May be irritant, therefore start with low concentration. For 30-minute regimen *see* p. 64 | Dithrocream range<br>Micanol range | Micanol 1%<br>Dithrocreme 0.1, 0.25, 0.5, 1% |
| *Retinoid*<br>Contraindicated in pregnancy and during lactation | Tazarotene (Zorac gel) | Tazarotene (Tazarac gel) |
| *Tar*<br>These clean refined tar preparations are suitable for home use. Messier, although more effective, formulations exist but are best used in treatment centres | | |

| Type of preparation and general comments | UK preparations | USA preparations |
|---|---|---|
| Bath additives | Polytar emollient<br>Psoriderm bath emulsion | Balnetar liquid |
| Scalp applications | Exorex lotion. Carbo-Dome cream<br>Psoriderm cream | Denorex Psoriasis overnight treatment<br>MG-217 2% ointment |
| Tar – salicylic acid combinations | Polytar<br>Alphosyl 2 in 1 lotion<br>Cocois ointment (*see* Keratolytics) | 10% Liquor carbonis detergens in Nivea oil |

**Preparations for venous ulcers**
Regardless of topical applications, venous ulcers will heal only if local oedema is eliminated. Remember that the surrounding skin is easily sensitized. To choose treatment for an individual ulcer see p. 156

| | | |
|---|---|---|
| *For cleansing* | Saline, potassium permanganate<br>(see Cleansing agents above)<br>Hydrogen peroxide solution (3%) | Saline, potassium permanganate<br>(see Cleansing agents)<br>Hydrogen peroxide solution (3%)<br>Bleach (sodium hypochlorite) $^1/_4$ cup to bathtub of water, or one tablespoon per quart for soaking – may bleach fabrics |
| *Low adherent dressings* | Tulle dressings – e.g. Bactigras<br>(contains chlorhexidine), Jelonet<br>(paraffin gauze)<br>Textiles – e.g. Mepitel | Telfa<br>Vaseline gauze (contains petrolatum) |
| *Enzymes* | | Enzymes (Elase ointment – contains fibrinolysin and deoxyribonuclease; Collagenase Santyl ointment – contains collagenase) |
| *Antiseptics* | Silver sulfadiazine – active against<br>*Pseudomonas* (Flamazine cream)<br>Silver nitrate aqueous solution (0.5%)<br>Cadexomer iodine (Iodosorb powder) | Silver sulfadiazine (Silvadene cream)<br>Nitrofurazone (Nitrofurazone solution)<br>Mupirocin (Bactroban ointment) |
| *Medicated bandages*<br>Beware of allergic contact reactions to parabens preservatives which are in most bandages | Zinc paste and calamine (Calaband)<br>Zinc paste and ichthammol (Ichthopaste)<br>Zinc oxide (Viscopaste PB7) | Zinc oxide<br>Dextranomer (Debrisan) – for absorbing exudates<br>Becaplermin (Regranex) – growth factor |
| *Other dressings* | Hydrocolloid (Granuflex, DuoDERM Extra Thin)<br>Calcium alginate (Kaltostat)<br>Hydrogels (Intrasite, Aquaform)<br>Polyurethane foam (Tielle)<br>Vapour-permeable film dressing (Opsite)<br>Activated charcoal with silver (Actisorb silver 200) | Hydrocolloid (Duoderm)<br>Vapour-permeable film dressing (Opsite, Tegaderm)<br>Hydrogel (Vigilon)<br>Calcium alginate<br>Biafin – recruits macrophages |

| Type of preparation and general comments | UK preparations | USA preparations |
|---|---|---|
| **Miscellaneous** | | |
| *5-Fluorouracil* | | |
| The treatment of individual lesions in patients with multiple actinic keratoses is tedious or impossible. For such cases 1–5% cream containing 5-fluorouracil is useful. It should be applied twice daily for 2–3 weeks. Patients should be warned about the inevitable inflammation and soreness which appear after a few days. Lesions on the scalp and face do better than those on the arms and hands | Efudix cream | Efudex cream 2% or 5% Fluroplex 1% cream Carac 0.5% cream |
| *Imiquimod* | | |
| Enhances the immune response to superficial BCC | Imiquimod 5% (Aldara) Applied 5 days per week for 6 weeks. The response is related to the degree of inflammation | Imiquimod 5% (Aldara) Applied 5 days per week for 6 weeks for treatment of superficial basal cell carcinomas. The response is related to the degree of inflammation. When used to treat actinic keratoses, apply 2 or 3 times per week for 16 weeks and wash off after 8 h |
| *Diclofenac* | | |
| For actinic keratoses | 3% Diclofenac sodium in sodium hyaluronate base (Solaraze). Applied twice daily for 60–90 days | 3% Diclofenac sodium in sodium hyaluronate base (Solaraze). Applied twice daily for 60–90 days |
| *Minoxidil* | | |
| May be used as a possible treatment for early male-pattern alopecia. The response is slow, and only a small minority of patients will obtain a dense regrowth even after 12 months. Hair regained will fall out when treatment stops – warn patients about this | Regaine liquid 2% or 5% – only on private prescription | Rogaine 2% solution Rogaine 5% solution for men |
| *Capsaicin* | | |
| A topical pepper that depletes substance P. Useful for the treatment of post-herpetic neuralgia. May itself sting. Apply up to 3–4 times daily after lesions have healed. May take 2–4 weeks to relieve pain | Axsain cream (0.075%) | Zostrix cream (0.025%) Capzasin HP cream (0.075%) Axsain cream (0.075%) |
| *Lidocaine/prilocaine* | | |
| A local anaesthetic for topical use. Applied on skin as a thick layer of cream under an occlusive dressing or on adult genital mucosa with no occlusive dressing. Read manufacturer's instructions for times of application | Lidocaine and prilocaine (EMLA cream) | Lidocaine 4% (ELA-Max) Lidocaine 2.5%/prilocaine 2.5% (EMLA cream) |

# Formulary 2  Systemic medication

We list here only preparations we use commonly for our patients with skin disease. **The doses given are the usual oral doses for adults**. We occasionally use some of these drugs for uses not approved by federal regulatory agencies. We have included some, but not all, of the side-effects and interactions; these are more fully covered in the *British National* *Formulary (BNF)* (UK) and *Physician's Desk Reference (PDR)* (USA) and the package insert. Physicians prescribing these drugs should read about them there, in more detail, and specifically check the dosages before treating their patients. If possible, systemic medication should be avoided in pregnant women.

| Main dermatological uses and usual adult doses | Adverse effects | Interactions | Other remarks |
|---|---|---|---|
| **Antibacterials** | | | |
| *Cefalexin and cefuroxime* Cephalosporins not inactivated by penicillinase. For Gram-positive and Gram-negative infections resistant to penicillin and erythromycin (cefalexin 250–500 mg four times daily; cefuroxine 250 mg twice daily) | Gut upsets Candidiasis Rarely, erythema multiforme or toxic epidermal necrolysis Transient hepatotoxicity Rarely nephrotoxic | Probenecid reduces excretion | Ten per cent of penicillin-allergic patients will react to this |
| *Ciprofloxacin* A 4-quinolone used for Gram-negative infections, especially *Pseudomonas*, and Gram-positive infections. First choice for skin infections in the immunosuppressed if the causative organism is not yet known (500 mg twice daily) | Gut upsets Occasionally hepatotoxic and nephrotoxic Haemolysis in those deficient in glucose-6-phosphate dehydrogenase | Antacids reduce absorption Enhances effects of warfarin and theophylline | Crystalluria if fluid intake is inadequate Care if renal impairment Avoid in pregnancy, breast feeding, children and epileptics |
| *Co-amoxiclav amoxicillin/clavulanate (Augmentin)* A broad-spectrum penicillin combined with clavulanic acid: use if organisms resistant to both erythromycin and flucloxacillin. Also for Gram-negative folliculitis (375 mg three times daily) | Gut upsets Candidiasis Rashes, especially in infectious mononucleosis | As for other penicillins | Use with care in hepatic or renal failure, pregnancy, and breast feeding Avoid in those allergic to penicillin |

| Main dermatological uses and usual adult doses | Adverse effects | Interactions | Other remarks |
|---|---|---|---|
| *Erythromycin*<br>**1** Acne vulgaris (250–500 mg twice daily)<br>**2** Gram-positive infections, particularly staphylococcal and streptococcal. Useful with penicillin allergy (250–500 mg four times daily) | Gut upsets<br>Rashes<br>Cholestatic hepatitis if treatment prolonged (reversible and most common with estolate salt) | Increased risk of toxicity if given with theophylline or carbamazepine<br>Potentiates effects of warfarin, ergotamine, ciclosporin , disopyramide, carbamazepine, terfenadine, astemizole, theophylline, cisapride digoxin and other drugs, metabolized by CYP3A4 | *P. acnes* now widely resistant to erythromycin<br>Avoid estolate in liver disease<br>Care when hepatic dysfunction<br>Excreted in human milk |
| *Flucloxacillin, dicloxacillin and cloxacillin*<br>Penicillins used for infections with penicillinase-forming staphylococci (250–500 mg four times daily) | Gut upsets<br>Morbilliform eruptions<br>Arthralgia<br>Anaphylaxis | Probenecid increases blood level<br>Reduces excretion of methotrexate | Accumulate in renal failure<br>Atopics may be at increased risk of hypersensitivity reactions<br>Avoid in those allergic to penicillin |
| *Metronidazole*<br>**1** Anaerobic infections (400 mg three times daily)<br>**2** Stubborn rosacea (200 mg twice daily)<br>**3** Trichomoniasis (200 mg three times daily for 7 days) | Gut upsets<br>Metallic taste<br>Candidiasis<br>Ataxia and sensory neuropathy<br>Seizures | Potentiates effects of warfarin, phenytoin and lithium<br>Drugs that induce liver enzymes (e.g. rifampicin, barbiturates, griseofulvin, phenytoin, carbamazepine, and smoking) increase destruction of metronidazole in liver and necessitate higher dosage<br>May have disulfiram-like effect with alcohol (headaches, flushing, vomiting, abdominal pain)<br>Co-administration with disulfiram may cause psychotic reactions | Use lower dose in presence of liver disease<br>Neurotoxicity more likely if central nervous system disease<br>Carcinogenic and mutagenic in some non-human models |
| *Minocycline*<br>A tetracycline used for acne and rosacea (50 mg/day or twice daily, or 100 mg/day in a modified release preparation) | Gut upsets<br>Dizziness and vertigo<br>Candidiasis<br>Deposition in bones and teeth of fetus and children<br>Deposition in skin and mucous membranes causes blue–grey pigmentation<br>Benign intracranial hypertension<br>Lupus erythematosus-like syndrome with hepatitis | May impair absorption of oral contraceptives<br>May potentiate effect of warfarin<br>Risk for benign intracranial hypertension from tetracyclines may increase with isotretinoin or acetretin | Avoid in pregnancy and in children under 12 years |

| Main dermatological uses and usual adult doses | Adverse effects | Interactions | Other remarks |
|---|---|---|---|
| *Tetracycline and oxytetracycline*<br>Acne and rosacea<br>(250–500 mg twice daily) | Gut upsets<br>Candidiasis<br>Rashes<br>Deposition in bones and teeth of fetus and children<br>Rare phototoxic reactions<br>Benign intracranial hypertension | Absorption impaired when taken with food, antacids and iron<br>Many impair absorption of oral contraceptives<br>May potentiate effect of warfarin<br>Risk for benign intracranial hypertension from tetracyclines may increase with isotretinoin or acetretin | Avoid in pregnancy and in children under 12 years<br>Should not be used if renal insufficiency |
| *Penicillin V*<br>(phenoxymethylpenicillin)<br>**1** For infections with Gram-positive cocci<br>(250–500 mg four times daily)<br>**2** Prophylaxis of erysipelas<br>(250 mg/day) | Gut upsets<br>Morbilliform rashes<br>Urticaria<br>Arthralgia<br>Anaphylaxis | Blood level increased by probenecid<br>Reduces excretion of methotrexate | Accumulates in renal failure<br>Atopics at increased risk of hypersensitivity reactions |
| **Antifungals**<br>*Terbinafine*<br>Dermatophyte infections when systemic treatment appropriate (as a result of site, severity or extent)<br>Usual first-choice systemic antifungal agent. Unlike itraconazole and fluconazole its action does not involve cytochrome P-450 dependent enzymes in the liver<br>Dose: 250 mg/day<br>Tinea pedis: 2–6 weeks<br>Tinea corporis: 4 weeks<br>Tinea unguium: 6 weeks to 3 months | Gut upsets<br>Headache<br>Rashes – including toxic epidermal necrolysis<br>Taste disturbance<br>Rarely, liver toxicity | Plasma concentration reduced by rifampicin<br>Plasma concentration increased by cimetidine | Avoid in hepatic and renal impairment and when breastfeeding<br>Not for use in pregnancy<br>Not yet recommended for children |
| *Griseofulvin*<br>Has largely been superseded by newer antifungals<br>Dermatophyte infections of skin, nails and hair<br>Not for *Candida* or pityriasis versicolor (500 mg/day microsize) | Gut upsets<br>Headaches, rashes, photosensitivity | Induces microsomal liver enzymes and so may increase elimination of drugs such as warfarin | Not for use in pregnancy, liver failure, porphyria or systemic lupus erythematosus<br>Men should not father children within 6 months of taking it<br>Absorbed better when taken with fatty foods |

| Main dermatological uses and usual adult doses | Adverse effects | Interactions | Other remarks |
|---|---|---|---|
| *Fluconazole*<br>1 Candidiasis<br>*Acute/recurrent vaginal* (single dose of 150 mg)<br>*Mucosal (not vaginal) conditions* (50 mg/day)<br>Oropharyngeal: 7–14 days<br>Oesophagus: 14–30 days<br>*Systemic candidiasis* – see manufacturer's instructions<br>2 Second-line treatment in some systemic mycoses (e.g. cryptococcal infections)<br>3 Dermatophyte infections (except of nails) and pityriasis versicolor (50 mg/day for 2–6 weeks) | Gut upsets<br>Rarely rashes<br>Angio-oedema/anaphylaxis<br>Liver toxicity<br>May be worse in AIDS patients | Hydrochlorothiazide increases plasma concentration<br>Rifampicin reduces plasma concentration<br>Potentiates effects of warfarin, ciclosporin and phenytoin<br>May potentiate effects of sulphonylureas leading to hypoglycaemia<br>May inhibit metabolism of astemizole causing serious dysrhythmias | Avoid in pregnancy<br>Hepatic and renal impairment<br>Use in children only if imperative and no alternative<br>Avoid in children under 1 year and when breastfeeding |
| *Itraconazole*<br>1 Candidiasis<br>*Vulvovaginal* (200 mg twice daily) for 1 day<br>*Oropharyngeal* (100 mg/day) for 15 days<br>2 Pityriasis versicolor (200 mg/day) for 7 days<br>3 Dermatophyte infections (100 mg/day)<br>Tinea pedis and manuum for 30 days<br>Tinea corporis for 15 days<br>Tinea of nails – an intermittent regimen can be used (200 mg twice daily for 1 week per month, continued for three or four cycles) | Gut upsets<br>Headache | Antacids reduce absorption<br>Rifampicin and phenytoin reduce plasma concentration<br>May potentiate effects of warfarin<br>May increase plasma levels of digoxin and ciclosporin<br>Inhibits metabolism of astemizole: this may lead to serious dysrhythmias | Avoid in hepatic impairment<br>Avoid in children, in pregnancy and when breastfeeding<br>Prescribe with caution to patients at risk of heart failure |
| *Ketoconazole*<br>Widespread pityriasis versicolor (200 mg/day for 14 days or 400 mg each morning for 3 days) | As with fluconazole but greater incidence of liver toxicity | Same as fluconazole<br>Decreased absorption if given with an acids or poton pump inhibitors | Seldom used in UK. Monitor liver function continually if used for longer than 14 days |
| *Nystatin*<br>1 Recurrent vulval and perineal candidiasis<br>2 Persistent gastrointestinal candidiasis in immunosuppressed patients (500 000 units three times daily) | Unpleasant taste<br>Gut upsets | | Not absorbed and when given by mouth acts only on mouth and bowel yeasts. Sugar in syrup may cause tooth decay |

| Main dermatological uses and usual adult doses | Adverse effects | Interactions | Other remarks |
| --- | --- | --- | --- |
| **Anthelmintics** | | | |
| *Albendazole* (400 mg/day for 3 days) | | | Both drugs available on a named patient basis |
| *Ivermectin* (12 mg. Single dose)<br>1 Cutaneous larva migrans<br>2 Filariasis<br>3 Cutaneous larva currens (*Strongyloides stercoralis*)<br>4 Scabies | | | |
| **Antivirals** | | | |
| *Aciclovir, famciclovir and valaciclovir* (for dosages see specialist literature) | | | |
| Famciclovir and valaciclovir are more reliably absorbed than aciclovir and need be taken only two or three times a day<br>1 Severe herpes simplex infections – primary or recurrent<br>2 Severe herpes zoster infections – use may reduce incidence of post-herpetic neuralgia<br>3 Prophylaxis for recurrent herpes simplex especially in the immunocompromised.<br>4 eczema herpeticum and chickenpox in the immunocompromised | Generally safe drug. Rapid gut upsets, transient rise in urea and creatinine in 10% of patients after intravenous use<br>Raised liver enzymes<br>Reversible neurological reactions<br>Decreases in haematological indices | Excretion may be delayed by probenicid<br>Lethargy when intravenous aciclovir given with zidovudine | Adequate hydration of patient should be maintained<br>Risk in pregnancy unknown<br>Reduce dose in renal impairment<br>No effect on virus in latent phase<br>Must be given early in acute infections to have maximum effect |
| **Antihistamines** | | | |
| All those listed here are H1-blockers though some dermatologists combine these with H2-blockers in recalcitrant urticaria | | | |
| *Non-sedative*<br>Used for urticaria and type I hypersensitivity reactions | Rarely sedate | Metabolized by CYP3A4 and to a lesser extent by CYP2D6 | Non-sedative antihistamines should be avoided, or used with caution in pregnancy and lactation |
| *Loratadine and desloratadine* (Loratadine, 10 mg/day; desloratadine, 5 mg/day) | | | Desloratidine to be used with caution in renal impairment |
| *Cetirizine and levocetirizine* (Cetirizine 10 mg/day; levocetirizine 5 mg/day) | | | Use half the usual dose when renal impairment |
| *Fexofenadine* (a metabolite of terfenadine) 60–180 mg/day | | | |

| Main dermatological uses and usual adult doses | Adverse effects | Interactions | Other remarks |
|---|---|---|---|
| *Sedative*<br>Urticaria, type I hypersensitivity including intravenous use in anaphylaxis (p. 362). Also used as antipruritic agents in atopic eczema, lichen planus | Sedation (promethazine > trimeprazine (alimemazine)> hydroxyzine> chlorphenamine = diphenhydramine = cyproheptadine)<br>Anticholinergic effects:<br>• dry mouth<br>• blurred vision<br>• urinary retention<br>• tachycardia<br>• glaucoma<br>Consider lower doses in the elderly | Potentiate effect of alcohol and central nervous system depressants<br>Potentiate effect of other anticholinergic drugs | Increased rate of elimination in children<br>Sedation may be useful in an excited itchy patient<br>Warn of risk of drowsiness when driving or operating dangerous machinery |
| *Chlorpheniramine*<br>(4 mg three or four times daily)<br>*Diphenhydramine*<br>(25–50 mg four times daily)<br>*Hydroxyzine*<br>(25 mg, nocte at first, but up to 100 mg four times daily if needed)<br>*Cyproheptadine*<br>(4 mg four times daily)<br>*Promethazine*<br>(10–25 mg/day to three times daily)<br>*Alimemazine* (Trimeprazine)<br>(10 mg two or three times daily) | | | Hydroxyzine particularly useful for pruritus |
| **Antiandrogens**<br>*Cyproterone acetate and ethinylestradiol*<br>(UK: Dianette; USA: not available)<br>**1** Acne vulgaris, unresponsive to systemic antibiotics, in women only<br>**2** Idiopathic hirsutism, one tablet (cyproterone acetate 2 mg, ethinylestradiol 35 mg) daily for 21 days, starting on fifth day of menstrual cycle and repeated after a 7-day interval. Treat for 6 months at least | As for combined oral contraceptives | Should not be given with other oral contraceptives | Contraindicated in pregnancy. Cyproterone acetate is an antiandrogen and if given to pregnant women may feminize a male fetus. For women of childbearing age, therefore, it must be given combined with a contraceptive (the ethinylestradiol component)<br>Also contraindicated in liver disease, disorders of lipid metabolism and with past or present endometrial carcinomas<br>Not for use in males or children |

| Main dermatological uses and usual adult doses | Adverse effects | Interactions | Other remarks |
|---|---|---|---|
| *Drospirenone and ethinyloestradiol* (USA: Yaz; UK: not available) | Hyperkalaemia | NSAIDS and ACE inhibitors increase risk of hyperkalaemia | Contraindicated if abnormal renal or hepatic function Drospirenone is an analogue of spironolactone. Avoid in pregnancy |
| *Spironolactone* 25–50 mg/day for idiopathic hirsutism Used in USA | Hyperkalaemia | Increases plasma concentration of digoxin | May feminize male fetus Avoid in pregnancy Causes gynaecomastia Avoid if renal or hepatic impairment |
| *Finasteride* 1 mg/day for male-pattern baldness | Impotence and decreased libido | | 5α-reductase inhibitor, reduces formation of dihydrotestosterone Not for use by women |
| **Immunosuppressants** *Azathioprine* For autoimmune conditions (e.g. systemic lupus erythematosus, pemphigus and bullous pemphigoid) often used to spare dose of systemic steroids (1–2.5 mg/kg/day). We strongly recommend checking thiopurine methyltransferase levels before starting treatment with azathioprine as homozygotes for the low-activity allele have a high risk of bone marrow suppression | Gut upsets Bone marrow suppression, usually leucopenia or thrombocytopenia Hepatotoxicity, pancreatitis Predisposes to infections, including warts and possibly also to skin cancers | Increased toxicity if given with allopurinol | See comment about the need to check for thiopurine methyltransferase levels (in first column) Weekly blood checks are necessary for the first 8 weeks of treatment and thereafter at intervals of not longer than 3 months Reduce dosage if severe renal impairment Avoid in pregnancy Possible increased risk of lymphomas |
| *Ciclosporin* 1  Severe psoriasis when conventional treatment is ineffective or inappropriate 2  Short-term (max. 8 weeks) treatment of severe atopic dermatitis when conventional treatment ineffective or inappropriate (2.5 mg/kg/day in two divided doses). See p. 68 for guidance in use | Hepatic and renal impairment Hypertension Gut upset Hypertrichosis Gum hyperplasia Tremor Hyperkalaemia Occasionally facial oedema, fluid retention and convulsions Hypercholesterolaemia Hypomagnesaemia | (See *BNF* and *PDR* for fuller details) (Use with tacrolimus specifically contraindicated) 1  Drugs that may increase nephrotoxicity • Antibiotics (aminoglycosides, co-trimoxazole) • Non-steroidal anti-inflammatory drugs • Melphalan 2  Drugs that may increase ciclosporin blood level (by cytochrome P-450 inhibition) | Contraindicated if abnormal renal function, hypertension not under control and concomitant premalignant or malignant conditions Monitor renal function and blood pressure as indicated on p. 68 |

| Main dermatological uses and usual adult doses | Adverse effects | Interactions | Other remarks |
|---|---|---|---|
| | | • Antibiotics (erythromycin, amphotericin B, cephalosporins, doxycycline, aciclovir)<br>• Hormones (corticosteroids, sex hormones)<br>• Diuretics (frusemide/furosemide thiazides)<br>• Other (warfarin, H2 antihistamines, calcium-channel blockers, ACE inhibitors, grapefruit juice)<br>3 Drugs that may decrease ciclosporin levels (by cytochrome P-450 induction)<br>• Anticonvulsants (phenytoin, phenobarbital, carbamazepine, sodium valproate)<br>• Antibiotics (isoniazid, rifampicin) | |
| *Methotrexate*<br>Severe psoriasis unresponsive to local treatment (initially, 2.5 mg test dose and observe for 1 week, then 5–20 mg once a week orally or intramuscularly) | Gut upsets<br>Stomatitis<br>Bone marrow depression<br>Liver or kidney dysfunction | Aspirin, probenecid, thiazide diuretics and some non-steroidal anti-inflammatory drugs delay excretion and increase toxicity<br>Antiepileptics, co-trimoxazole, and pyrimethamine increase antifolate effect<br>Toxicity increased by ciclosporin and acitretin. Co-administration of folate does not antagonize the effect of methotrexate on psoriasis and may confer protective effects (p. 67) | Full blood count and liver function tests before starting treatment, and then weekly until therapy is stabilized. Thereafter test every 2–3 months<br>Avoid in pregnancy<br>Reduce dose if renal or hepatic impairment<br>Folinic acid (folic acid – USA) given concomitantly prevents bone marrow depression<br>Reduced fertility in males<br>Traditionally, the development of hepatic fibrosis has been detected with a liver biopsy before treatment and periodical biopsies thereafter. Need for liver biopsy is being replaced by serial measurement of serum procollagen III aminopeptide. Elderly may be more sensitive to the drug |

| Main dermatological uses and usual adult doses | Adverse effects | Interactions | Other remarks |
|---|---|---|---|
| **Corticosteroids** *Prednisone and prednisolone* Acute and severe allergic reactions, acute eczemas, severe erythema multiforme, connective tissue disorders, pemphigus, pemphigoid and vasculitis (5–80 mg/day or on alternate days) Withdrawal should be gradual for patients who have received systemic corticosteroids for more than 3 weeks or those who have taken high doses | Impaired glucose tolerance Redistribution of fat (centripetal) Muscle wasting, proximal myopathy Osteoporosis and vertebral collapse Aseptic necrosis of head of femur Growth retardation in children Peptic ulceration Euphoria, psychosis or depression Cataract formation Precipitation of glaucoma Increase in blood pressure Sodium and water retention Potassium loss Skin atrophy and capillary fragility Spread of infection Iatrogenic Cushing's syndrome | Liver enzyme inducers (e.g. phenytoin, griseofulvin, rifampicin) reduce effect of corticosteroids Carbenoxolone and most diuretics increase potassium loss as a result of corticosteroids Corticosteroids reduce effect of many antihypertensive agents and drugs that affect glucose metabolism | 1 Before long-term treatment screen: • Chest X-ray • Blood pressure • Weight • Glycosuria • Electrolytes • Consider the need for a bone density scan • Tuberculin skin test (USA) • Past history of peptic ulcer, cataracts/glaucoma, and affective psychosis 2 During treatment check blood pressure, weight, glycosuria and electrolytes regularly. Patients can carry a steroid treatment card or wear a labelled bracelet. Always bear in mind the possibility of masked infections and perforations 3 Long-term treatment has to be tapered off slowly to avoid adrenal insufficiency 4 Do not use for psoriasis or long-term for atopic eczema 5 Consider the need for adjunctive treatment for prevention of osteoporosis |
| **Retinoids** *Acitretin* Severe psoriasis, resistant to other forms of treatment (may be used with PUVA, p. 66), palmoplantar pustulosis, severe ichthyoses, Darier's disease, pityriasis rubra pilaris (0.2–1.0 mg/kg/day) Acitretin is not recommended for children except under exceptional circumstances | 1 *Mucocutaneous* (common) Rough, scaly, dry-appearing skin and mucous membranes Chafing Atrophy of skin and nails Diffuse thinning of scalp and body hair Curly hair Exuberant granulation tissue (especially toe nail folds) Disease flare-up Photosensitivity | Avoid concomitant high doses of vitamin A Possible antagonism to anticoagulant effect of warfarin Increases plasma concentration of methotrexate Increases hepatotoxicity of methotrexate | All women of childbearing age must use effective oral contraception for 1 month before treatment, during treatment and for at least 2 years after treatment (see specialist literature for details) Patients should sign a consent form indicating that they know about the danger of teratogenicity Should not donate blood during or for 2 years after stopping the treatment (teratogenic risk) |

| Main dermatological uses and usual adult doses | Adverse effects | Interactions | Other remarks |
|---|---|---|---|
| | **2** *Systemic*<br>Teratogenesis<br>Diffuse interstitial skeletal hyperostosis<br>Arthralgia, myalgia and headache<br>Benign intracranial hypertension<br>**3** *Laboratory abnormalities*<br>Haematology:<br>↓ White blood cells<br>↑ Erythrocyte sedimentation rate<br>Liver function tests:<br>↓↑ Bilirubin<br>↑ AST/ALT<br>↑ Alkaline phosphatase (abnormal in 20% of patients)<br>Serum lipids:<br>↑ Cholesterol<br>↑ Triglycerides<br>↑ High-density lipoprotein (abnormal in 50% of patients) | | Regular screening should be carried out to exclude:<br>1 Abnormalities of liver function<br>2 Hyperlipidaemia<br>3 Disseminated interstitial skeletal hyperostosis<br>Avoid if renal or hepatic impairment |
| *Isotretinoin* (13 *cis*-retinoic acid)<br>Severe acne vulgaris, unresponsive to systemic antibiotics (0.5–1.0 mg/kg/day for 16 weeks) (p. 169) or to total dose of 120 mg/kg | (See Acitretin)<br>Almost all patients experience cheilitis. Other common side-effects are aches and pains, epistaxis, dry skin, dry eyes and occasional change in night vision | Avoid concomitant high doses of vitamin A<br>Possible antagonism to anticoagulant effect of warfarin<br>Increases plasma concentration of methotrexate<br>Increases hepatotoxicity of methotrexate | Females of childbearing age must take effective contraception for 1 month before treatment is started, during treatment, and for 3 months after treatment is stopped; check pregnancy test(s) before starting treatment and monthly. Maximum 4 weeks supply of drug to be administered only on receipt of negative pregnancy test. Females should sign a consent form which states the dangers of teratogenicity (see p. 169 for USA recommendations)<br>Before starting a course of isotretinoin, patients and their doctors should know about the risk of the appearance or worsening of depression. The drug should be stopped immediately if there is any concern on this score (see p. 169)<br>Avoid in renal or hepatic impairment<br>Blood tests as for acitretin |

| Main dermatological uses and usual adult doses | Adverse effects | Interactions | Other remarks |
|---|---|---|---|
| **Drugs acting on the central nervous system (CNS)** | | | |
| *Amitriptyline* | | | |
| **1** Depression secondary to skin disease **2** Post-herpetic neuralgia (50–100 mg at night; start with 10–25 mg in the elderly) | Sedation, anticholinergic effects, cardiac dysrhythmias Confusion in the elderly Postural hypotension Jaundice Neutropenia May precipitate seizures in epileptics | Potentially lethal CNS stimulation with monoamine oxidase inhibitors Increases effects of other CNS depressants and anticholinergics Metabolism may be inhibited by cimetidine | Avoid in the presence of heart disease or hypertension Use small doses at first to avoid confusion in the elderly Warn about effects on skills such as driving |
| *Doxepin* | | | |
| Antidepressant with sedative properties sometimes used for antipruritic effect 10–50 mg at bedtime or twice daily | See amitriptyline | See amitriptyline | Avoid in breastfeeding Potent H1 antihistamine |
| *Diazepam* | | | |
| Anxiety – often associated with skin disease (2–5 mg three times daily) | Sedation Impaired skills (e.g. driving) or ataxia Dependence (withdrawal may lead to sleeplessness, anxiety, tremors) | Potentiates effects of other CNS depressants including alcohol Breakdown inhibited by cimetidine and propranolol Liver enzyme inducers (e.g. phenytoin, griseofulvin, rifampicin) increase elimination | Use for short spells only (to avoid addiction) Avoid in pregnancy and breastfeeding Use with care in presence of liver, kidney or respiratory diseases, and in the elderly |

**Biological therapies**

These are agents that block specific molecular steps in disease pathogenesis. In the UK they are licensed for the treatment of severe psoriasis, which has either failed to respond to standard systemic therapy, or for patients who are intolerant of standard systemic therapy. 'Biologics' either target TNF-α or T cells and antigen-presenting cells

| | | | |
|---|---|---|---|
| *Tumour necrosis factor α* | | | |
| TNF-α targeting biologics | Predispose to infection and malignancies. May reactivate TB and hepatitis B. May exacerbate heart failure and demyelinating conditions | Avoid concomitant use with live vaccines Avoid with anakinra (IL-1 inhibitor) | Occasionally, and paradoxically elicits new psoriasis |
| *Etanercept* (Enbrel) | | | |
| **1** Psoriasis as above **2** Psoriatic arthritis. Subcutaneous injection 25 mg, twice weekly, increasing to 50 mg depending on response. Maximum treatment 24 weeks | Injection site reactions Rare lupus syndrome | | A recombinant human TNF-α receptor fusion protein, which binds soluble and membrane-bound TNF-α Screen for TB pretreatment |

| Main dermatological uses and usual adult doses | Adverse effects | Interactions | Other remarks |
|---|---|---|---|
| *Infliximab* (Remicade)<br>**1**  Psoriasis as above<br>**2**  Psoriatic arthritis.<br>IV infusion, 5 mg/kg at weeks 0, 2, 6 and then 8-weekly intervals | Hypersensitivity reactions, particularly 1 or 2 h after 1st or 2nd infusion | | A human/mouse chimeric monoclonal IgG antibody to TNF-α. Binds and forms stable complexes with circulating and membrane-bound TNF-α<br>Caution in hepatic and renal impairment<br>Screen for infections and TB pretreatment<br>May induce neutralising antibodies |
| **T-cell inhibitors**<br>*Efalizumab* (Raptiva)<br>Psoriasis as above<br>Subcutaneous injection 0.7 then 1 mg/kg/week<br>Discontinue after 12 weeks if poor response | Influenza-like symptoms. Exacerbation of psoriasis and risk of 'new forms' and rebound flare when drug is discontinued. Thrombocytopenia (monitor platelets before and during treatment). Injection site reactions | Discontinue 8 weeks before and until 2 weeks after vaccination with live or live-attenuated vaccines | A humanized murine antibody to CD11a. Inhibits T-cell trafficking, activation and keratinocyte binding<br>Avoid if history of malignancy |
| *Alefacept* (Amevive)<br>15 mg IM once weekly for 12-week course<br>Requires baseline and weekly monitoring of CD4 T-cell counts. Hold dose if <250 cells/μL, DC if count <250 cells/μL for more than 1 month<br>TB test before starting | Injection site reactions, cough, myalgias, nausea | No live vaccines | Not licensed for use in UK<br>Fusion protein of human LFA-3 and Fc portion of IgG<br>Blocks the interaction of accessory molecules LFA-3 and CD2 needed for T-cell activation<br>Monitor for lymphopenia, malignancy, infections, liver enzyme changes and cardiovascular troubles |
| **Miscellaneous**<br>*Adrenaline (epinephrine) injection*<br>Emergency treatment for acute anaphylaxis 0.5 mg (0.5 mL of 1 in 1000 solution given as a slow subcutaneous or, rarely, intramuscular injection. May be repeated after 10 min if necessary)<br>An Epipen is a convenient way in which patients can carry adrenaline with them for self-injection if needed | Tachycardia<br>Cardiac dysrhythmias<br>Anxiety<br>Tremor<br>Headache<br>Hypertension<br>Hyperglycaemia<br>Hypokalaemia | If given with some beta-blockers may lead to severe hypertension | Do not confuse the different strengths<br>Give *slowly*, subcutaneously or intramuscularly, but *not* intravenously, except in cardiac arrest |

| Main dermatological uses and usual adult doses | Adverse effects | Interactions | Other remarks |
|---|---|---|---|
| *Dapsone*<br>Leprosy, dermatitis herpetiformis, vasculitis, pyoderma gangrenosum (50–150 mg/day) | Haemolytic anaemia<br>Methaemoglobinaemia<br>Headaches<br>Lethargy<br>Hepatitis<br>Peripheral neuropathy<br>Exfoliative dermatitis<br>Toxic epidermal necrolysis<br>Agranulocytosis<br>Aplastic anaemia<br>Hypoalbuminaemia | Reduced excretion and increased side-effects if given with probenecid | Regular blood checks necessary (weekly for first month, then every 2 weeks until 3 months, then monthly until 6 months and then 6-monthly)<br>Not felt to be teratogenic, but should not be given during pregnancy and lactation if possible. For dermatitis herpetiformis, a gluten-free diet is preferable at these times<br>Avoid in patients with glucose-6-phosphate dehydrogenase deficiency (screen for this, especially in USA) |
| *Hydroxychloroquine*<br>Systemic and discoid lupus erythematosus, polymorphic light eruption: 200–400 mg/day, maintaining level at lowest effective dose. Must not exceed 6.5 mg/kg body weight/day (based on the ideal/lean body weight and not on the actual weight of the patient) | Retinopathy which may cause permanent blindness<br>Corneal deposits<br>Headaches<br>Gut upsets, pruritus and rashes<br>Worsening of psoriasis<br>Vivid dreams<br>Patients with porphyria cutanea tarda may develop acute chemical hepatitis | Should not be taken at the same time as other antimalarial drugs<br>May raise plasma digoxin levels<br>Potential neuromuscular toxicity if taken with gentamicin, kanamycin, or tobramycin<br>Bioavailability decreased if given with antacids | In the UK, before treatment, patients should be asked about their visual acuity (not corrected with glasses). If it is impaired, or eye disease is present, assessment by an optometrist is advised and any abnormality should be referred to an ophthalmologist. The visual acuity of each eye should be recorded using a standard reading chart. In the USA all patients should have a pretreatment ophthalmological assessment with evaluation of visual fields, and examinations every 6–12 months. In addition, patients can check visual fields and acuity with special charts at home<br>Discontinue drug if any change occurs<br>Reduce dose with poor renal or liver function<br>Best avoided in the elderly and children<br>Do not give automatic repeat prescriptions<br>Prefer intermittent short courses to continuous treatment if possible |

| Main dermatological uses and usual adult doses | Adverse effects | Interactions | Other remarks |
|---|---|---|---|
| *8-Methoxypsoralen (methoxsalen)* Used usually with UVA as PUVA therapy (p. 66) Severe psoriasis, vitiligo, localized pustular psoriasis, cutaneous T-cell lymphoma; rarely, lichen planus, atopic dermatitis Tablets: 0.6–0.8 mg/kg body weight taken as a single dose 1–2 h before exposure to UVA Liquid (Ultra Capsules) (USA): 0.3 mg/kg body weight taken 1 h before exposure to UVA | Nausea Itching Photoxicity Catracts Lentigines Ageing changes of skin Hyperpigmentation Cutaneous neoplasms | Avoid other photosensitizers (Chapter 18) | The following should checked before treatment • *Skin* Examine for premalignant lesions and skin cancer • *Eyes* Check for cataracts. Fundoscopic examination of retina. Visual acuity • *Blood* Full blood count, liver and renal function tests and antinuclear factor test • *Urine analysis* Eyes should be protected with appropriate lenses for 24 h after taking the drug Protective goggles must be worn during radiation If feasible, shield face and genitalia during treatment Patients must protect skin against additional sun exposure after ingestion Monitor eyes for development of cataracts Try to avoid maintenance treatment, more than 250 treatments and a cumulative dose of more than 1000 joules/cm$^2$ (skin cancer risk) |

# INDEX

Note: page numbers in *italics* refer to figures, those in **bold** refer to tables